Fundamentals of
AUDIOLOGY
FOR THE SPEECH-LANGUAGE PATHOLOGIST

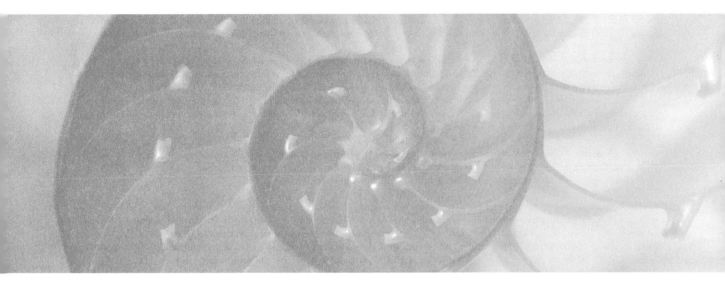

Deborah R. Welling, AuD, CCC-A, FAAA
Associate Professor and Director of Clinical Education
Department of Speech-Language Pathology
Seton Hall University
South Orange, New Jersey

Carol A. Ukstins, MS, CCC-A, FAAA
Educational Audiologist
Newark Public Schools
Newark, New Jersey

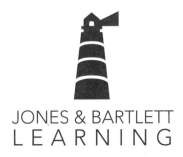

JONES & BARTLETT
LEARNING

World Headquarters
Jones & Bartlett Learning
5 Wall Street
Burlington, MA 01803
978-443-5000
info@jblearning.com
www.jblearning.com

Jones & Bartlett Learning books and products are available through most bookstores and online booksellers. To contact Jones & Bartlett Learning directly, call 800-832-0034, fax 978-443-8000, or visit our website, www.jblearning.com.

Production Credits

Executive Publisher: William Brottmiller
Editorial Assistant: Sean Fabery
Production Editor: Joanna Lundeen
Marketing Manager: Grace Richards
VP, Manufacturing and Inventory Control: Therese Connell

Composition: Aptara®, Inc.
Cover Design: Kristin E. Parker
Photo Research and Permissions Coordinator: Amy Rathburn
Cover and Front Matter Image: © Mircea BEZERGHEANU/ShutterStock, Inc.
Printing and Binding: Edwards Brothers Malloy
Cover Printing: Edwards Brothers Malloy

To order this product, use ISBN: 978-1-4496-6030-7

Library of Congress Cataloging-in-Publication Data
Welling, Deborah R., author.
 Fundamentals of audiology for the speech-language pathologist / by Deborah R. Welling and Carol A. Ukstins.
    p. ; cm.
 Includes bibliographical references and index.
 ISBN 978-1-4496-5731-4—ISBN 1-4496-5731-1
 I. Ukstins, Carol A., author. II. Title.
 [DNLM: 1. Hearing Disorders—therapy. 2. Hearing—physiology. 3. Hearing Disorders—diagnosis.
 4. Speech-Language Pathology—methods. WV 270]
 RF290
 617.8—dc23
                                    2013019682
6048
Printed in the United States of America
17 16 15 14 13   10 9 8 7 6 5 4 3 2 1

I dedicate this book to my mother, Regina, who had to maneuver, without a rudder, the waters of managing a child with hearing loss. To my sister, Barbara, who inspired me to pursue audiology. To my husband, Bill, for the days, months, and years of seeing me through this project. Thank you for your support.

—Deborah R. Welling

I dedicate this text to Dr. Susan Rezen, the person who taught me to love audiology, and to never say "Oops!" behind an audiometer. To my family: my husband, Jim, and my children, Nyasia, John, and Elizabeth, who have been a constant source of encouragement through the processes of this manuscript. To my mother, Joyce, who taught me that I could do anything.

—Carol A. Ukstins

Together, we dedicate this book to Dr. Annette Zaner, mentor and friend, who brought us together more than 20 years ago, never imagining that we would still be working together 20 years later.

Contents

CHAPTER 17 **Acute, Subacute, and Nursing Home/Long-Term Care Facilities 291**
Carol A. Ukstins and Deborah R. Welling

Foreword

Audiology and speech-language pathology are two professions that share a common bond—to prevent, identify, diagnose, and treat communication disorders. We work together so that persons with speech, language, swallowing, or hearing impairments can participate fully in society. Developed from a similar origin, the disciplines have evolved over the decades to become highly specialized fields that require those who enter each of these professions to achieve mastery of vast amounts of knowledge and significant skills. Yet there is substantial knowledge in each profession that is highly relevant to the other. Speech-language pathologists (SLPs) must understand the impact of hearing problems on the speech and language skills of their clients. Audiologists must consider the communication needs of their clients when assessing hearing and providing hearing rehabilitation services. In their daily work, SLPs focus on improving communication and swallowing whereas audiologists focus on hearing. Yet, these domains are so deeply interrelated that each discipline must be cognizant of a person's abilities in all of these areas in order to assist the person in the most effective manner. Regardless of the age, diagnosis, or ability level of a particular client, an SLP must always be knowledgeable about the individual's auditory abilities in order to make an appropriate diagnosis and design an effective treatment plan.

In this unique text, the authors have compiled information that is essential knowledge for both the student of speech-language pathology and the practicing clinician. For graduate students, this text will highlight the need to understand the risk of hearing loss in varied populations, the signs of hearing loss, and how disorders of audition impact our clients' abilities to either develop or maintain communication. For clinicians in the field, this text will serve as a valuable resource on the SLP's bookshelf, regardless of work setting. As a speech-language pathologist,

I've relied on the expertise of audiologists countless times throughout my career in my work with individuals with communication disorders. When I was working in early intervention, one of the first questions I asked parents who were concerned about their child's language development was about the results of any hearing testing. An audiological evaluation must be completed on any child suspected of a language or speech difficulty before a diagnosis can be made. On my caseload I had many children with Down syndrome who were at high risk for conductive hearing loss, so I worked very closely with an audiologist and otolaryngologist to ensure that these children could maximally benefit from their therapy programs. When I worked in home care with adults with aphasia, I often counseled these patients and their families about the value of using auditory amplification and the need for regular visits to the audiologist to monitor hearing status and troubleshoot problems with hearing aids. In my private practice, I worked closely with audiologists to help understand the auditory processing difficulties experienced by my pediatric clients with language disorders. I had many conversations with an audiology colleague on how to interpret the results of auditory processing assessments and how we could work together to make recommendations so that our clients could maximally benefit from their intervention programs. From these conversations, I also learned how to make classroom environments more "listener friendly" for all learners, not just those with language-learning difficulties.

Deborah Welling and Carol Ukstins have compiled information from experts in various segments of the field in order to provide the reader with a sound understanding of the principles of hearing development and disorders and the impact of these topics on speech-language pathology practice. Collaboration is a persistent theme that is seen throughout the text and refers not just to collaboration between SLPs and audiologists, but among all members of healthcare and educational teams. The authors open the text with a discussion of a way to think about teaming, which is very pervasive in the literature right now—the concept of interprofessional collaboration. Welling and Ukstins and their contributing authors return to this topic consistently throughout the book and provide concrete examples of how SLPs can educate team members about hearing and communication.

The text is organized into three sections: first, the authors address the basics of sound and hearing to provide a firm foundation for the topics that follow; then issues related to assessment and identification of hearing impairment and rehabilitative strategies are discussed; and finally, topics related to hearing issues across the lifespan and in varied work settings are addressed. The text begins with fundamental information on the development of hearing and principles of auditory assessment, including understanding of key case history data useful for diagnosis and intervention planning. A variety of audiological tests are summarized in a style that communicates the type of information that is provided by each assessment and how to understand and apply the data obtained. The text then covers assistive technology both for children and adults and includes key information on laws, standards, and guidelines related to hearing and hearing loss for all work settings.

The final chapters provide an exhaustive treatment of hearing issues across the lifespan and provide information for clinical practice in all work settings. The section begins with a summary of hearing development and provides a detailed description of the role of hearing issues in the early intervention years. Clinicians working in school systems will find the chapter on audiology services in schools to be of great value. The text can serve as a resource for ensuring that all children are provided with optimal hearing conditions to support learning. The chapter on central auditory processing provides information to help the SLP wade through the confusing and sometimes conflicting information on identification and

management of this complex disorder. Those working with adults in a healthcare setting will find the information on management of hearing issues key to maximizing communication for their patients. Hearing loss occurs frequently in elderly populations and can be a central cause of a communication disorder or be an accompanying problem. SLPs will find very helpful, practical strategies advocated by the authors, including checklists and strategies for doing in-services in healthcare settings. In addition, the authors give beneficial suggestions for educating health professionals and family members about the impact of a hearing problem on a patient's daily life.

On a personal note, Dr. Deborah Welling has been helping me understand audiology since we were both graduate students at Queens College of the City University of New York several decades ago. I was enrolled in the speech-language pathology cohort and she was in the audiology cohort. Our groups spent little classroom time together, but we commiserated about our heavy workloads and how we struggled in our clinical practica. Dr. Welling and her audiology colleagues were so skilled in using the technical equipment in the audiology booth that my fellow SLP students and I relied on their expertise when we were enrolled in audiology clinic and trying to figure out how to conduct masking. I still have trouble interpreting all of those abbreviations on an audiogram, but I know I can continue to turn to her for advice. It's gratifying to see how her career has developed, and serendipitous that we are both colleagues once again, this time at Seton Hall University, across the river in New Jersey.

Theresa E. Bartolotta, PhD, CCC-SLP

Director of Assessment for Academic Affairs,
Office of the Provost

Associate Professor of Speech-Language
Pathology

Seton Hall University

South Orange, New Jersey

Introduction

Fundamentals of Audiology for the Speech-Language Pathologist is a manuscript forged as a true interdisciplinary text designed by a group of professionals with a sincere interest in training the speech-language pathologist in the essential components of audiology practices. For the student, it is our hope that this text provides a solid foundational understanding of the hearing mechanism, audiological equipment and procedures, and the diagnosis and (re)habilitation of hearing loss. For the practicing speech-language pathologist, *Fundamentals of Audiology for the Speech-Language Pathologist* should be viewed as a reference to use when seeking guidance in the management of hearing loss. It is not, however, intended to take the place of consulting one-on-one with colleagues in audiology, but rather to use as a tool to aid in asking the right questions. In order to maintain a text that is equal in both breadth and depth, much of the technical jargon used throughout the field of audiology has been replaced with easy-to-understand text providing the speech-language pathologist with an adequate understanding of audiometric concepts without getting bogged down in terminology.

When considering the demands of a career as a speech-language pathologist, your role in performing measures of hearing sensitivity or working with individuals with hearing loss may or may not have crossed your mind. However, both fall (within guidelines) under the scope of practice as a speech-language pathologist. Clearly, then, in order to perform screening measures and interpret test data, a certain level of understanding must be achieved regarding a range of audiologic procedures and concepts. The purpose of this manuscript is not to convert the speech-language pathologist into an audiologist but rather to provide the professional with the necessary information, resource tools, and understanding to competently perform the roles and responsibilities as outlined in the scope of practice.

Through this clear presentation of audiometric measures and practices, it is our goal to provide the clinician with the resources in hand to properly assist in the service provision for patients of all ages with hearing loss so that through the therapeutic processes, families do not leave your office without a clear understanding of hearing loss; patients with hearing loss achieve the highest possible clinical/therapeutic outcomes; and, not one more child with hearing loss is misdiagnosed.

Fundamentals of Audiology for the Speech-Language Pathologist is your starting point on an exciting journey. From the basics of hearing science and anatomy of the ear, through the essential principles of evaluation, to the habilitation of infants and the rehabilitation of the elderly patient, at journey's end, you will find your reward: to make a difference in the lives of individuals with hearing loss.

About This Textbook

When considering the demands of a career as a speech-language pathologist, your role in performing measures of hearing sensitivity or working with individuals with hearing loss may or may not have crossed your mind. Further, as previously discussed, both fall (within guidelines) under the scope of practice as a speech-language pathologist. Clearly then, in order to perform screening measures and interpret audiometric test data, a certain level of understanding must be achieved regarding a range of audiologic procedures and concepts. The purpose of this text is not to convert the speech-language pathologist into an audiologist, but rather to provide the professional with the necessary information, resource tools, and understanding to competently perform the roles and responsibilities. To that end, this text will address the concepts of hearing evaluation, hearing loss, technology, and rehabilitation as they pertain specifically to your needs as a communication disorders service provider. The extensive underlying mathematical and neurological processes related to the evaluation of hearing is best left to the practicing audiologist. However, you are always encouraged to research further into a concept should your specific practices necessitate such knowledge.

In order to facilitate a clear understanding of the necessary elements of audiology, the reader will find the following headings throughout much of this text as discussion of testing procedures and practices unfolds. The goal of each section is described as follows.

What You Need To Know

This section contains a basic overview of the particular procedure, some of the key terminology used, and a more general answer to the question "why do we do this?". Excessive technological information detail is not discussed.

How It Works

This section provides more specific information regarding the procedure and what it is, a discussion of objective versus subjective measures, and the yield of the procedure. In some cases, the materials used are also referenced.

Technically Speaking

This section provides a more in-depth technical, anatomical, and/or physiological basis for each particular area discussed. Additional depth and detail are added for those with a keen interest in the particular topic.

Methodologies

Very simply, this section explains the process and/or procedures by which the examiner obtains the data derived, including testing instructions and steps taken for obtaining such data. As appropriate, this section also contains information regarding how the results of the given test or procedure fits in with the larger test battery.

Acknowledgments

We would like to thank those professionals who assisted in the creation of this text. Without the efforts of the following individuals, we would not have realized our goal to create a text that exemplifies a true collaborative effort. It is with gratitude that we recognize Karen Kushla, Donna Merchant, Arsen Zartarian, Christina Perigoe, Marietta Paterson, Nancy Schneider, Cheryl DeConde Johnson, Ralph Moscarella, Tena McNamara, and Annette Hurley. We extend our sincere appreciation to our colleagues Nina Capone Singleton and Natalie Neubauer for their expertise and input throughout this project. We would also like to thank Amanda Russo and Mary Carlson for their tireless energy and efforts. May the knowledge you have gained assist you in becoming great professionals. Finally, we would like to recognize Neil Bauman, Curator of The Hearing Aid Museum, not only for his contribution to this text, but for his efforts to keep a portion of audiology history alive for generations to come.

About the Authors

Deborah R. Welling, AuD, CCC-A, FAAA is an associate professor and director of clinical education in the Department of Speech-Language Pathology at Seton Hall University. Dr. Welling earned her bachelor of arts degree in communication arts and sciences from Hofstra University, her master's degree in audiology from Queens College of the City University of New York, and her doctoral degree in audiology from the University of Florida.

Dr. Welling is a member of the American Speech-Language-Hearing Association (ASHA); a fellow of the American Academy of Audiology (AAA); and a member of the New Jersey Speech-Language-Hearing Association (NJSHA), for whom she has served as Vice-Chair of the Higher Education Committee.

Prior to her role as an associate professor and director of clinical education, Dr. Welling spent many years in direct clinical service provision and supervision, with extensive experience in the behavioral assessment of the very young and difficult-to-test populations. It was during this time period that she met her coauthor, Carol Ukstins.

Dr. Welling has also had extensive involvement with interdisciplinary screening and evaluation processes in the early intervention, preschool, and school-aged populations, with an emphasis on (central) auditory processing assessment.

Since joining the faculty at Seton Hall University, Dr. Welling has been teaching undergraduate and graduate-level courses that cover anatomy and physiology of the auditory system, fundamentals of sound (acoustics), basic and advanced audiologic measurement and interpretation, and aural habilitation and rehabilitation. In addition, she provides clinical and academic advising and mentoring for undergraduate- and graduate-level students.

Carol A. Ukstins, MS, CCC-A, FAAA is an educational audiologist who is currently serving as the Auditory Impairments Program Specialist for The Newark Public Schools, the largest school system in the State of New Jersey. She holds a bachelor's degree in communication sciences and disorders from Worcester State College (1987), a master's degree in audiology from Syracuse University (1989), and advanced certification in assistive technology (2010). She is a member of the American Speech-Language-Hearing (ASHA) association and a fellow of the American Academy of Audiology (AAA).

With more than 20 years of experience in audiology, she has worked in hospital and community healthcare centers. Alongside her coauthor, Deborah Welling, she has worked extensively with a wide range of difficult-to-test populations including the very young and those with multiple disabilities.

She currently works in the public school sector with Deaf and hard of hearing students, providing support throughout the district to students with both hearing impairment and central auditory processing deficits. The parent of two children with hearing loss; she speaks with both professional and personal knowledge on the impact of hearing loss.

Contributors

Annette Hurley, PhD, CCC-A
Associate Professor
Department of Communication Disorders
LSU Health Sciences Center
New Orleans, Louisiana

Cheryl DeConde Johnson, EdD, FAAA
Board Certified in Audiology with Pediatric Audiology
    Specialty Certification
The ADEvantage Consulting
Adjunct Assistant Professor
University of Arizona
Tucson, Arizona

Karen J. Kushla, ScD, CCC-A/FAAA
Adjunct Professor
School of Communication Disorders and Deafness
Kean University
Union, New Jersey

Tena L. McNamara, AuD, CCC-A/SLP
Assistant Professor
Department of Communication Disorders
    and Sciences
Eastern Illinois University
Charleston, Illinois

Donna M. Goione Merchant, AuD, CCC, FAAA
NJ Certified Teacher of the Deaf/Hearing Impaired
NJ Certified Teacher of the Handicapped
Private Practice Audiologist
Assistant Professor
Montclair State University
Montclair, New Jersey

Ralph Moscarella, MA, CCC-A, FAAA
Educational Audiologist
Newark Public Schools
Newark, New Jersey
Audiologist-Private Practice
Audiology Associates of Freehold
Freehold, New Jersey

Marietta M. Paterson, EdD, CED
Director, Education of the Deaf
Associate Professor
Department of Speech and Hearing Sciences
The University of Southern Mississippi
Hattiesburg, Mississippi

**Christina Barris Perigoe, PhD, CED, CCC-SLP,
LSLS-Cert. AVT**
Coordinator
Graduate Program in Early Oral Intervention
Associate Professor
Department of Speech and Hearing Sciences
The University of Southern Mississippi
Hattiesburg, Mississippi

Nancy G. Schneider, MA, CCC-A, FAAA
Audiologist
Little Falls, New Jersey

Arsen Zartarian, Esq.
President
New Jersey Association of School Attorneys
Deputy General Counsel
The Newark Public Schools
Newark, New Jersey

Reviewers

Vishwa Bhat, PhD, CCC-A, F-AAA
Associate Professor
Department of Communication Disorders and Sciences
William Paterson University
Wayne, New Jersey

Rieko M. Darling, PhD, FAAA, CAAA
Associate Professor of Audiology
Department of Communication Sciences and Disorders
Western Washington University
Bellingham, Washington

Dean Mancuso, AuD
Assistant Professor of Audiology
Department of Otolaryngology / Head and Neck Surgery
Columbia University Medical Center
New York City, New York

Anne D. Olson, PhD
Associate Professor
Department of Communication Sciences and Disorders
University of Kentucky
Lexington, Kentucky

Donna Pitts, AuD, CCC-A
Assistant Professor
Department of Speech-Language Pathology
Loyola University Maryland
Baltimore, Maryland

Chapter 1

The Speech-Language Pathologist in Audiology Services: An Interprofessional Collaboration

Carol A. Ukstins, MS, CCC-A, FAAA
Educational Audiologist
Office of Special Services
Newark Public Schools

Deborah R. Welling, AuD, CCC-A, FAAA
Associate Professor and Director of Clinical Education
Department of Speech-Language Pathology
Seton Hall University

Key Terms

Behavioral procedure
Best practice
Deaf
Diagnostic audiometry
Evidence-based practice
  (EBP)

False negative response
False positive response
Hard of hearing
Interprofessional
  collaboration
Nonbehavioral procedure

Response to intervention
  (RTI)
Screening procedure
Sensitivity
Specificity

Objectives

- Understand the requirements of the speech-language pathologist as it relates to audiologic services
- Discuss the difference between screening versus diagnostic service provision, and the information they provide
- Discuss the concept of collaboration and understand its importance
- Become familiar with terminology related to persons with hearing loss

Introduction

Speech-language pathology is an exciting profession. Listed as number 28 on *U.S. News & World Report*'s list of best jobs for 2013 (Graves, 2012), the field encompasses science, technology, and the humanities. It involves patient care from diagnosis to rehabilitation, working with all ages from infants to geriatrics. The speech-language pathologist (SLP) may find him- or herself working in a wide range of settings, including medical, educational, rehabilitative, and industrial. Perhaps one of the most exciting aspects of a career in speech-language pathology is the flexibility to work in such a wide range of settings and with an even wider range of individuals and disabilities without ever having to change your field. Throughout this rewarding career, it is quite likely that the speech-language pathologist will eventually have the opportunity to work with an individual who is hard of hearing or deaf. It is perhaps even more likely that the SLP will work with multiply impaired individuals with a wide variety of comorbidities, one of which may be hearing loss.

Working with such individuals requires that speech-language pathologists have a secure understanding of their own scope of practice as well as what it means to practice in an interprofessionally collaborative manner. Other elements critical to successful practice and interventions include best practice guidelines, evidence-based practice principles, and response to intervention. These topics will be addressed in this chapter.

Interprofessional Collaboration

The literature contains a variety of definitions related to **interprofessional collaboration**; some of them are unnecessarily extensive and complicated. At the heart of interprofessional collaboration, whether in the educational area or in clinical practice, is the concept of collaboration, which ". . . conveys the idea of sharing and implies collective action oriented toward a common goal, in a spirit of harmony and trust, particularly in the context of health professionals" (D'Amour, Ferrada-Videla, Rodriguez, & Beaulieu, 2005). Some of the potential benefits of interprofessional collaboration include increased coordination of service provision, better outcomes for the patient, higher satisfaction on the part of the professional, and time and cost efficiency.

Successful interactions among communication disorders service providers demonstrate the importance of having a collaborative relationship in health care, and the devastating effects that may result from its absence. If a child is referred for a speech-language evaluation because she is not speaking clearly and there is no communication between the speech-language pathologist and the audiologist, a hearing loss may go undiagnosed; unfortunately, this can and does happen. It is likely that many professionals who have worked in the field of communication disorders have encountered this scenario. The lack of interprofessional collaboration for this child can result in impaired speech-language development, academic progress, social interactions, vocational choices, and more.

The broader view of interprofessional collaboration sheds light on the fact that it is not only speech-language pathologists and audiologists whose professional areas are interrelated, but also those of occupational therapists, physical therapists, and recreational therapists (De Vries, 2012). As described by De Vries (2012), the skills required for effective interprofessional teamwork include understanding one's own and others' professions, mutual respect, cooperation, communication, coordination, assertiveness, shared responsibility, and autonomy (Banfield & Lackie, 2009; Hall, 2005; Lidskog, 2007). Although successful collaboration is clearly a complex process, fully understanding one's own scope of practice is an integral part of collaboration.

We emphasize again to the reader the importance of collaborating and working as a team, striving always to improve the quality of patient care. We also strongly encourage clinicians to be cognizant of their professional roles and responsibilities; not only in terms of their scope of practice and the knowledge and skills acquisition (KASA) standards, but also in terms of their ethical obligations.

Scope of Practice for the Speech-Language Pathologist

When the speech-language pathologist's job responsibilities include performing audiological procedures, the professional is cautioned to fully understand what is and what is not within their scope of practice. A sound understanding of how to perform a thorough hearing screening, as well as interpret audiometric data and manage the needs of a hard of hearing/deaf individual in your care, is an integral part of the speech-language pathologist's responsibilities.

The American Speech-Language-Hearing Association (ASHA) defines the scope of practice for the field of speech-language pathology. In its 2007 document titled *Scope of Practice in Speech-Language Pathology*, ASHA presents an official policy that specifies the breadth of practice within the profession of speech-language pathology. We will point out significant passages of this policy statement that are pertinent to your roles and responsibilities with the hard of hearing/deaf individual.

The speech-language pathologist addresses typical and atypical communication and swallowing in a variety of areas, such as speech, sound production, resonance, voice, fluency, language, cognition, and feeding and swallowing. As clearly pointed out in the "Professional Roles and Activities" section of this document, the potential etiologies of these communication and swallowing disorders include, among others, auditory problems such as hearing loss and deafness. It is quite noteworthy to point out that the other potential etiologies that appear on this list, such as neonatal complications, respiratory compromise, and genetic disorders, are also potential causes of hearing loss. The professional roles and activities of the SLP include, further, not only assessment, diagnosis, and treatment planning, but also prevention, advocacy, education, administration, and research (ASHA, 2007, p. 6). With these responsibilities in mind, knowing how to perform an air conduction screening is transparently inadequate. Although the speech-language pathologist's practice does not necessitate the scope and depth of knowledge required of the audiologist, an understanding that is broader and deeper than air conduction audiometry is a must.

Moving on to the document's section describing "Clinical Services," the speech-language pathologist provides services that include "screening individuals for hearing loss or middle ear pathology using conventional pure-tone air conduction methods (including otoscopic inspection), otoacoustic emissions screening, and/or screening tympanometry" (p. 7). However, the role of the SLP does not stop there; on the contrary, being competent to screen and interpret the results might be considered merely scratching the surface. The following list is an excerpt from *Scope of Practice in Speech-Language Pathology* (ASHA, 2007, p. 7) that includes additional examples of services within the SLP scope of practice:

5. Collaborating with other professionals (e.g., identifying neonates and infants at risk for hearing loss, participating in palliative care teams, planning lessons with educators, serving on student assistance teams) . . .

8. Providing intervention and support services for children and adults diagnosed with auditory processing disorders . . .

10. Counseling individuals, families, coworkers, educators, and other persons in the community regarding acceptance, adaptation, and decision making about communication and swallowing;

11. Facilitating the process of obtaining funding for equipment and services related to difficulties with communication and swallowing;

12. Serving as case managers, service delivery coordinators, and members of collaborative teams (e.g., individualized family service plan and individualized education program teams, transition planning teams);

13. Providing referrals and information to other professionals, agencies, and/or consumer organizations;

14. Developing, selecting, and prescribing multimodal augmentative and alternative communication systems, including unaided strategies (e.g., manual signs, gestures) and aided strategies (e.g., speech-generating devices, manual communication boards, picture schedules);

15. Providing services to individuals with hearing loss and their families/caregivers (e.g., auditory training for children with cochlear implants and hearing aids; speechreading; speech and language intervention secondary to hearing loss; visual inspection and listening checks of amplification devices for the purpose of troubleshooting, including verification of appropriate battery voltage);

16. Addressing behaviors (e.g., preservative or disruptive actions) and environments (e.g., classroom seating, positioning for swallowing safety or attention, communication opportunities) that affect communication and swallowing;

17. Selecting, fitting, and establishing effective use of prosthetic/adaptive devices for communication and swallowing (e.g., tracheoesophageal prosthesis, speaking valves, electrolarynxes; *this service does not include the selection or fitting of sensory devices used by individuals with hearing loss or other auditory perceptual deficits, which falls within the scope of practice of audiologists; ASHA, 2004);*

Reproduced from American Speech-Language-Hearing Association. (2007). Scope of Practice in Speech-Language Pathology. http://www.asha.org/policy/SP2007-00283/

The knowledge and skills set necessary for the speech-language pathologist to competently perform these duties is indescribably greater than just knowing how to conduct a hearing screening. Moreover, the responsibility does not end here. This manuscript also elaborates on the responsibilities as they relate to prevention and advocacy, education, administration, and research; each of these areas requires a solid understanding of the normal and abnormal auditory system, and the role each plays in communication development and abilities.

The complete document can be found by going to www.asha.org/policy/SP2007-00283.htm.

Diagnostic Audiometry Versus Hearing Screening Procedures

The difference between **diagnostic audiometry** and hearing **screening procedures** can sometimes be confusing. Simply put, a diagnosis of hearing status cannot be made based on a screening procedure; it can be made only as a result of a complete evaluation. A screening is generally a less time-intensive procedure, sometimes taking only 1 minute, whereas a diagnostic assessment is a comprehensive and time-consuming process that starts with a thorough case history and incorporates multiple behavioral, physiologic, and electrophysiologic measures. The hearing screening can identify only those individuals who appear likely to have a hearing loss, whereas the diagnostic assessment can confirm and delineate the type and severity of auditory disorder as well as provide possible recommendations for remediation.

Principles of Screening

A screening can be defined as a means to separate apparently healthy individuals from those for whom there is a greater probability of having a disease or condition, and then to refer the latter for appropriate diagnostic testing (ASHA, 1994). All screening methods should be scrutinized using two criteria when determining the process of pass and fail—sensitivity and specificity. These terms relate to the screening test's ability to accurately separate those who have a given disorder (in this case hearing loss) from those who do not. **Sensitivity** represents the percentage labeled positive on a test that truly have the target condition; **specificity** represents the percentage labeled negative who are truly free of the condition (ASHA, 1997). Table 1.1 provides an illustration of sensitivity and specificity possibilities.

In the case of air conduction hearing screenings, one critically important consideration is the intensity (or loudness) level used to do the screening. When the decibel level is set inappropriately low (too soft), a larger number of individuals will fail the screening. The individuals who failed under this very strict condition, but really *do not* have a hearing loss, are **false positive responses** (B in Table 1.1). This scenario actually might identify all individuals who really do have a hearing loss (high sensitivity); unfortunately, it also *wrongly* identifies many who really do not have a loss (low specificity).

If, on the other hand, the test intensity is set at a higher (too loud) decibel level, a larger number of individuals might pass under this inappropriately lenient condition. Those who pass under this condition but really *do* sustain hearing loss are **false negative responses** (C in Table 1.1). This scenario will correctly identify all of those cases that truly *do not* have a hearing loss (high specificity); however, the false negative responses represent the individuals who truly *do* have a hearing loss and were—quite unfortunately—not identified (low sensitivity).

The percentages of individuals who fall into each category shown in Table 1.1 for a given hearing screening event will depend largely on the parameters set, but they may also depend on other logistical concerns such as cost in time and money (McPherson, Law, & Wong, 2010; Peterson & Bell, 2008). Ideally, a screening protocol will be established that achieves sensitivity (true positive responses; A in Table 1.1) and specificity (true negative responses; D in Table 1.1) that are as high as possible. We must recognize, however, that real-life circumstances and considerations preclude the statistical perfection that would result in having a protocol that correctly separates out, with 100% accuracy, those who have the disorder from those who do not. We believe it is a reasonable goal to institute a hearing screening protocol that will minimize the false negatives as much as is possible and reasonable. Thus, no individual who actually sustains a hearing loss will miss out on the opportunity for follow-up and intervention.

Behavioral Versus Nonbehavioral Procedures

The numerous procedures used in the audiologic test battery include both behavioral and nonbehavioral types. Very simply stated, a **behavioral procedure** requires the client to actively participate in the task; thus, these types of tests are considered subjective. An example of a behavioral task is when pure tone audiometry is performed and the client is

Table 1.1 Sensitivity and Specificity

	Disease Positive	Disease Negative
Test Positive	A	B
Test Negative	C	D

required to raise his or her hand each time a beep is heard. A **nonbehavioral procedure** does not require the active participation of a client and, in fact, can be performed while the individual is asleep or sedated; thus, this type of task is referred to as objective.

Both behavioral and objective test measures are employed in various combinations in order to determine the type and extent of hearing loss. It is important to understand that the most comprehensive and useful diagnostic information is obtained when a test battery approach, utilizing both subjective and objective techniques, is employed. Thus, even when assessing infants, it is desirable to obtain corroboration of hearing loss by using a combination of behavioral and nonbehavioral test types.

Your Friendly Neighborhood Audiologist

As mentioned at the beginning of this chapter, never underestimate the power of collaboration. As sister fields, speech-language pathology and audiology both fall under the umbrella of ASHA; no matter where you find yourself practicing, you have a network of colleagues whom you can use as resources on a routine, daily basis. These individuals should never be hard to find in acute care medical facilities because those settings often have speech and hearing departments or otolaryngology departments where the audiologists are located. Subacute and nursing home facility employees may have a more difficult time locating the audiologist employed by the facility, possibly the result of limited hours of consultation. Within school systems there are fewer professionals employed as *educational audiologists*, but they can usually be accessed through local, county, regional, or state departments. National and state speech-language-hearing association conventions are an excellent venue for networking opportunities, as are continuing education workshops and national/international symposiums. Regardless, it is professionally beneficial that you will always be able to network with an audiologist when working with an individual with hearing loss.

A Word on Terminology

As a service provider to the patient diagnosed with hearing loss, it is important not only to understand the "technical" implications of certain terms, but also to be sensitive to the fact that some of these terms might carry unpleasant connotations and may also be considered offensive to some individuals.

Deaf

Deaf is the preferred terminology for a person presenting with a hearing loss of such significant degree that benefit derived from hearing aids is minimal. Manual communication and speech reading are the primary means of communication for these individuals. Many prefer not to attempt using amplification of any type. The archaic term *deaf and dumb* is considered offensive. In fact, in many European languages the term meant, as it did in English, not only "deaf and mute" but "deaf and stupid"—incapable of speech and, hence incapable of being educated (Power, 2006). Deaf individuals who choose not to use spoken language are technically considered *mute*. Unfortunately, a common definition of mute implies decreased mental aptitude, which is not the case for most deaf individuals. Today, deaf people find it insulting to be called "deaf and dumb."

Hard of Hearing

Hard of hearing is the preferred terminology for a person presenting with a hearing loss who can derive benefit from hearing aids and uses aural/oral speech for communication; for example, someone who can use a standard telephone (Zak, 1996). The term *hearing impaired* is felt to draw attention away from the person as an individual and focus directly on the disability itself.

Putting the Person First

Current terminology supports the view of "person first" when referring to an impairment or disability. According to *The Language Used to Describe Individuals with Disabilities*, disabilities are the person and they do not define the person, so do not replace person-nouns with disability-nouns (Folkins, 1992). Emphasis should be on the individual; this means that referring to someone as "hearing impaired", and similarly, "aphasic" or "autistic", should be avoided.

Resources for Best Practice, Evidence-Based Practice, and Response to Intervention

The practicing speech-language pathologist is held to high ethical standards by ASHA to provide the best quality service possible to his or her patients. Although a job description or a policies and procedures manual will provide guidance for the speech-language pathologist in specific practice settings and situations, there are several overlying concepts that will provide guidance in the quality of your services. Whether it is in the form of a hearing screening using state-of-the-art technology or evaluating the articulation of a child with developmental disabilities, holding yourself accountable for quality service should be at the forefront of your clinical practice.

Best Practice

Considered by many to be a buzzword, the term **best practice** describes the development of a standard of practice or process that can be used as a benchmark across a profession; best practices provide a clear expression of professional roles and responsibilities (English, 1991). Best practice refers to a clinical process or testing technique that is judged to be scientifically sound and that consistently yields results of better quality than those achieved with other procedures. Best practices are never static, but are ever-changing as improvements in therapeutic intervention and technology are discovered. Best practices are not mandated legislative regulations, but rather guidelines used as effective measures for a standard of practice.

To this end, ASHA's practice policy documents, along with other cardinal documents of the Association, are written for and by ASHA members and approved by its governance to promulgate best practices and standards in the professions of audiology and speech-language pathology (ASHA, n.d.). As current or future members of ASHA, the vast Association resources that are available and at your disposal through the ASHA website (see www.asha.org/policy/about/) include documents in the following categories:

- *Preferred Practice Patterns*—the informational base for providing quality patient/client care and a focus for professional preparation, continuing education, and research
- *Scope of Practice*—an outline of the parameters of each of the professions
- *Guidelines*—current best practice procedures based on available evidence
- *Position Statements*—public statements of ASHA's official stand on various issues
- *Knowledge and Skills*—the knowledge and set of skills required for a particular area of practice
- *Technical Reports*—supporting documentation and research for an ASHA position statement

- *Relevant Papers*—supporting and related professional documents
- *Standards/Quality Indicators*—documents related to certification accreditation, and professional standards
- *Ethics*—includes the *Code of Ethics* (by which all members and certificate holders are bound) and supporting documents
- *Bylaws*—the bylaws of ASHA, the ASHFoundation, and the ASHA PAC

Evidence-Based Practice

Entire textbooks and courses are devoted to the study of **evidence-based practice (EBP)**. As such, this section is not intended—in any way—to provide thorough coverage of the topic or what it entails. It is important, however, to highlight the importance of employing EBP principles to the clinician's practice. Therefore, the purpose of this section is merely to define and describe EBP, and to provide resources for you to further investigate this topic on your own.

EBP is the foundational component of research from Dr. David Sackett, considered a pioneer in the area of evidence-based practice. Evidence-based practice can be defined as the conscientious, explicit, and judicious use of current best evidence in making decisions about the care of the individual patient. It means integrating individual clinical expertise with the best available external clinical evidence from systematic research (Sackett & Rosenberg, 1996).

For the speech-language pathologist, EBP is the integration of clinical knowledge, the value a patient places on his or her therapy session, and research evidence into the decision-making process for patient care. You might think of this as being a three-legged stool that will collapse if any of those legs are missing. Knowledge of clinical practice is based on the clinician's collective experiences, education, and clinical skills. However, an integral part of EBP is also the patient. The nature of the disability, concern regarding therapeutic outcome, expectations, and values of the therapy session all play a large role in EBP. Best practices, as discussed in the previous section, are included as well because data regarding patient outcomes is usually found in clinically relevant research that has been conducted using sound methodology (Sackett, 2000).

The evidence of therapeutic progress by itself does not determine the level of therapeutic effectiveness, but it can help support the patient care process. The full integration of all three areas into clinical decisions increases the opportunity for effective clinical outcomes and quality of life. Evidence-based practice requires the clinician to constantly develop new skills, including efficient literature searching and the ability to effectively evaluate clinical literature, which serves to hone clinical practices.

A plethora of resources for EBP are available through the ASHA website at http://www.asha.org/members/ebp/. A guide to the steps in the EBP process, EBP tutorials, and a list of evidence-based systematic reviews on a broad range of topics are only a few of the many educational tools available through the website. Students and practicing clinicians alike are encouraged to explore the information available.

Response to Intervention

The roots of **response to intervention (RTI)** are in the educational realm. Stemming from the release of the No Child Left Behind Act, it is a systematic methodology of providing assistance to children who are experiencing educational difficulty to prevent academic failure. The design of RTI is to provide interventions, frequent measurements of progress, and a spectrum of increasingly intensive research-based instructional interventions for those children who continue to demonstrate difficulty in a specific academic area. The design of RTI is based on the premise of keeping children out of the arena of special education by intervening when academic difficulties are noted, rather than waiting for the child to fail and then be referred to the Child Study Team for evaluation. RTI is viewed by many to be an alternative to the "discrepancy model," in which cognitive ability, measured by psychological measures of intelligence (i.e., IQ testing) and their academic achievement are compared and a determination of a specific type of learning disability is made. The model of RTI is thought by many to be a better alternative to the individualized education program (IEP) generated through a referral and evaluation process of special education. Its premise is that through the collaboration of all stakeholders in the educational process, a child struggling to succeed can be provided with the appropriate interventions while remaining in the general education population. Figure 1.1 demonstrates the continuum of the RTI service provision model within the general education setting.

Although RTI is clearly and specifically written into No Child Left Behind as a process that now must take place prior to referring a child for special education and related services, much controversy surrounds the RTI model. Proponents of RTI support this multitier model of academic

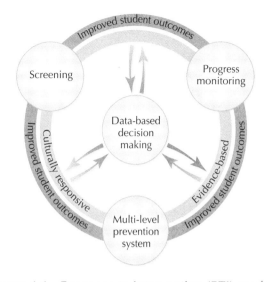

Figure 1.1   Response to Intervention (RTI) model.
Reproduced from National Center on Response to Intervention (June 2010). What is Response to Intervention (RTI). Washington, DC: U.S. Department of Education, Office of Special Education Programs, National Center on Response to Intervention.

assistance in the general education setting focusing on the early design of interventions for those struggling in the mainstream of education. Merging special education into the general education classroom provides the least restrictive environment (LRE) for these students and allows them the best possible services. By having clear standards, useful measurements, and sound instructional practices within the classroom, academic performance is enhanced. Designing a program that exposes these students to the general education setting with their nondisabled peers will result in improvement in academic achievement and overall educational success (Batsche et al., 2005).

Opponents claim that RTI simply identifies low achieving students rather than students with learning disabilities. Poor supports in the process of RTI result in students continuing in a program that is not working to meet their needs. General education teachers cannot always provide the necessary modifications to instruction, or cannot do it systematically. Opponents claim that the main flaw in RTI is that through this intervention model we are asking the student to change when it is the instruction that must change (Batsche, Kavale, & Kovaleski, 2006). The RTI model assumes full cooperation of all stakeholders in the process and that the process itself is clearly defined and implemented.

The devil is in the details. The success of RTI will depend on whether highly trained professionals appropriately implement it—and this is likely to be a problem.

Summary

The role of the speech-language pathologist in servicing patients with hearing loss is clearly defined in the ASHA *Scope of Practice in Speech-Language Pathology*. Through the effective measures of hearing screening, application of best practice methods, and being proactive in interprofessional collaboration, this process can and will serve the deaf or hard of hearing individual in the most effective therapeutic ways possible. This can only be done when the speech-language pathologist is clear about his or her role as a professional, has a strong understanding of the premise behind the screening measure used to identify potential hearing loss, and keeps his or her professional practices current based on research and trends within the field of speech-language pathology.

Discussion Questions

1. Describe the difference between a diagnostic evaluation and a screening measure.
2. Specificity and sensitivity are the two components of screening measures. Describe how each plays a role in setting the parameters of screening. How do they affect the four quadrants of your screening results?
3. What are the three components to evidence-based practice (EBP)? How does the patient's investment in their therapy play an important role in EBP?
4. What is response to intervention (RTI)? Describe a scenario in which RTI would work well for a student. Describe a scenario in which RTI would not work well for a student.

References

American Speech-Language-Hearing Association (ASHA). (1994). *Audiologic screening*. Available from http://www.asha.org/policy.

American Speech-Language-Hearing Association (ASHA). (1997). *Guidelines for audiologic screening*. Available from http://www.asha.org/policy.

American Speech-Language-Hearing Association (2004). *Scope of practice in audiology*. Available from http://www.asha.org/policy.

American Speech-Language-Hearing Association (ASHA). (2007). *Scope of practice in speech-language pathology*. Available from http://www.asha.org/policy/SP2007-00283.htm.

American Speech-Language-Hearing Association (ASHA). (n.d.). *About ASHA practice policy*. Available from http://www.asha.org/policy/about/.

Banfield, V., & Lackie, K. (2009). Performance-based competencies for culturally responsive interprofessional collaborative practice. *Journal of Interprofessional Care*, 23 (6): 611–620.

Batsche, G., Elliot, J., Graden, J. L., Grimes, J., Kovaleski, J. F., Prasse, D., et al. (2005). *Response to intervention: Policy considerations and implementation*. Alexandria, VA: National Association of State Directors of Special Education.

Batsche, G., Kavale, K., & Kovaleski, J. (2006). Response to intervention: Competing views. *Assessment for Effective Intervention*, 32: 6–20.

D'Amour, D., Ferrada-Videla, M., Rodriguez, L. S., & Beaulieu, M. (2005). The conceptual basis for interprofessional collaboration: Core concepts and theoretical frameworks. *Journal of Interprofessional Care*, Supplement 1: 116–131.

De Vries, D. R. (2012). *Therapists value of interprofessional collaboration*. Available from http://condor.cmich.edu/cdm/ref/collection/p1610-01coll1id/3631.

English, K. (1991). Best practice in educational audiology. *Language, Speech, and Hearing Services in Schools*, 22: 283–286.

Folkins, J. (1992). *Resource on person-first language: The language used to describe individuals with disabilities*. Available from http://www.asha.org/publications/journals/submissions/person_first/.

Graves, J. A. (2012, Dec. 18). The best jobs of 2013. *U. S. News & World Report*. Available from http://money.usnews.com/money/careers/articles/2012/12/18/the-best-jobs-of-2013.

McPherson, B., Law, M. M. S., & Wong, M. S. W. (2010). Hearing screening for school children: Comparison of low-cost, computer-based and conventional audiometry. *Child: Care, Health and Development*, 36(3): 323–331.

Peterson, M. E., & Bell, T. S. (2008). *Foundations of audiology: A practical approach*. Upper Saddle River, NJ: Pearson Education.

Power, D. (2006). Googling "deaf": Deafness in the world's English-language press. *American Annals of the Deaf*, 151(5): 513–518.

RTI, Differentiated Instruction, and Their Marriage, The Foundation. Available from: http://www.sagepub.com/upm-data/40757_omeara_ch1.pdf.

Sackett, D. *Evidence-based Medicine: How to Practice and Teach EBM*. 2nd edition. Edinburgh: Churchill Livingstone, 2000.

Sackett, D. L., & Rosenberg, W. M. C. (1996). Evidence-based medicine—What it is and what it isn't. *BMJ: British Medical Journal (International Edition)*, 312(7023): 71–72.

Zak, O. (1996). *Zak's politically incorrect glossary*. Available from http://www.zak.co.il/d/deaf-info/old/zpig.html#hoh.

Chapter 2

Sound and Hearing

Karen J. Kushla, ScD, CCC-A/FAAA
Adjunct Professor
School of Communication Disorders and Deafness
Kean University

Key Terms

Acceleration
Acoustics
Auditory labyrinth
Basilar membrane
Bel
Boyle's law
Broca's area
Conductive hearing loss
Decibel (dB)
Decibel hearing level (dB HL)
Decibel sensation level (dB SL)
Decibel sound pressure level (dB SPL)
Displacement
Elastic
Endocochlear electrical potential

Endolymph
Equilibrium
Eustachian tube
External auditory meatus
Force
Helicotrema
Impedance-matching transformer
Incus
Inertia
Inner hair cells
Linear scale
Logarithmic scale
Malleus
Mass
Membranous labyrinth
Mixed hearing loss
Organ of Corti

Osseous labyrinth
Ossicles
Outer ear
Outer hair cells
Oval window
Pars flaccida
Pars tensa
Pascal (Pa)
Perilymph
Pinna
Pressure wave
Propagation
Pure tone
Rarefaction
Round window
Saccule
Scala media
Scala tympani

Scala vestibuli
Semicircular canals
Sensorineural hearing loss
Simple harmonic motion
  (SHM)
Sound
Stapedius muscle
Stapes

Tectorial membrane
Tensor tympani muscle
Tonotopic organization
Transducer
Traveling wave theory
Tympanic membrane
Uniform circular motion
Utricle

Vector
Vestibular labyrinth
Vestibular membrane
Vestibule
Wavelength
Wernicke's area

Objectives

- Describe the characteristics of sound
- Define and apply the concept of simple harmonic motion to periodic sounds
- Describe the characteristics of the decibel and why it is used
- Describe sound transduction through the auditory system

Introduction

This chapter will review the key concepts needed to understand what, how, and why we hear. The general characteristics of sound are presented so the reader can understand how changes in sound pressure affect what we hear. Special attention is paid to the description of sound intensity and its measurement. The structure and function of the outer, middle, and inner ear are also described to demonstrate how sound travels through the auditory system up to the brain.

General Characteristics of Sound

Sound is all around us, although it may be too faint for us to hear or too intense for us to listen to for any length of time. In the 1700s, the British philosopher George Berkeley asked the question, "If a tree falls in the forest and no one is around to hear it, does it make a sound?" Of course it does, unless it falls on another planet with a rarefied atmosphere, in which case there is no sound.

The study of sound is a branch of physics called **acoustics**. **Sound** itself is a physical phenomenon that is described as the movement or **propagation** of a disturbance (i.e., a vibration) through an elastic medium (e.g., air molecules) without permanent displacement of the particles.

There are three prerequisites for production of sound: (1) a source of energy (e.g., a force), (2) a vibrating object that generates an audible pressure wave, and (3) a medium of transmission (e.g., air). However, a receiver of these prerequisites of sound production is optional.

As human beings, we produce sound primarily in air, so let's begin our discussion of the prerequisites with the medium of transmission we call air. Air molecules are not static; in fact, they are moving constantly in random fashion. This random movement at high speeds is called **Brownian motion**, named for Robert Brown (1773–1858), a Scottish botanist who described this motion, which results from the impact of molecules found within a gas or liquid. Brownian motion causes these air molecules to collide with each other and with whatever is in their path—walls, furniture, people. These molecules are **elastic**—that is, the objects exhibit a tendency to resist deformity and return to their rest position—so there is no change in their shape when they bump into each other and/or other objects. These collisions produce pressure. Although we may not be able to feel that pressure, it is there. You feel this pressure whenever air is set into motion, such as on a windy day or when we speak.

A source of energy, such as a force, is the next prerequisite. **Force** is a push or a pull on an object, and is a **vector**; that is, it has both magnitude (some amount greater than zero) and direction. Force is mathematically determined to be the product of mass times acceleration ($\mathbf{F} = ma$). Air molecules have **mass** (the quantity of matter present). Mass is not identical to weight because weight is affected by gravitational forces; however, for our purposes, mass and weight are the same. Because air molecules have mass, they obey Newton's laws of motion, the first of which states that all bodies remain at rest or in a state of uniform motion unless other forces act in opposition. (This property is called **inertia**.) The amount of inertia an object (e.g., an air molecule) has is directly proportional to its mass; the greater an object's mass, the greater its inertia. An outside force must be applied to change this tendency. **Acceleration** is the speed (distance traveled per unit time) of an object per unit time, which is represented mathematically as length/(time)^2. When a force is applied to the air particles by a moving object, the air particles will travel in the direction of the force. The amount of this distance is proportional to the magnitude of the applied force—a large force will cause the object to travel much further than a small force. Therefore, the greater the force applied to the object, the greater the distance the object travels by that force; in addition, the restoring force is proportional to the displacement (i.e., the object obeys Hooke's law, named for Robert Hooke [1635–1703], an English experimental philosopher who first described this action).

Finally, we need an object that is capable of vibrating. Air molecules happen to vibrate quite well, and can be set into vibration easily to produce a **pressure wave**. For example, if we strike a tuning fork on a hard surface to set its tines into vibration, the air molecules surrounding the tuning fork tines are also set into vibration, creating this pressure wave. This initial impact starts movement of the air molecules away from rest (**displacement**) in the same direction of the force. This pressure wave displaces air molecules near the tuning fork tines; these displaced air molecules further displace other air molecules adjacent to the pressure wave, which displace adjacent air molecules, and so on. Therefore, the wave motion is propagated, or transferred, through the air to the human ear.

When the air molecules reach the maximum point of displacement, their motion is momentarily halted because of inertia (i.e., air molecules follow Newton's first law of motion, which states that objects at rest will remain at rest unless acted upon by a force). Once the force is removed, the restoring force of elasticity returns the displaced air molecule to a resting state called **equilibrium**. When the

air molecules return to their resting state, the void left by their former positions are filled by the adjacent air molecules, which then displace the adjacent air molecules in the opposite direction (i.e., the air molecules follow Newton's third law, which states that for any action there is an equal and opposite reaction). The elastic medium is not displaced over an appreciable distance; rather, the air molecules vibrate to and fro about their average equilibrium positions away from the source of energy.

Elasticity in the tuning fork tine allows for this displacement, but also generates a restoring force that momentarily stops the movement at the point of maximum amplitude away from the rest position. The restoring fork pushes the tuning fork tines back to their rest position, but inertia carries the tines past the rest position. By overshooting the rest position, the tines then are pushed toward the opposite maximal position; the restoring force builds up in the other direction, and the tuning fork tines return to the rest position once again. The tuning fork tines overshoot the rest position, the restoring force builds up again, and the pattern repeats; this alternating pattern of inertia and elasticity creates one full cycle of vibration. As you can see, inertia and the restoring forces vary continuously during each cycle; inertia is strong when the restoring force is weak, and vice versa. This interplay between the two forces enables the vibration to persist until other external forces (for example, friction, which causes a gradual decay in vibratory amplitude) overcome the tuning fork tines' mass and elasticity and the energy dissipates. Although the air molecules are displaced from their rest position at various points throughout the cycles of vibration, they continue to vibrate at the same frequency as the tuning fork.

As air molecules vibrate, waves of pressure fluctuations are created and travel through the elastic medium. (However, the molecules themselves move only a short distance.) As this vibratory disturbance (and not the air molecules themselves) propagates through the air, the atmosphere goes through alternating periods of increased and decreased air particle density and, consequently, of high and low pressure. Because air molecules are able to flow easily, they flow from regions of higher pressure to regions of lower pressure. The density (concentration) of these air particles alternately increases and decreases relative to their conditions at rest (i.e., when there is no vibration and the molecules are in equilibrium). For a fixed volume of vibrating air molecules, increased concentration (density) of air particles results in increased air pressure; this is called **Boyle's law** (after Robert Boyle [1627–1691], British physicist and

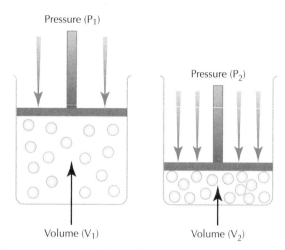

Figure 2.1   Boyle's law illustrated.

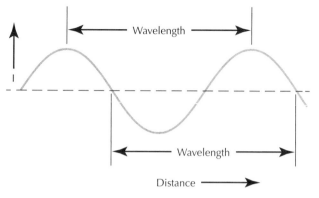

Figure 2.2   Wavelength.

chemist), which states that the pressure and volume of a gas are inversely proportional if kept at a constant temperature (see Figure 2.1).

Because the initial force is a vector, it causes an outward movement of the tuning fork tines toward a positive displacement, which causes the surrounding air molecules to be crowded together. The force of displacement is passed from molecule to molecule; this displacement creates areas of increased pressure and density of air molecules that are called **condensation** (also known as **compression**). When the tines return toward equilibrium because of elasticity, the force on the surrounding medium is relieved, and the air molecules also return toward their position of equilibrium. This "thinning" of air molecules creates areas of decreased air pressure and density (**rarefaction**). The distance between two successive condensations (i.e., from a point on one wave to the same point on the next cycle of the wave) is called the **wavelength** of the sound wave. The wavelength represents the length of the disturbance created by the wave in a medium (see Figure 2.2). Wavelength is measured in units of length (e.g., meters), and is represented by the Greek letter lambda (λ).

Sound in air moves in the same (or opposite) direction of the force; in other words, this pressure wave moves longitudinally. In a longitudinal wave, air molecules approach and recede from each other to create variations in pressure so that the wave movement is parallel to the force. The air molecules do not move far from their rest positions; instead, they move a short distance in either direction from rest but do not move forward with the wave itself. To demonstrate longitudinal waves at home, have a friend hold one end of a Slinky

(the metal ones work best), and you hold the other end. Pinch a few of the coils together and then release them. The energy released will travel down the Slinky toward the other end, and then return to you until the energy is overcome by friction and dies. In a transverse wave, on the other hand, the air molecules vibrate at right angles to the direction of wave propagation. To demonstrate transverse waves, fill a deep, wide bowl with water, and place a feather (or float a cork) on the water surface. (The fluid tension will keep the feather or the cork floating on the water's surface because the water has greater density than either the feather or the cork.) Drop a small object (e.g., a pebble or a penny) into the bowl; the feather or cork will bob up and down. This movement is perpendicular to the direction of wave propagation.

Simple Harmonic Motion and Sound

In acoustics, when air particles are set into motion by a force to produce changes in pressure, areas of condensation and rarefaction alternate. If these areas of alternating condensation and rarefaction occur at a steady rate of change, the resultant pressure wave is said to be a **pure tone** (also known as those little beeps you hear during a hearing test), which moves in **simple harmonic motion (SHM)** and is represented graphically by a sine wave. Although pure tones rarely occur in nature, they result when sound waves are propagated through an elastic medium and complete the same number of complete cycles of vibration per unit time. Examples of pure tones include tuning forks and pendulums, both of which produce vibrations that move in SHM (see Figure 2.3).

Characteristics of SHM

The basic attributes of a sound wave—period, frequency, amplitude, and phase are explained through SHM. When pure tones move in SHM, they take the same amount of

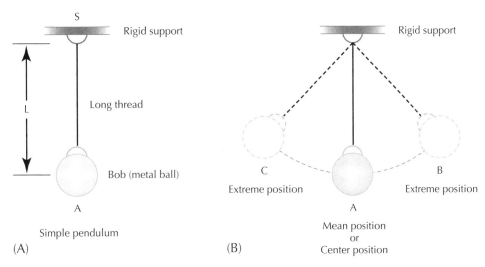

Figure 2.3   Example of simple harmonic motion.

time to complete each cycle of vibration. In other words, pure tones are periodic. A period (p) is a physical characteristic that describes the amount of time it takes to complete one full cycle of vibration, and is measured in units of time (usually seconds [s] or milliseconds [ms]). Frequency (f) is the inverse of the pure tone's period and is a physical characteristic that describes the number of complete cycles of vibration that occur per unit time (**Figure 2.4**). Frequency

is measured in units called Hertz (Hz), in honor of Heinrich Hertz (1857–1894), a German physicist who contributed to the field of electromagnetism through his description of wave movement. Only one frequency is described in a pure tone (e.g., 1000 Hz).

Pitch and frequency are not synonymous. Because frequency is a physical characteristic, it depends on the mass of the vibrating object, its overall size, and so on; in general,

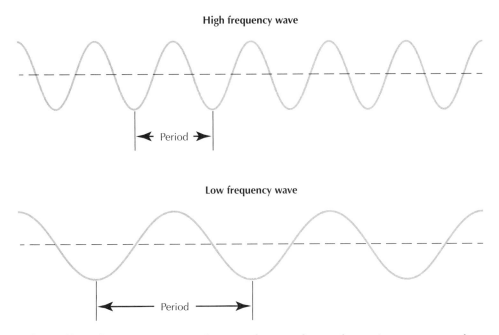

Figure 2.4   High- and low-frequency waves. The waveform at the top has twice as many cycles and its period is half as long as the wave at the bottom; therefore, the upper wave is one octave above the bottom wave.

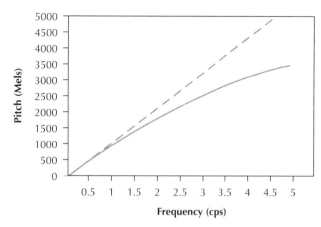

Figure 2.5 This graph shows the relationship between frequency (x-axis, in units of cycles per second, cps) and pitch (y-axis, in units of Mels). At lower frequencies, frequency (dashed line) and pitch (solid line) have nearly a 1:1 relationship, but at higher frequencies, pitch differs from frequency.

the larger the vibrating object, the more slowly that object will vibrate. Pitch, on the other hand, is a percept (a psychological correlate), and is related to the listener's perceptual response to frequency. We might also think of pitch as a relative term; that is, if you ask whether a certain sound is high pitch or low pitch, the question that would arise is: higher or lower than what? Pitch is measured in Mels. The Mel scale is a psychophysical scale of pitch perception; 1000 Mels is the pitch equal to a 1000-Hz tone at a particular intensity. Figure 2.5 shows the relationship between pitch and frequency.

As a sound wave travels through an elastic medium like air, we can calculate how far it travels through one complete cycle of vibration. This is called the wavelength (λ), and is measured in units of length (e.g., meters). We can also determine the speed (velocity) of the sound wave if we know how far it travels per unit time. The velocity of air at standard room temperature and pressure (20° Celsius at sea level) is approximately 344 m/s. (In gases such as air, temperature plays an important part in how fast sound travels. Sounds travel faster through liquids and fastest along solids because the greater elasticity and density of these media increase the velocity of conduction.) How fast the sound wave moves depends on the density and elastic properties of the medium through which it is moving, and is independent of pressure as long as air temperature is constant. Therefore, a faint sound travels at the same velocity as a loud sound. We can calculate the wavelength λ of a 1000-Hz sound wave very easily if we know the velocity of sound;

because velocity divided by frequency equals wavelength, 344 m/s ÷ 1000 cycles/s = 0.344 m (approximately 1 foot). (Note: Do not confuse the velocity of sound wave propagation with the velocity of particle movement; particles vibrating in SHM constantly change velocity, moving with maximum velocity over their rest position.)

Amplitude (**A**) is another vector quantity that describes both magnitude and direction of wave displacement from rest. Amplitude is a derived unit of measurement that describes the distance from an object's rest position by a vibrating body or the magnitude of pressure change that occurs by that object's motion. The greater the distance caused by vibration is from the point of rest, the greater the amplitude. In general, the greater the amplitude, the louder the pure tone sounds. Amplitude can be described by both physical parameters and psychophysical percepts. Loudness is the percept of intensity and depends on how our inner ears (specifically, the cochlea) interpret how much sound pressure is presented over our tympanic membranes (eardrums). The human ear happens to be very sensitive to changes in sound pressure, so small changes in pressure (i.e., intensity) will result in either an increase or a decrease in loudness sensation. Intensity is a derived unit of measurement that describes the amount of acoustic energy (i.e., sound) that passes through a unit of area in a given time span. A pure tone's intensity is measured by the amplitude of its sine wave, and varies with time. The human ear is capable of hearing a wide range of sound intensities.

SHM is usually depicted as a sine wave, with peaks (i.e., compressions) and troughs (i.e., rarefactions). If we were to cut that sine wave in half and move the trough directly beneath the peak, we would form a circle. If an air molecule were to move around the circumference of that circle at a constant rate, we could describe that movement as projected **uniform circular motion**. The air molecule's displacement along that circumference varies with the passage of time in the same way during a cycle of movement as long as the frequency of the sine wave is constant. This brings us to our last characteristic of SHM: phase. Phase is that portion of a cycle that has elapsed at any instant in time, relative to some arbitrary starting point, that is, the relative timing of compressions and rarefactions of an object moving in SHM. Because of this relationship between SHM and projected uniform circular motion, phase is measured in degrees (from 0° to 360°). **Figures 2.6** and **2.7** depict the relationship between these concepts.

Why is phase important? If two sound waves of the exact same frequency are exactly in phase, their amplitudes add

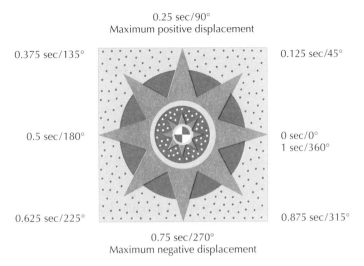

0.25 sec/90°
Maximum positive displacement

0.375 sec/135°

0.125 sec/45°

0.5 sec/180°

0 sec/0°
1 sec/360°

0.625 sec/225°

0.875 sec/315°

0.75 sec/270°
Maximum negative displacement

Figure 2.6 Relationship between simple harmonic motion, projected uniform circular motion, phase, and degrees in a sine wave.

together and result in a doubling of intensity; if these sound waves are slightly out of phase, their amplitudes add together, but the resultant intensity ranges from not quite doubled to almost zero. If two sound waves are exactly out of phase, their amplitudes add together to cancel; no sound is produced because there is no change in sound pressure. This is how noise-cancellation headphones work—a sound wave exactly opposite the generating wave is produced so that their amplitudes cancel.

The Decibel: Measure of Relative Intensity

What Is a Decibel?

Earlier I noted that intensity is the physical measure of what we perceive as the loudness of a sound. A sound's intensity is measured in acoustic (sound) pressure. Pressure is created when a force is distributed over an area; mathematically,

pressure = force/area. (Force is the product of mass and acceleration; its unit of measurement is the dyne.) When we measure sound intensity, we are measuring the force of that sound wave's vibration over a given unit of area. The greater the change in air pressure, the greater the intensity of sound. The unit of measurement that describes sound pressure is the **Pascal** (Pa), named in honor of Blaise Pascal (1623–1662), a French mathematician; 1 Pa = 10 dynes/cm². Normal human hearing sensitivity ranges from 0.0002 dynes/cm² to 2000 dynes/cm². Although it is possible to measure sound pressure in units of dynes/cm², it would force us to use very large numbers to describe a person's hearing sensitivity (e.g., 10,000,000,000,000 dynes/cm²).

When we describe sound pressure using Pascals, we are using what is called a linear (or integral) measuring scale (also known as an absolute scale)—there is a true zero point, each increment on the scale is equal to every other increment, and you can sum incremental units by addition.

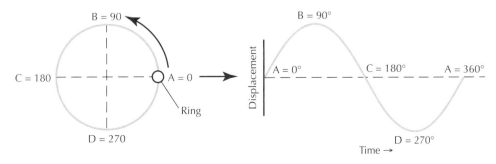

Figure 2.7 Relationship among simple harmonic motion, phase, and projected uniform circular motion.

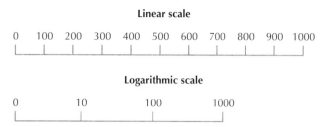

Figure 2.8 Relationship between linear and logarithmic scales.

An example of a **linear scale** is a ruler like a yardstick; you can't have a negative distance, and each increment (e.g., 1 inch) is equivalent. A better measurement scale to use for intensity, however, is a logarithmic (ratio) scale. A **logarithmic scale** is a relative scale where there is no zero point (you must define what zero is), the zero point does not represent the absence of what is being measured, and each successive unit is larger than the one preceding it; therefore, each increment is not equal, and represents increasingly large numerical differences. A logarithmic scale compresses the potentially very large numbers used in a linear scale into much more manageable increments to use. See **Figure 2.8**, which illustrates the incremental differences between linear and logarithmic scales.

Why do we use a logarithmic scale for intensity? It has been known since the 19th century that the logarithmic scale corresponds nicely to how intensity differences are perceived in the human ear. Equal increases in sensation (in this case, loudness) are obtained by multiplying the stimulus by a constant factor. Although this doesn't work for all intensities to which the ear is sensitive, it is accurate enough to be practical.

The unit of measurement used to describe human intensity differences is the **Bel** (named in honor of Alexander Graham Bell [1847–1922], the Scottish American inventor and teacher of oral speech to the deaf). The Bel is a relative measurement of intensity that expresses the ratio of a measured sound intensity to a relative sound intensity. In other words, this very large range of human hearing (on the order of 10^{14} dynes/cm^2) is compressed so that smaller numbers are used. By using the Bel we bring the range of intensities heard from 10^{14} units to a range of 0 to 14 however, this is so far to the other extreme that it is absurd! The scale of the Bel has been compressed so much that fractions must be used to reflect the desired accuracy of measurement of intensity (e.g., an intensity of 4.5 Bels). To minimize the use of decimals we can use a smaller unit of measurement, the decibel

(literally, one-tenth of a Bel). The **decibel (dB)** is a much more useable unit of measurement of intensity because the range of human hearing on the decibel scale becomes whole numbers and ranges between 0 dB and 140 dB.

The decibel expresses a ratio between the measured sound pressure and a relative sound pressure (defined at 0.0002 dynes/cm^2, which happens to be the softest sound a person with normal hearing sensitivity can hear), using logarithms. In its simplest form, a logarithm is the same as an exponent, which indicates how many times a number is multiplied by itself. Take the equation $10 \times 10 = 100$. The number 10 is multiplied by itself. We can also express this equation as $10^2 = 100$; in this case, the number 10 is the base and the number 2 is the exponent. If we wanted to express the second equation logarithmically, we can also say $\log_{10} 100 = 2$. The number 10 is still the base, the number 2 is still the exponent, and the number 100 is still the product of the multiplication of 10×10. We just rearranged how we expressed the multiplication problem using logarithms. To multiply logarithms with the same base number, you add their exponents; to divide logarithms with the same base number, you subtract their exponents.

We also use decibels to denote intensity for another reason: We can describe intensity either in units of power (used in acoustics) or sound pressure (dB SPL, used in the measurement of hearing sensitivity). (Because we are primarily interested in changes in sound pressure—e.g., running speech—this discussion will be limited to audiometric applications.) In audiology, intensity level refers to the changes in sound pressure level, as measured in dynes/cm^2. Because decibels are based on relative differences in intensities, a reference value (standard) must be provided, which is the threshold of human hearing (equal to 0.0002 dynes/cm^2 in units of sound pressure). We can calculate sound intensity in decibels using the following formula:

$$dB\ SPL = 20 \log_{10} (P_o/P_r)$$

where P_o = measured sound pressure and P_r = recognized reference point (0.0002 dynes/cm^2).

To illustrate how we use this equation, let's say that our measured sound pressure (P_o) is equivalent to our reference pressure (P_r = 0.0002 dynes/cm^2). We can then substitute these values into the equation to get:

$$dB\ SPL = 20 \log_{10} (0.0002\ dynes/cm^2 \div 0.0002\ dynes/cm^2)$$
$$= 20 \log_{10} (1) = 0$$

To what power do we raise 10 to equal 1? The answer is zero (0) because $10^0 = 1$, and anything multiplied by 0 is equal

Table 2.1 Relationship of Measured Pressure to Intensity

Measured Pressure (dynes/cm²)	Intensity (dB SPL)
0.0002	0 (minimum audible sound)
0.002	20
0.02	40
0.2	60
2.0	80
20.0	100
200.0	120
2000.0	140

to 0. Therefore, a sound stimulus that is minimally audible has an intensity of 0 dB SPL.

As you can see from Table 2.1, a tenfold increase in sound pressure (a linear measure) yields a 20 dB increase in intensity (a logarithmic measure).

Intensity versus Loudness

Intensity, like frequency, is a physical property of an acoustic signal. The loudness—the subjective, psychological sensation of intensity—of a signal is related to its intensity; however, this relationship between loudness and intensity is not linear. At a given intensity, loudness perception varies with sound frequency because the human auditory system is designed to receive the middle frequencies with much less intensity than is needed for extremely high and low frequencies. Just as frequency has a perceptual correlate (pitch), intensity also has perceptual correlates: the phon (a unit of equal loudness) and the sone (an arbitrary unit of loudness). The phon level roughly matches intensity (in dB SPL) at a frequency of 1000 Hz. Frequencies in the range of 1000 Hz to 6000 Hz are detected at the lowest sound pressure levels, whereas very low and very high frequencies require greater sound pressure levels to pass the threshold of hearing. Figure 2.9 shows how equal loudness changes over a range of frequencies, that is, the minimum audibility needed at each frequency. (However, lower frequencies span the range of loudness with a smaller range of perceptual intensities than do the higher frequencies.) The sone, on the other hand, is defined as the loudness of a 1000-Hz tone set at 40 dB above threshold. The sensation of loudness increases more slowly than the actual increase in intensity for normal auditory systems; in pathologic systems, the abnormally rapid growth of loudness is called

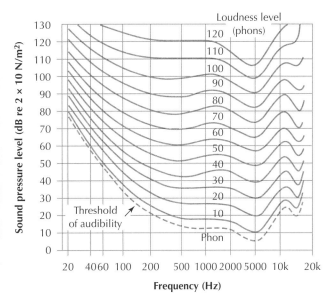

Figure 2.9 The heavy line on a phon curve also represents the 0 dB HL line on an audiogram. This is also known as a Fletcher–Munson curve, named for the researchers (H. Fletcher and W.A. Munson) who developed the scale.

Modified from Fletcher, H., & Munson, W.A. (1933). Loudness: its definition, measurement and calculation. Journal of the Acoustical Society of America, 5, 82–108.

recruitment. This phenomenon usually occurs in those individuals who have sensorineural (especially cochlear) hearing loss. The scales used in acoustics are shown in Table 2.2.

Which Decibel Should I Use?

The decibel symbol is often qualified with a suffix that indicates which reference quantity has been used. We have seen how the decibel (in units of sound pressure level, dB SPL) expresses a ratio of measured sound pressure to a reference sound pressure. Indeed, we use dB SPL to indicate the intensity of a sound stimulus. However, when we measure an individual's auditory sensitivity, it is more useful to compare that threshold intensity to the softest intensity the

Table 2.2 Relative Scales Used in Acoustics

	Name	Unit
Physical Properties	Frequency	Hertz (Hz)
	Intensity	Decibel (dB)
Psychological Properties	Pitch	Mel (scaling)
	Loudness	Sone (scaling) Phon (equal)

average person with normal hearing sensitivity can hear. Therefore, we use a different decibel—in terms of hearing level (dB HL)—to show this deviation from what is considered to be "normal hearing." The decibel in units of hearing level (dB HL) is used audiometrically to show the degree of hearing impairment, and its reference level varies with frequency according to a minimum audibility curve (as was shown in the discussion of phon).

Therefore, at each frequency, the average of the softest intensity heard by young adults is denoted as 0 dB HL (also known as audiometric zero), to which we can compare an individual's auditory sensitivity. We denote these comparisons on a graph called an audiogram, which plots the intensity (in units of dB HL) for each test frequency (in units of Hz). Another common reference that is used audiometrically is the individual's auditory threshold for a stimulus. A threshold is defined as the level at which a stimulus (e.g., a pure tone or speech) is so soft that it is perceived 50% of the time it is presented. The intensity in decibels above an individual's threshold is called the sensation level (SL), and is denoted as dB SL. We often use dB SL when denoting speech audiometric testing; just as we can determine speech intensity (in dB HL), we can also test speech understanding at intensity levels above threshold (in dB SL).

Anatomy and Physiology of Hearing

Sound is audible to us only if we have an auditory system that is capable of utilizing the physical characteristics of sound—that is, a sound's frequency (or frequencies), intensity, and phase(s)—to understand the world around us. Our hearing is sensitive enough to hear very faint sounds (e.g., leaves rustling on the ground from a gentle breeze), yet can appreciate and identify the different instruments comprising a symphony orchestra at much higher intensities. This section will describe the different parts of the ear—the outer, middle, and inner ear—to see how sound waves travel from the ambient air into the outer ear and then are funneled through the middle and inner ear up to the brain.

The ear itself is described as a **transducer**—it changes one form of energy (in this case, acoustic energy) to another form (fluid/electrical) via mechanical energy of the middle ear. This transduction of sound enables the ear to analyze the various physical parameters (frequency, intensity, phase, and duration) to perceive in the brain what the ear has heard.

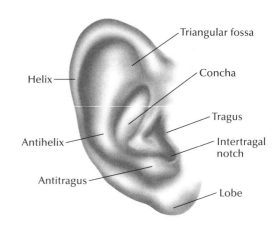

Figure 2.10   The outer ear.

The Outer Ear

We most often think of our ears as just what is visible, the outer ear. The **outer ear** (**Figure 2.10**) comprises two structures, the **pinna** (or auricle) and the **external auditory meatus** (ear canal). The pinna is the visible part of the auditory system and is shaped like a funnel; it is composed of skin overlaying stiffer cartilage along with a fleshier lobe, and is attached to the cranium by ligaments. The pinna has several landmarks, such as the concha (depression in the lower center of the pinna) and the helix (auricular rim). Its funnel-like shape gives rise to the pinna's basic function: to collect and send sound waves through the ear canal. The pinna also assists in sound localization and helps to protect the entrance to the external auditory canal.

The external auditory meatus is a tube that runs from the pinna to the eardrum (**tympanic membrane**). It is approximately 6 mm in diameter and about 23–29 mm long in adults, is lined with epithelium (skin) and tiny hairs (cilia), and contains glands in the cartilaginous portion that produce earwax (cerumen). Cerumen is waxy and somewhat sticky, which helps to keep the ear canal moisturized and clean of debris that could accumulate. The external auditory canal has two main functions: (1) to protect the delicate middle and inner ears from foreign bodies that could damage these structures; and (2) with the concha, to boost (that is, increase) the amplitude of high-frequency sounds. The concha and external auditory meatus have a natural resonant frequency to which they respond best, and each structure increases the sound pressure at its resonant frequency by approximately 10 to 15 dB. This increase in amplitude is helpful in discriminating fricative consonants such as /s, z, ʃ, and ʒ, all of which have acoustic energy above 2000 Hz. This boost of high-frequency sounds also enables us to localize the source of sounds, because high-frequency sounds have short wavelengths that cannot travel around the head. (In contrast, low-frequency sounds have longer wavelengths, which enable them to travel around the head.) Differences in sound wavelengths help to create timing differences between the ears and give us cues to where sounds are located.

The Middle Ear

The external auditory meatus terminates medially at the tympanic membrane, which acts as the anatomic boundary between the outer and middle ear. The tympanic membrane is comprised of multiple layers of tissue: the lateral epithelial layer, the medial membranous layer, and the fibrous layer sandwiched between the epithelial and membranous layers. These layers are both concentric and radial. The medial layer of the eardrum is a membranous layer that is contiguous with the membranous lining of the middle ear cavity and consists of a small air-filled cavity lined with a mucous membrane, which forms the link between the air-filled outer ear and the fluid-filled inner ear. The tympanic membrane has a more compliant, smaller section called the **pars flaccida**, which is located superiorly, and a stiffer, larger section called the **pars tensa**, located inferiorly.

The **ossicles**—malleus (hammer), incus (anvil), and stapes (stirrup)—are the smallest bones in the human body. These three bones, which fit very easily on a dime, are among the hardest-working bones in the body. The **malleus**, less than a centimeter in length, is embedded slightly into the tympanic membrane at its manubrium; as the tympanic

membrane vibrates from sound energy impinging on it, the malleus moves at the same vibratory speed. The **incus** is the middle bone, attaching to both the malleus and the stapes. It is also less than a centimeter in length, and has two processes, the short crus, which is fitted into a recess in the wall of the tympanic membrane, and the long crus, which is attached to the head of the stapes. The **stapes** looks like a stirrup, with two crura and a footplate, which fits very neatly over the oval window of the cochlear wall and helps to push the acoustic energy into the inner ear. The ossicles are suspended in the middle ear cavity by ligaments, which permit movement of the ossicles.

The ossicular chain acts like an **impedance-matching transformer**. The middle ear compensates for loss of sound energy when going from air to a fluid medium through two primary mechanisms: the difference in area between the tympanic membrane and the oval window (the tympanic membrane is about 17 times the size of the oval window) and the incudomalleolar joint between the malleus and long process of the incus, which forms a complex lever system that helps to amplify sounds traveling through the middle ear space to the inner ear (Figure 2.11). The area difference between the tympanic membrane and oval window recovers almost 25 dB of sound energy; the difference in length between the malleus and long process of the incus adds another 5 dB of sound energy. Together, almost 30 dB of sound energy are added to the system in order to compensate for the impedance mismatch between the air-filled middle ear and the fluid-filled inner ear. However, the ability of the middle ear system to amplify the sound pressure depends on the signal's frequency; little amplification occurs for frequencies below 100 Hz or above 2500 Hz. The outer ear, however, amplifies sound energy by about 20 dB for frequencies between 2000 Hz and 5000 Hz. Taken

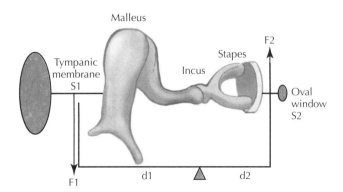

Figure 2.11   Schematic of the ossicular lever system and size differential between the tympanic membrane S1 and oval window S2.

together, this range of frequencies corresponds to the range of frequencies in human speech that are most important for communication.

Also found in the middle ear cavity is the **Eustachian (auditory) tube**, which has two important functions: (1) to equalize air pressure between the middle ear cavity and the nasopharynx and (2) to help drain fluids that might accumulate in the middle ear into the nasopharynx. You may be familiar with the stuffed feeling in your ears when you take off or land in an airplane. The Eustachian tube is at work, equalizing the air pressure in the middle ear.

If the Eustachian tube is not functioning well, fluids can build up in the normally air-filled middle ear space, which compromises the ossicular chain movement. Additional sound pressure is needed to overcome this lack of ossicular movement, leading to a hearing loss caused by problems with sound conduction (i.e., a conductive hearing loss). This disorder, called otitis media (middle ear infection), is often caused by an upper respiratory infection and/or allergies and occurs most often in young children due to the immature angle of the Eustachian tube in comparison to adults (see **Figure 2.12**). Acute otitis media is usually caused by a bacterial infection and often presents with an elevated temperature (Rosenfield et al., 2004). In many cases, this condition goes away on its own without treatment with antibiotics, but on occasion fluid will remain in the middle ear space because the Eustachian tube walls stick to each other and create a vacuum, which pulls the fluid from the skin cells lining the middle ear. This fluid is called effusion. The presence of effusion may result in a temporary loss of sound intensity (i.e., a conductive hearing loss). To remedy this situation, an otolaryngologist (ear–nose–throat surgeon) may surgically insert a tympanostomy (pressure-equalizing) tube into the eardrum. This tube helps to ventilate the middle ear space, thereby giving the dysfunctional Eustachian tube a chance to heal so that the middle ear cavity is once again aerated normally.

Finally, there are two muscles found in the middle ear, the **stapedius** and the **tensor tympani**. The stapedius muscle contracts bilaterally in response to high-intensity sounds to stiffen the ossicular chain, which protects the inner ear from intense sounds. This contraction of the stapedius muscle results in attenuation of sound pressure reaching the inner ear. Depending on the frequency of the sound, there is a 15- to 20-dB decrease in sound pressure because the middle ear efficiency in transmitting sound energy is in the range of 75–120 dB SPL. This reflex is consensual, so that when either ear is stimulated appropriately, the muscles in both ears contract. It is also important for reducing the upward spread of masking of high frequencies by low-energy sounds because the effect is greatest at frequencies less than 2000 Hz. This information is used clinically with the electroacoustic measurement called the stapedial reflex, which measures the intensity needed to cause contraction of the stapedius muscle. This contraction fatigues because prolonged exposure to high-intensity environments may decrease the degree to which the stapedius contracts, which lessens the effectiveness at damping loud sounds.

The other muscle, the tensor tympani, runs parallel to the Eustachian tube and assists in its function. When the tensor tympani contracts, it pulls on the malleus to draw the tympanic membrane inward, which increases the pressure in the middle ear and Eustachian tube. The tensor veli palatini muscle then contracts to open the Eustachian tube.

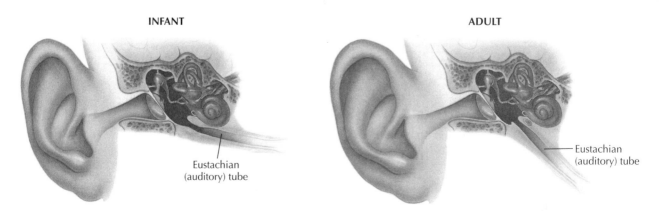

INFANT

ADULT

Eustachian (auditory) tube

Eustachian (auditory) tube

Figure 2.12   The angle difference between infant and adult Eustachian tubes.

The Inner Ear

The inner ear consists of the **auditory** and **vestibular labyrinths**, which are intricate pathways in the petrous portion of each temporal bone. Within the auditory and vestibular labyrinths are two labyrinths: the **osseous labyrinth**, which is a channel in the bone, and the **membranous labyrinth**, which consists of soft-tissue, fluid-filled channels within the osseous labyrinth containing the end-organ structures of the hearing and vestibular systems. The auditory labyrinth is called the **cochlea** and is the sensory end-organ of hearing; the **semicircular canals** are the sensory end-organ of balance. These two end-organs are connected via the **vestibule**, which houses the **saccule** and **utricle**.

The cochlea is a fluid-filled space within the temporal bones and is a snail-shaped, spiral canal. It has two 5/8 turns that, when straightened out, measure about 3.5 cm in length. Within each membranous duct are three chambers—the **scalae vestibuli**, **media**, and **tympani**—that are filled with fluid. **Perilymph**, which has a higher concentration of sodium ions (Na^+) than potassium ions (K^+), circulates through the scalae vestibuli and tympani, while **endolymph**, which has a higher concentration of K^+ than Na^+, is found in the scala media. This difference in ionic concentration between endolymph and perilymph gives rise to an endocochlear electrical potential ("cochlear battery") of about +80 mV in the scala media, which helps to conduct neural transmission of sound. The base of the cochlear duct is the **basilar membrane**, whereas the membranous roof is called the **vestibular membrane**. Two tissue-covered openings are found on the cochlea: the **oval window** (which is covered by the stapes footplate) is between the basilar membrane and scala vestibuli, and the **round window** is between the scala tympani and middle ear. The membranous portion is slightly smaller than the bony portion; the point where the scalae vestibuli and tympani communicate is called the **helicotrema**.

Within the cochlear duct is the **organ of Corti**, containing the sensory cells of hearing, which lies on the basilar membrane. These mechanoreceptor cells are shaped like hair and are called, appropriately, hair cells. The **outer hair cells**, of which there are about 15,000, form three rows shaped like a *W* and have their nerve fibers embedded into the **tectorial membrane**, a gel-like membrane that forms the roof of the basilar membrane. Because the basilar and tectorial membranes have different pivot points, vibration of the basilar membrane causes the cilia of the outer hair cells to bend, which alternately hyperpolarizes and depolarizes the nerve fibers of the eighth cranial nerve (CN VIII, auditory portion). Figure 2.13 shows the movement of the tectorial

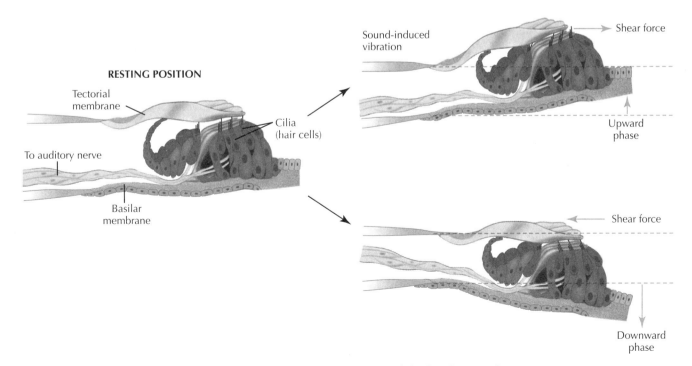

Figure 2.13   Shearing action of the hair cells and movement of the basilar membrane.

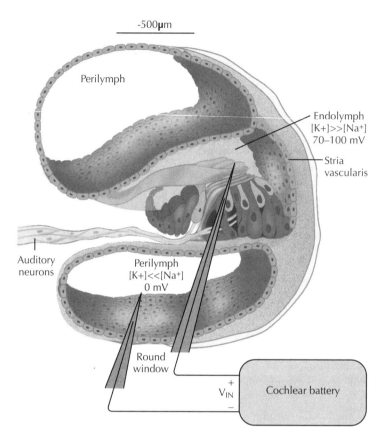

Figure 2.14   Cross-section of the cochlear duct showing membranous structures.

membrane in response to hair-cell polarization; Figure 2.14 depicts the electrochemical response of hair-cell polarization within the cochlea. The lengths of the outer hair cells increase at this point of maximum amplitude so that a vigorous electrical response is created by the incoming stimulus. The overall effect of this change of amplitude is a more precise analysis of stimulus frequency due to the different characteristic frequencies of the auditory nerve fibers, which are arranged **tonotopically**. Near the oval window, at the base, the nerve fibers in the hair cells are attuned to higher frequencies; at the apex, toward the center of the cochlea, the hair cells are attuned to low-frequency sounds. Outer hair cells are tuned especially to sound intensity; in essence, they act like transducers, changing fluid energy into electrical energy. In fact, this cochlear transduction of sound is similar to that of a microphone, which changes acoustic energy to electrical energy, and is referred to as the cochlear microphonic. This transduction function is described as the shearing force and is applied to the cilia in response to the acoustic stimulation, giving rise to electrical (i.e., receptor) potentials. Fewer than 10% of the outer hair cells are neurologically

connected to the brain, but they enhance the cochlear mechanical response to vibrations so that we are able to hear lower-intensity sounds. Outer hair cells also generate their own vibrations, both spontaneously and by using an evoking stimulus; we can measure these sounds (called otoacoustic emissions) clinically to determine cochlear function.

Inner hair cells, in contrast, are far fewer in number (about 3,500 altogether), and form a row in proximity of the tectorial membrane, near the modiolus (bony core) of the cochlea. However, more than 90% of these hair cells are neurologically connected to the brain via nerve fibers—they preferentially encode sound clarity.

The basilar membrane is where the cochlea begins its analysis of both frequency and intensity of incoming sound signals; in essence, the basilar membrane is where the incoming complex sound wave is transformed into simple sine waves similar to Fourier analyses. The stapes footplate rocks back and forth in the oval window, which establishes a wave within the scala vestibuli. Inward displacement of the perilymph at the oval window is matched by the outward displacement of the fluids via the round window due to increased pressure. This perilymph wave displaces the scala media, setting up a wave on the basilar membrane that moves from the base to the apex. The vibrations of the basilar membrane progress dynamically as the incoming traveling waves move from the cochlear base toward the helicotrema at the apical end. The primary physical feature of the basilar membrane that accounts for the direction in which the traveling wave progresses is the stiffness gradient of the basilar membrane—the greater stiffness in the basal portion of the cochlea opposes displacement when stimulated by low-frequency sound, and forces the wave to travel further up the cochlea toward the apex to a region having less stiffness and less opposition to low-frequency vibration. Thus, more of the basilar membrane is stimulated by low-frequency sounds. However, high-frequency sounds displace the basilar membrane only near the basal end, at the oval window, and do not travel further toward the apex. This basilar membrane displacement pattern increases gradually in amplitude until the point of maximum amplitude is reached, and then decreases abruptly. There is also a stronger mechanical/electrical response to low- and moderate-intensity sounds; this is called the cochlear amplifier. Although we are uncertain how intensities are encoded in the cochlea, it is thought that the relative rate of nerve impulse spikes transmits this information to the brain (see Zemlin, 1998, pp. 486–487).

The **traveling wave theory** of sound transduction (proposed by Georg von Bekesy [1899–1972], and for which he received the Nobel Prize for Physiology in Medicine in 1961) through the cochlea describes how higher-frequency sounds are analyzed (Zemlin, 1998). This theory does not account for all basilar membrane mechanics, however, because the membrane itself is not displaced sharply enough to distinguish low-frequency sounds by place of stimulation. As noted in Zemlin (1998), Ernest Glen Wever hypothesized in 1937 and published in 1949 that low-frequency sounds are determined by the number of clusters of firing nerve fibers in synchrony with the low frequency; high-frequency sounds are analyzed through place theory (because neurons cannot fire at high frequencies) and/or volley theory (which describes cooperation of neurons in neural transmission of high frequencies).

Retrocochlear Pathway and Auditory Cortex

The auditory nerve fibers fire in an all-or-nothing fashion, needing only about 2 ms to rise to maximum amplitude of neural firing. They are arranged on the basilar membrane in a tonotopic fashion—nerve fibers at the apical end of the cochlea respond preferentially to low-frequency stimuli, and high-frequency sounds are encoded at the base. Similarly, the auditory nerve is tonotopically arranged so that low-frequency sounds are found in the core of the auditory nerve and high-frequency sounds are arranged around the periphery. Thus, the brain obtains information regarding frequency of the incoming sound. In addition to frequency coding, the neural fibers of the auditory nerve also encode intensity for sounds with frequencies less than 5000 Hz; neural firing approximates the period of the stimulus waveform.

Neural firing of the auditory portion of the eighth cranial nerve generates action potentials; this electrical signal then travels from the cochlea to the auditory cortex in the temporal lobe. Although most of these fibers travel up to the auditory cortex to form the ascending (afferent) pathways, some neural fibers travel from either the brainstem or auditory cortex to form the descending (efferent) pathways. All auditory nerve fibers terminate at the level of the ipsilateral cochlear nucleus, where frequency and timing information about the auditory stimulus are further encoded. Although some neural pathways are ipsilateral and project into the next structure along the central auditory pathway (**Figure 2.15**), the superior olivary complex (in the medulla), most of these afferent pathways are contralateral (opposite side) so that the nerve fibers decussate (cross over) to the opposite superior olivary complex. Therefore, auditory information from both ears is represented in each ear, which enables us to localize sounds in space and to improve speech perception because ipsilateral fibers are excitatory and contralateral fibers are inhibitory. (Low-frequency stimuli are encoded for differences in timing, whereas high-frequency stimuli are encoded for differences in latency.) Other structures along the afferent auditory pathway include the lateral lemniscus (at the level of the pons), the inferior colliculus (in the midbrain, where decussation occurs), and the medial geniculate body (at the level of the thalamus), where all ascending fibers terminate before radiating into the appropriate cortex (in this case, the auditory cortex). Tonotopic organization of frequency to place is preserved throughout the afferent auditory pathway, which preserves the redundancy of speech.

The auditory cortex is located in the temporal lobes of the brain, and is divided into three basic areas: primary, secondary, and tertiary cortices. The primary auditory cortex, the first cortical region of the auditory pathway, is tonotopically arranged in a fashion similar to that found in the cochlea and

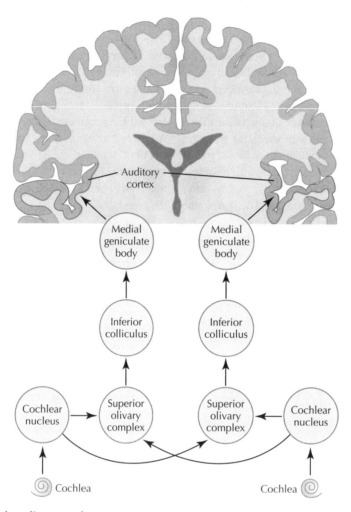

Figure 2.15 The central auditory pathway.

is largely responsible for discrimination of frequency and intensity of the incoming auditory stimulus. The location of a sound stimulus in space is also identified in the primary auditory cortex. The secondary and tertiary auditory cortices are largely responsible for language production, processing, and perception, and include **Broca's area** (inferior frontal gyrus), where motor production of language is located and where processing of sentence structure, grammar, and syntax is located, and **Wernicke's area** (in the lower temporal lobe), where speech perception is located. In addition, other areas within the brain—the superior temporal gyrus (where morphology and syntactic processing occur in the anterior section, and integration of syntactic and semantic information in the posterior section), the inferior frontal gyrus (working memory and syntactic processing), and the middle temporal gyrus (lexical semantic processing)—contribute to language comprehension. In almost all right-handed individuals, the left hemisphere is usually dominant,

with bilateral activation occurring for syntactic processing; this is true for most left-handed individuals also. The right hemisphere is important in processing suprasegmental features like prosody and melodic contours.

Although the retrocochlear auditory pathway is primarily sensory and contains afferent pathways from the cochlea up to the auditory cortex, a complex efferent system is also present containing descending neural fibers that correspond closely to the ascending auditory fibers. These efferent fibers connect the auditory cortex to the central auditory pathway and to the cochlea, and are thought to inhibit neural activity along this pathway to increase neural activation at lower brain centers. This inhibitory feedback improves stimulus processing by decreasing background noise that may interfere with the stimulus.

Figure 2.16 provides an overview of the process of sound transduction through the auditory system.

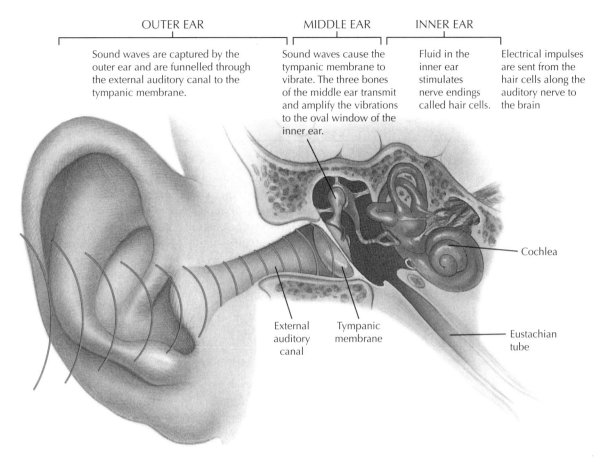

OUTER EAR   MIDDLE EAR   INNER EAR

Sound waves are captured by the outer ear and are funnelled through the external auditory canal to the tympanic membrane.

Sound waves cause the tympanic membrane to vibrate. The three bones of the middle ear transmit and amplify the vibrations to the oval window of the inner ear.

Fluid in the inner ear stimulates nerve endings called hair cells.

Electrical impulses are sent from the hair cells along the auditory nerve to the brain

Cochlea

External auditory canal

Tympanic membrane

Eustachian tube

Figure 2.16   An overview of the process of sound transduction through the auditory system.

Hearing Loss: An Error of Sound Transduction

Hearing loss may occur at any point along the auditory pathway. When damage occurs in the outer and/or middle ears, a conductive hearing loss is the result. Some examples of **conductive hearing loss** include outer ear disorders such as microtia (small or absent pinna) and atresia (lack of external auditory meatus), and middle ear disorders such as otitis media with or without effusion (fluid in the middle ear space) and otosclerosis (fixation of the stapes footplate to the oval window of the cochlea). Disorders affecting the outer and/or middle ear are usually amenable to medical and/or surgical intervention to correct the problem. Conductive hearing loss results in the decrease of sound intensity reaching the cochlea; typically, clarity of speech is preserved in conductive hearing loss because the cochlea is unaffected. However, chronic conductive hearing loss can also affect speech perception because of alterations in the normal inertial mechanisms of the middle ear, which affect conduction of sound through bone.

Those whose hearing loss is found in the inner ear have sensorineural hearing loss. **Sensorineural hearing loss** occurs due to damage to the cochlea and/or retrocochlear pathway, resulting in alterations of perception of sound frequency and intensity. In addition to a decrease of sound intensity, sensorineural hearing loss also results in a loss of speech clarity due to damage to the neural fibers located in the cochlea. Examples of sensorineural hearing loss include acoustic trauma from noise, tumors on CN VIII, ototoxic agents like loop diuretics, systemic neural diseases like diabetes mellitus, hypoxia (lack of oxygen), meningitis (both bacterial and viral, leading to inflammation of the meninges covering the brain), and Ménière's disease (which results in an increase of endolymph fluid in the cochlea, leading to fluctuating hearing loss, aural fullness, and/or vestibular dysfunction). Sensorineural hearing loss may also result from the normal aging process (presbycusis), leading to both cochlear and retrocochlear dysfunction, and which usually results in poorer speech understanding due to damage to the cochlea and higher auditory centers.

When both conductive and sensorineural components are present in hearing loss (e.g., an individual with sensorineural hearing loss develops otitis media), a **mixed hearing loss** results. Mixed hearing loss may result from complications of middle ear surgery, otosclerosis, and the like. Medical/surgical intervention may limit the conductive portion of the hearing loss, but the sensorineural component of the loss is still present.

Summary

Sound is defined as the movement of a disturbance through an elastic medium (such as air molecules) without permanent displacement of the particles. There are three prerequisites for production of sound: (1) a source of energy such as a force, (2) a vibrating object that generates an audible pressure wave, and (3) a medium of transmission. Sounds may be described by their frequency, intensity, and phase, all of which are physical characteristics that are measureable. Sound moves through the human ear in stages—the outer ear (which collects sound), the middle ear (which acts as a transducer to change acoustic energy to fluid energy via mechanical energy), and then the inner ear (which sends frequency and intensity information up to the brain via the central auditory pathway). Errors in sound transduction result in hearing loss. If the error is found in the outer or middle ear, a conductive hearing loss results; if the error is in the inner ear or central auditory pathway, a sensorineural hearing loss results.

Discussion Questions

1. List the characteristics of sound.
2. What is simple harmonic motion?
3. How are the characteristics of frequency and pitch related?
4. How are intensity and loudness related?
5. Why do we use the decibel to describe sound intensity?
6. For each part of the ear, identify the type of energy used for sound transduction.
7. What is the primary function of the middle ear?
8. In the inner ear, name the end-organs of hearing and balance.
9. What does the term *tonotopic organization* mean regarding cochlear function?

References

Rosenfeld, R. M, Culpepper, L., Doyle, K. J., Grundfast, K. M., Hoberman, A., Kenna, M. A., et al. (2004). Clinical practice guidelines: Otitis media with effusion. *Otolaryngology—Head and Neck Surgery, 130*(5): S95–S118. Available from http://oto.sagepub.com/content/130/5_suppl/S95.

Zemlin, W. R. (1998). Hearing. In: *Speech and hearing science: Anatomy and physiology* (4th ed., pp. 414–511). Boston: Allyn & Bacon.

Recommended Readings

Bear, M. F., Connors, B. W., & Paradiso, M. A. (2001). The auditory and vestibular system. In: *Neuroscience: Exploring the brain* (2nd ed., pp. 351–395). Philadelphia: Wolters Kluwer/Lippincott Williams & Wilkins.

Bess, F. H., & Humes, L. E. (2008). *Audiology: The fundamentals* (4th ed.). Philadelphia: Wolters Kluwer/Lippincott Williams & Wilkins.

Denes, P. B., & Pinson, E. N. (1993). *The speech chain: The physics and biology of spoken language* (2nd ed.). New York: W. H. Freeman.

Deutsch, L. J., & Richards, A. M. (1979). *Elementary hearing science*. Baltimore, MD: University Park Press.

Ferrand, C. T. (2007). *Speech science: An integrated approach to theory and clinical practice* (2nd ed.). Boston: Pearson/Allyn & Bacon.

Hixon, T. J., Weismer, G., & Hoit, J. D. (2008). Acoustics. In: *Preclinical speech science: Anatomy, physiology, acoustics, and perception* (pp. 317–355). San Diego: Plural.

Krizman, J., Skoe, E., & Kraus, N. (2010). Stimulus rate and subcortical auditory processing of speech. *Audiology & Neurotology, 15*: 332–342. Available from http://www.karger.com/Article/FullText/289572.

Martin, F. N., & Clark, J. G. (2012). *Introduction to audiology* (11th ed.). Boston: Allyn & Bacon.

Raphael, L. J., Borden, G. J., & Harris, K. S. (2011). *Speech science primer: Physiology, acoustics, and perception of speech* (6th ed.). Philadelphia: Lippincott Williams & Wilkins.

Chapter 3

Audiometric Equipment

Deborah R. Welling, AuD, CCC-A, FAAA
Associate Professor and Director of Clinical Education
Department of Speech-Language Pathology
Seton Hall University

Carol A. Ukstins, MS, CCC-A, FAAA
Educational Audiologist
Office of Special Education
Newark Public Schools

Key Terms

Air conduction pathway
American National
  Standards Institute
  (ANSI)
Audiometer
Auditory brainstem
  response (ABR)
Bone conduction oscillator
Bone conduction pathway

Circumaural earphones
Diagnostic
Electronystagmography
  (ENG)
Insert earphones
Otoacoustic emissions
  (OAEs)
Otoscope
Screening

Speech-picture audiometer
Sound booth
Supra-aural earphones
Tympanometer
Videonystagmography
  (VNG)
Visual reinforcement
  audiometry (VRA)

Objectives

- Be familiar with the equipment and technology used in the assessment of the ear and hearing
- Understand the impact that the test environment may have on the assessment of auditory function
- Understand the need for routine calibrations and the time frame within which each must be completed
- Understand and discuss the need for universal precaution

Introduction

The practice of audiology involves the use of an extensive array of equipment; perhaps it's that technical aspect of the field that attracted some to pursue the profession in the first place. From diagnostic equipment to screening tools, from conventional hearing aids to cochlear implants, the audiologist spends much of his or her day immersed in technology. Specialized equipment and a prescribed noise-controlled environment are of paramount importance for successful administration and accurate interpretation of results. In this chapter we will give an overview of the variety of equipment used in routine practice and the requirements to ensure their proper functioning is maintained.

Audiology Sound Booth

The testing environment in which audiometric procedures are performed is critically important. The presence of background noise can interfere with the client's ability to hear and respond to sound and, therefore, must be kept to specified levels in order to ensure accuracy of the test results. In order to ensure that the background noise in a test setting is acceptable and does not exceed acceptable levels, the **American National Standards Institute (ANSI)** has established guidelines that are to be adhered to (ANSI/ASA S3.1-1999 [R2008]).

Complete **diagnostic** evaluations of auditory function are typically performed in sound-treated acoustic environments specifically designed to meet the standards just discussed. **Figure 3.1** shows an example of a typical hearing test suite (**sound booth**) used for such evaluations. Routine calibrations are performed to ensure that these environments continue to meet the maximum permissible levels as summarized. Unfortunately, not all assessments have the benefit of a sound-controlled environment, as is most often the case when a speech-language pathologist (or audiologist) is required to do a hearing screening in a typical school setting. When in this situation (that is, when the environment has not been calibrated and certified as meeting ANSI specifications for background noise levels), the tester must make every effort to ensure that the test is being conducted in the quietest environment possible, using insert earphones or other noise-reducing earphones if available. When the background noise–controlled conditions cannot be met and no noise-reducing earphones are available, extreme caution must be used in the interpretation of any results.

Audiometer

The **audiometer** could be considered the most important piece of equipment that is used to measure hearing sensitivity. Audiometers range in complexity from a very simple

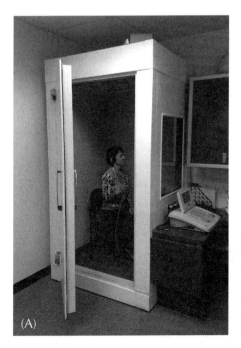
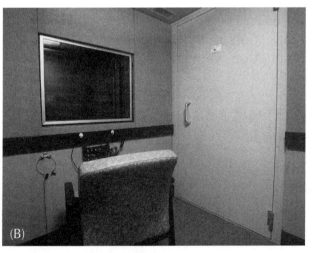

Figure 3.1 **(A)** Audiometric test booth. **(B)** Patient side of audiometric test suite.

or bone conduction oscillator). The intensity selector (either a dial or push button), calibrated to decibels in hearing level (dB HL, in accordance with the most recent ANSI/ASA S3.6-2010 specifications for audiometers), potentially spans from a low of −10 dB HL through a maximum of +120 dB HL; this range will vary depending on the frequency selected, transducer used (earphones or bone conduction vibrator), and whether the equipment being used is of the screening or diagnostic type. Another important feature that all audiometers must have is the presentation switch, often referred to as the interrupter, which turns the test tone on so that the signal is presented to the patient. Lastly, most audiometers also have a second channel of operation in order to introduce simultaneous signals to both ears.

Diagnostic Audiometer

A diagnostic audiometer is used in a clinical setting; it enables the audiologist to perform all basic audiometric procedures, including air conduction and bone conduction testing, basic speech audiometry, specialized speech audiometry tests (e.g., those performed during an auditory processing assessment), masking, and sound field testing.

The typical diagnostic audiometer (Figure 3.3), used for pure tone air conduction testing, has a frequency range that includes the octaves of 125, 250, 500, 1000, 2000, 4000, and 8000 Hz and the interoctave frequencies of 750, 1500, 3000, and 6000 Hz. Some specialized audiometers include the frequencies between 8000 and 20,000 Hz. The intensity range typically spans from a low of −10 dB HL through a maximum possible upper limit of approximately 120 dB HL, with the frequencies in the lower and higher ends of the frequency range having reduced upper intensity limits. As mentioned previously, frequency ranges and intensity limitations depend on the specific make and model of equipment used.

The diagnostic audiometer also has a speech circuit capable of being connected to external sources, such as a CD player or other electronic components. Thus equipped, the audiologist can perform basic as well as specialized speech audiometry procedures as part of a variety of assessment types including, but not necessarily limited to, the basic audiologic evaluation, hearing aid assessment and follow-up, auditory processing evaluations, and cochlear implant candidacy evaluations.

Portable/Screening Audiometer

The portable audiometer (Figure 3.2), as its name suggests, is easily carried from place to place and can connect to a

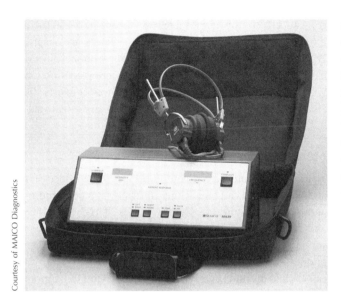

Courtesy of MAICO Diagnostics

Figure 3.2   Maico portable audiometer.

portable or **screening** device (see Figure 3.2) to the elaborate equipment used in diagnostic and clinical settings (see Figure 3.3). Regardless of the sophistication of the machine in question or the variety of test procedures it is capable of performing, all audiometers have a few basic components in common.

All audiometers must have a frequency dial that allows the selection of each of the various frequencies used during the hearing test. The frequencies most commonly available include the octaves from 125 Hz through 8000 Hz, with some audiometers going to 12,000 Hz and higher. The output selector (either a dial or push button) allows the tester to choose the transducer (earphones, insert earphones, speaker,

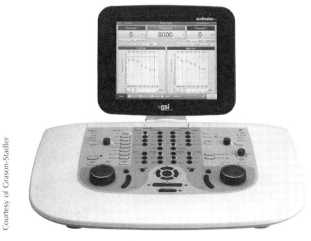

Courtesy of Grason-Stadler

Figure 3.3   Grason-Stadler AudioStar diagnostic.

conventional electrical outlet. The portability and ease of use make it an ideal equipment choice for the speech-language pathologist who must perform hearing screenings in a variety of settings as part of their diagnostic and/or treatment services.

The typical portable screening audiometer is capable of air conduction and often bone conduction testing as well as some form of masking. Less common, but available, are speech circuits for the administration of basic speech audiometry measures as well.

Speech-Picture Audiometer

Screening the very young child and the special needs patient can be a challenge. Conditioning such a patient to raise their hand or otherwise respond to a tonal stimulus can be difficult, if not impossible, in many instances, due to the abstract nature of the task. The **speech-picture audiometer** seeks to overcome this dilemma. Its design allows the testing of hearing using familiar words in a picture-pointing task of a familiar scene (e.g., a farm or playground). Although the result obtained using such equipment should not be the sole or primary basis for a diagnosis, it can be extremely valuable when used as a supplement in the diagnosis and treatment of hearing loss. The Maico Pilot, shown in **Figure 3.4**, is an example of a speech-picture audiometer.

Earphones and Other Sound Transducers

A transducer is simply a device that transforms energy from one form to another form. An audiometer, whether screening or diagnostic, gets its power supply from an electrical socket. When we plug in the audiometer and turn it on, the power it receives is electrical. We connect sound transducers to the audiometer to change the electrical energy into sound or acoustic energy. There are several types of transducers, including standard earphones, insert earphones, noise reduction earphones, a bone conduction vibrator, and speakers. Each of these devices converts the electrical energy from the audiometer into an acoustic signal capable of being perceived by the individual.

Standard Earphones

Standard earphones are a common type of transducer for audiometers and can be of either the supra-aural or circumaural type. **Supra-aural earphones** of types TDH-39, TDH-49, and TDH-50 are most common. Supra-aural earphones have some advantages when compared with circumaural earphones. They are relatively lightweight and sit on top of rather than around the ear; therefore, they tend to be more comfortable, and achieving proper placement on the client is quick and easy. This latter aspect makes them an ideal choice when performing hearing screenings with a portable audiometer. **Figure 3.5** shows a pair of supra-aural earphones.

The other earphones that can be used with the audiometer are **circumaural earphones**. As shown in **Figure 3.6**, these earphones are larger, heavier, and as a result may be less comfortable than the supra-aural type. Additionally, proper placement is not as quick and easy. The advantage, however, is that the circumaural earphones are more efficient at

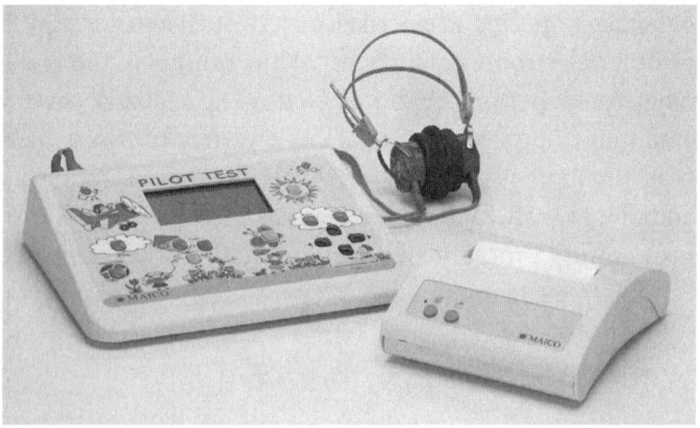

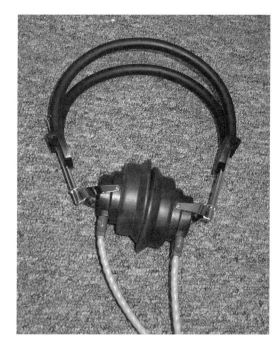

Figure 3.4 Maico speech-picture audiometer.

Figure 3.5 Supra-aural earphones.

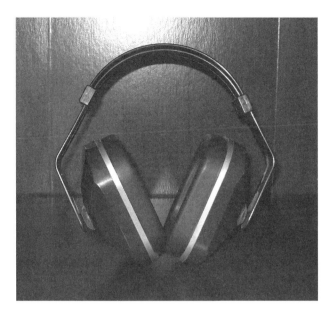

Figure 3.6   Circumaural earphones.

reducing unwanted ambient sound (Brannstrom & Lantz, 2010), and therefore they may be a good choice in screening environments where background noise is a problem and interferes with the hearing screening process.

Insert Earphones

A newer development in transducers (newer than the standard earphone) is the **insert earphones**. These devices, shown in Figure 3.7, are not as simple, easy, or expedient to use when trying to achieve proper placement; however, there are some clear advantages to the use of insert earphones. Performing a hearing test (screening or otherwise) on a client who has a unique condition known as a collapsible ear canal is a clear case in point. With such a client, the

use of standard earphones exerts pressure sufficient to cause the external auditory ear canal to close off and results in what appears to be a hearing loss; however, the observed hearing loss is an artifact and simply the result of the tragus collapsing over, and closing off, the opening to the external ear canal. When insert earphones are used instead, the ear canal is held open and reliable hearing test results can be obtained. There is also evidence (Wright & Frank, 1992) that insert earphones are better at reducing the impact of unwanted ambient noise when doing a hearing test in an environment that is less than the ideal sound-treated room; for example, trying to do a hearing screening in a noisy school setting.

Bone Conduction Oscillator

Another type of sound transducer used in audiometric testing is the **bone conduction oscillator**. Unlike earphones and insert earphones that convey sound to the external ear canal and use the **air conduction pathway** for transmission through the entire auditory system, the bone conduction oscillator uses the **bone conduction pathway**. With the air conduction pathway, sound enters the outer ear canal, goes through the middle ear, and then gets sent to the inner ear and beyond. In contrast, the bone conduction pathway directly stimulates the organ of hearing in the inner ear, thus bypassing the outer and middle ears completely. An example of the sensation of a bone-conducted sound is when you put your fingers over your ears and then speak—you hear yourself through bone conduction. A bone conduction oscillator is shown in Figure 3.8.

Figure 3.7   Etymotic ER3A insert earphones.

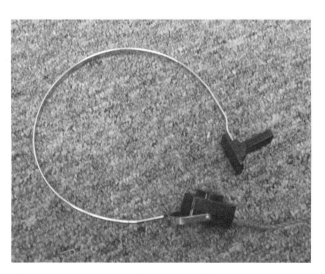

Figure 3.8   Bone conduction oscillator.

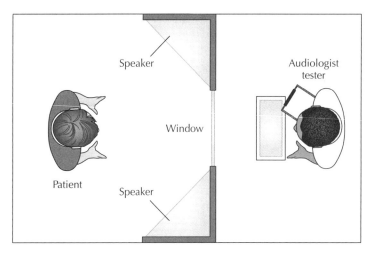

Figure 3.9 A room arrangement for sound field testing with speakers.

Speakers

Figure 3.9 illustrates how speakers are typically set up in an audiometric test suite.

Several situations may either preclude the use of earphones or insert earphones, or simply require additional test procedures that can only be accomplished with speakers. Examples of such situations include the testing of a very young infant or child who either cannot or will not accept earphones, or when we want to assess how someone hears while wearing their hearing aids or other assistive device, which cannot be accomplished by using earphones.

Visual Reinforcement Audiometry (VRA) Boxes

Especially appropriate for testing very young (either chronologically or developmentally) children is the **visual reinforcement audiometry (VRA)** system arrangement in the sound field. VRA systems (see Figure 3.10) use either boxes that contain animated toys and lights, just lights, or computer monitors displaying favorite characters or animation. The VRA technique will be discussed further in Chapter 5.

Otoscope

An **otoscope** is used to perform an otoscopic inspection (see Figure 3.11A). This device consists of a handle and a head, providing a magnifying lens and light source for visual inspection of the tympanic membrane and external ear canal. A variety of different sizes of specula attach to the otoscope, which are designed to fit different sizes of ear canals (see Figure 3.11B).

Tympanometer

A **tympanometer** is used to test middle ear function through a process known as tympanometry. Unlike audiometry, which allows the audiologist to make a statement regarding hearing sensitivity, tympanometry assesses the physical condition of the conductive system and helps to determine if a medical referral is necessary. Tympanometers are available as diagnostic units (see Figure 3.12A) as well as screening units (see Figure 3.12B).

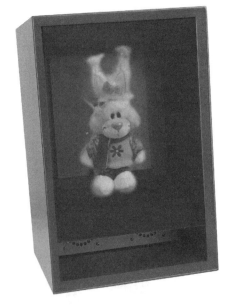

Courtesy of Interacoustics A/S

Figure 3.10 An example of an animated light-up toy used in visual reinforcement audiometry.

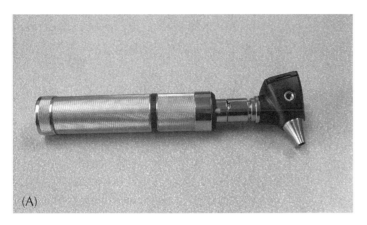
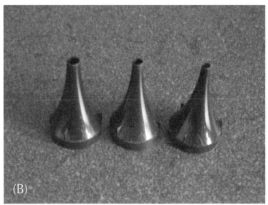

Figure 3.11   **(A)** Otoscope. **(B)** Various sizes of specula used with an otoscope.

Otoacoustic Emissions

A normal, healthy cochlea is capable of producing as well as receiving sound. The sound produced is known as **otoacoustic emissions (OAEs)**, and their existence in a normal, healthy cochlea provides the foundation for the audiometric procedure known by the same term. The sound that is emitted can be measured and recorded using equipment specifically designed for this purpose. **Figure 3.13** shows a picture of the Maico Titan Scan OAE system, which can be used as a screening, diagnostic, or combination device.

Auditory Brainstem Response

After sound travels beyond the outer, middle, and inner ear it reaches the level of the brainstem. The **auditory brainstem response (ABR)** refers to the physiologic activity that occurs at various structures of the auditory nervous system in response to a sound. This response can be objectively measured and recorded using a procedure known as ABR audiometry. An example of the type of equipment used to record these tracings is shown is **Figure 3.14**. As with the OAE equipment, both screening and diagnostic systems are available.

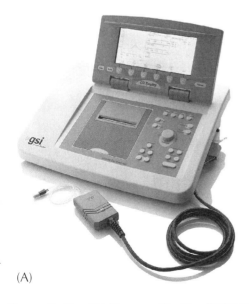
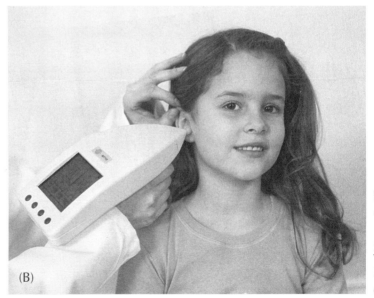

Courtesy of Grason-Stadler

Courtesy of Interacoustics A/S

Figure 3.12   **(A)** Grason-Stadler (GSI) TympStar diagnostic tympanometer. **(B)** Interacoustic screening tympanometer.

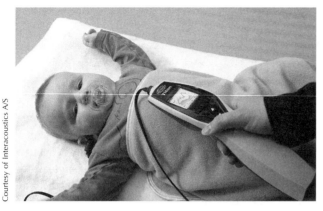

Figure 3.13 Maico otoacoustic emissions testing equipment.

Electronystagmography/ Videonystagmography

A symptom of an abnormal balance (vestibular) system is the presence of involuntary eye movement, which is known as nystagmus. The procedures of choice to establish the cause are **electronystagmography (ENG)** and **videonystagmography (VNG)**. The difference between these two is that the ENG makes its recordings from surface electrodes placed around the eyes, whereas the VNG uses an infrared video system. An example of an ENG/VNG system can be seen in Figure 3.15.

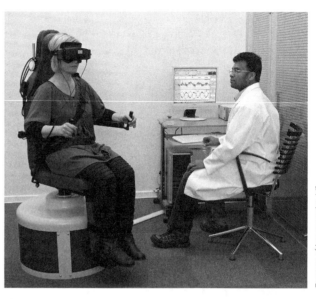

Figure 3.15 Interacoustics videonystagmography (VNG) equipment.

Tympanometer/Otoacoustic Emissions Hybrid

A hybrid that combines tympanometry with otoacoustic emissions is shown in Figure 3.16. Such devices are very convenient because they can facilitate a quick and reliable screening by combining the two procedures into one

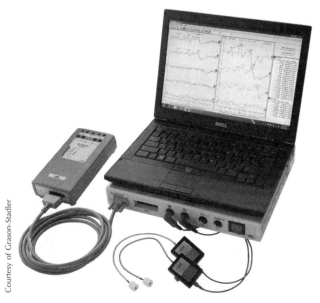

Figure 3.14 Grason-Stadler (GSI) Audera auditory brainstem response (ABR) audiometry test equipment.

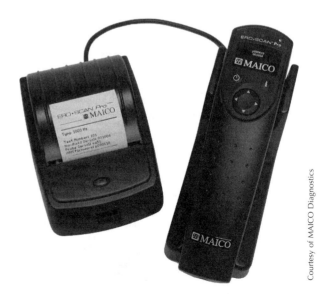

Figure 3.16 Maico Eroscan Pro combination otoacoustic emissions (OAE) and tympanometer testing equipment.

automatic sequence. This may be of particular interest to the speech-language pathologist or audiologist who needs to screen for hearing loss in the very young child or special needs population.

Auditory Brainstem/ Otoacoustic Emission Hybrid

The Early Hearing Detection and Intervention (EHDI) programs have spurred the development of hybrid devices used for newborn infant hearing screening in hospitals nationwide. Such devices combine auditory brainstem response (ABR) technology with otoacoustic emission capabilities. They allow for quick and effective objective hearing screenings. Their primary use is with infants in newborn nurseries and neonatal intensive care units (NICUs). An example is shown in **Figure 3.17**.

Calibration Requirements

It is within the scope of practice of the speech-language pathologist (SLP) to perform certain screenings prior to the evaluation and treatment of clients, so ensuring the calibration (electroacoustic as well as daily functional) of the equipment to be used for the screening is mandatory. As a speech-language pathologist, the maintenance of

audiometric equipment may or may not be given to you as a responsibility by your supervisor. However, as a professional routinely using audiometric tools (whether diagnostic or screening), you must be aware of the maintenance requirements of the equipment in your possession.

Electroacoustic Calibration

The routine electroacoustic calibration of the test equipment is required by the American Speech-Language-Hearing Association (ASHA) to be completed annually by an agency or a business specifically contracted by the individual facility to do so. This agency or business typically provides services of calibration, maintenance, and the sale of audiological equipment. Calibration is necessary to ensure the validity and accuracy of the results obtained and includes measurement of the background noise levels in the sound booth or other environment used for audiometric testing, and calibration of the audiometric equipment itself. To ensure that proper electroacoustic calibration has been completed on the equipment in use, search for a sticker with a calibration date and agency name on each piece of equipment; the SLP merely needs to verify that the date of the last calibration is within one calendar year of the date of the screening.

Daily Biological Calibration/Listening Checks

In addition to annual electroacoustic calibration, daily functional (visual) inspections, performance checks, and bioacoustic (listening) measurements must be conducted to verify the equipment performance before use (ASHA, 2005). The functional inspection, performed each day prior to use, is quickly and easily accomplished by plugging in the machine, making sure it turns on, putting on the standard earphones (or inserting the insert earphones), and performing a listening check on oneself to make certain that the equipment is subjectively functioning appropriately. A daily biometric calibration sheet should be available to record the date and initials of the staff member completing this daily responsibility.

Accurate results require equipment that is functioning appropriately. If the equipment's electroacoustic calibration sticker is out of date or if any mechanical or functional problem is suspected as a result of the daily biological/listening check, misdiagnosis of hearing loss can occur. Equipment problems should be identified to the supervisor in charge so that repair or replacement of equipment is done in a timely manner. Any equipment suspected of malfunction should be removed from clinical use immediately.

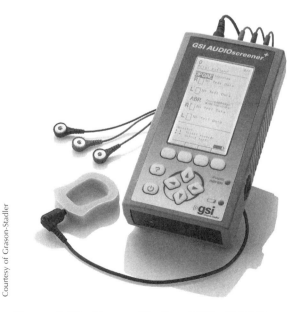

Courtesy of Grason-Stadler

Figure 3.17 Grason-Stadler (GSI) AUDIOscreener otoacoustic emissions (OAE) and auditory brainstem response audiometry (ABR) equipment.

Universal Precautions

Universal precautions are a set of procedures and practices designed to help protect healthcare workers and patients alike from a wide range of pathogens. Instrumentation coming into physical contact with the patient must be cleaned and disinfected after each use. According to the Occupational Safety and Health Administration (OSHA) 29 CRF standard 1910.1030, all human blood and certain human body fluids are to be treated as if they are already known to be infectious for human immunodeficiency virus (HIV), hepatitis B virus (HBV), and other bloodborne pathogens. Therefore, in agreement with the recommendations of the Centers for Disease Control and Prevention (CDC), standard precautions should be taken as the foundation for preventing transmission of infectious agents during the care of all patients, regardless of their diagnosis or presumed infection status.

The recommendations of ASHA are in agreement with these statements; the 2004 guidelines for Manual Pure-Tone Audiometry state that adherence to universal precautions and appropriate infection control procedures should be in place. The use of disposable acoustically transparent earphone covers or disposable insert earphone tips is recommended. Hand washing should be routine for the audiologist (or SLP) between patients (ASHA, 2005).

For specific information, recommendations, and guidelines, the readers are referred to Siegel et al., 2007.

Disclosure of Cleaning Materials

In many facilities, staff members are required to complete a Disclosure of Cleaning Materials document, sometimes known as GreenClean. The purpose of such disclosure is for the facility to manage and monitor the use of toxic chemical compounds within the confines of the agency. The speech-language pathologist is advised to familiarize him- or herself with the policies of his or her place of employment regarding the completion of such forms. Liquid cleaning solutions for ultrasonic cleaners as well as wipes and sprays used on therapy tables and equipment may all fall under the guidelines of disclosure.

Summary

Performance of a hearing evaluation or screening requires specific equipment denoted for the purpose of audiological evaluation. Although each piece of equipment is unique in its function, all equipment is necessary for the comprehensive evaluation of hearing sensitivity across all ages and groups. A well-equipped audiology facility will be able to perform a wide range of testing, some of which the speech-language pathologist will be employed to perform, other of which is outside of the speech-language pathologist's scope of practice.

Many of the terms used is this chapter will become second nature in the evaluation of hearing sensitivity. As you begin to use this "new language of audiology" fluently, you will gain a clear understanding of each piece of equipment, its testing procedure, and how the interpretation of results plays a role in managing the patient with hearing loss.

Discussion Questions

1. What are the advantages of testing hearing in a sound booth vs. a therapy room?
2. How is a tympanometer different from an audiometer?
3. What is the difference between a screening tool and a diagnostic tool?
4. Why are universal precautions important?
5. What are the two types of calibration? How are they the same? How are they different?

References

American National Standards Institute. (2008). *Maximum permissible ambient noise levels for audiometric test rooms.* ANSI/ASA S3.1-1999 (R2008). New York: Author.

American National Standards Institute. (2010). *American National Standards specification for audiometers.* ANSI S3.6-2010. New York: Author.

American Speech-Language-Hearing Association (ASHA). (2005). *Guidelines for manual pure-tone audiometry.* Available from http://www.asha.org/policy.

Brannstrom, K. J., & Lantz, J. (2010). Interaural attenuation for Sennheiser HDA 200 circumaural earphones. *International Journal of Audiology*, 49: 467–471.

Occupational Safety and Health Administration (OSHA). *Occupational Safety and Health standard; Toxic and hazardous substances, bloodborne pathogens,* 29CRF1910.1030 (b).

Siegel, J. D., Rinehart, E., Jackson, M., Chiarello, L., & the Healthcare Infection Control Practices Advisory Committee. *2007 guideline for isolation precautions: Preventing transmission of infectious agents in healthcare settings.* Available from http://www.cdc.gov/ncidod/dhqp/pdf/isolation2007.pdf.

Wright, D. C., & Frank, T. (1992). Attenuation values for a supra-aural earphone for children and insert earphones for children and adults. *Ear and Hearing,* 13(6): 454–459.

Chapter 4

Case History Assessment and the Process of Differential Diagnosis

Deborah R. Welling, AuD, CCC-A, FAAA
Associate Professor and Director of Clinical Education
Department of Speech-Language Pathology
Seton Hall University

Carol A. Ukstins, MS, CCC-A, FAAA
Educational Audiologist
Office of Special Education
Newark Public Schools

Key Terms

Comorbidity
Congenital
Dementia

Differential diagnosis
"Look, play, talk"
Look-alike diseases

Pseudohypacusis

Objectives

- Gain an understanding of ways to obtain a thorough case history
- Identify etiologies of hearing loss for various age categories across the lifespan
- Understand the process of a differential diagnosis
- Gain an understanding of conditions that may mimic or occur comorbidly with hearing loss

Introduction

There are many components to the diagnostic process, the very first of which is to conduct a comprehensive case history. The importance of conducting a meticulous history cannot be overestimated because the keen clinician will frequently be able to establish a differential diagnosis based on the case history information. The differential diagnosis is the process by which one disorder is distinguished or differentiated from another disorder, despite presenting with many of the same symptoms and characteristics. As pointed out by Kenneth E. Sack in his compelling 2012 article "Taking Away the Diagnosis," which was about a patient of his who had previously been misdiagnosed by a colleague, the test results can *confirm or refute* a diagnosis, but they rarely *make* the diagnosis. An individual's test results must be considered in the context of the case history and other information, not in isolation.

This chapter will focus on the various components of the case history and how to collect and glean information for the purpose of developing a differential diagnosis. As we hope readers will discover for themselves, careful and systematic case history taking will frequently facilitate the diagnostic process. Remember, the watch word is *thoroughness*.

Case History

There are several different steps that will assist the clinician in constructing thorough background information and current patient status. In the following sections we will briefly describe each of these components.

Patient Interview

There are several ways for a clinician to gather patient history information. One common method is to obtain or create a form that either a patient can be asked to fill out on his or her own or the clinician can fill out interview style. Regardless of which method works best for the individual clinician, the patient and/or family member should be encouraged to describe the primary problem or complaint in his or her own words.

An example of a commercially available case history form is the Speech-Language-Hearing Case History Form created by and available through Super Duper Publications (see this chapter's appendix). Although this particular tool is geared toward children, it provides the clinician with a rather comprehensive framework with which to conduct the case history interview. Another example of a thorough case history tool, geared toward the population from birth to age 3 years, is in the appendix to the chapter on Hearing Issues in the Early Intervention Years in this textbook.

There are many similar forms available geared toward various age ranges (from birth to geriatric) and special needs populations. Clinicians are encouraged to seek out an appropriate form to either use or modify depending on their specific needs, or they may wish to create one of their own. Whether using a premade form as is, modifying, or creating one's own, the clinician needs to take many considerations into account in the process. Most notably, it is incumbent on us as professionals to explore multiple ways of asking for the same information. It has been the experience of these authors that a patient does not necessarily willfully withhold information; rather, there are times when either the person doesn't fully understand the question being asked or we perhaps are not being clear in the way we are asking the question. As a result, the challenge for the clinician is to find multiple ways of asking certain key questions so as to elicit the necessary case history information.

In the sections that follow we present a variety of complications that have the potential to cause hearing loss across the life span. It is important to recognize that what we present here is not an exhaustive listing of the etiologies of hearing loss; this is meant as a guide only. It also is important to bear in mind that the most successful approach may be a collaborative one. It behooves us as professionals to work together in a cooperative manner by sharing our own expertise and seeking the expertise from other professionals so they may assist us in arriving at an accurate diagnosis in the most timely manner possible.

Prenatal, Perinatal, and Neonatal Complications

There are many potential complications during the prenatal, perinatal, and neonatal stages of development that can have significant deleterious effects on auditory development. These may be of genetic or nongenetic origin. According to information available from the American Speech-Language-Hearing Association (ASHA), some 75% of **congenital** hearing loss, or hearing loss present at birth, is genetic in origin. Clearly, therefore, a familial history of hearing loss or other communication disorder is significant and important to ascertain from the patient and/or family. Additionally, late onset hearing loss also can be genetic in origin (JCIH, 2007).

Some of the remaining approximately 25% of nongenetic prenatal issues may include maternal infections such as cytomegalovirus (CMV) infection, rubella (German measles), and herpes simplex virus. Other nongenetic etiologies of hearing loss include human immunodeficiency virus (HIV)/acquired immune deficiency syndrome (AIDS), Rh factor incompatibility, and fetal alcohol syndrome disorder (FASD), to name just a few. Prematurity and low birth weight are also of potential concern because these factors are known etiologies of congenital sensorineural hearing loss in children (Morzaria, Westerberg, & Kozak, 2004).

Some of the perinatal complications that can affect auditory development include lack of oxygen, prolonged labor, and jaundice. The neonatal period may include complications and infections such as those that occur, for example, as a result of CMV, Rh factor incompatibility, or any other condition that requires the infant to remain hospitalized beyond the discharge time of a normal, healthy infant. Remember, any of these complications has the potential to cause hearing loss, and perhaps more importantly, the onset does not necessarily have to occur or manifest immediately.

The literature provides an abundance of evidence regarding potential causes of and contributors to auditory dysfunction, which in turn may result in delayed and/or disordered speech, language, communication abilities, and overall academic achievement. It bears reiteration that the keen clinician will try to pose questions in an open-ended fashion, phrased in multiple different ways, in order to develop the fullest and most accurate differential diagnosis possible.

Toddler/Childhood Complications

If a baby has failed the newborn infant hearing screening, the absolute necessity for a full audiological evaluation is rather obvious, in order to rule out or confirm the presence of a hearing loss. What may not be quite so obvious is that if a baby passes the newborn infant hearing screening, but there is concern on the part of the parent (or primary caregiver), a full audiologic assessment is a must as well. Dismissal of concerns by a pediatrician or anyone else should not deter the family from pursuing the issue and following through with getting a complete evaluation. Again, there are numerous causes of late and progressive onset hearing loss, and a child can pass a hearing screening at one point in time yet still develop an abnormal auditory condition at a later date. As such, readers are directed to Appendix 1 of the *Year 2007 Position Statement: Principles*

and Guidelines for Early Hearing Detection and Intervention Programs (Joint Committee on Infant Hearing, 2007) for a more detailed listing of risk indicators associated with permanent congenital, delayed-onset, or progressive hearing loss in childhood.

Other childhood concerns and complications are numerous. Given that otitis media is reported to be one of the most common infectious diseases of childhood (Elmorsky et al., 2010; Ghonaim, El-Edel, Basiony, & Al-Zahrani, 2011; Sheer, Swarts, & Ghadiali, 2012), a thorough medical history is critical. Some of the questions may include whether there is a history of ear infections, allergies, or other symptoms or sequelae of middle ear pathology; use of medications; history of trauma; or medical or surgical treatment of any type. Should any significant medical history be reported to have occurred, it is prudent for the clinician to seek signed permission (from the patient, parent, or legal guardian) to contact the treating physician or other healthcare worker involved, in order to get a fuller understanding of the given condition. Collaborating with other healthcare providers can help the clinician better understand the patient's condition and, as previously stated, assist in arriving at an accurate diagnosis in the timeliest manner possible. Earlier diagnosis allows for earlier intervention, and earlier intervention may lead to more successful outcomes.

Lastly, some areas of exploration for a child might include behaviors of inattentiveness, listening to the television "too loud," any difficulty responding to questions or directions, any academic and/or reading problems in school, and whether there has been excessive noise exposure (such as MP3 use). Any area where concern is raised, obviously, should be explored further.

Adults/Geriatrics

An adult (as well as older children) can be asked to describe the hearing problems and other accompanying symptoms that they may be experiencing. Some questions about the hearing loss could include:

- How long has the difficulty been noticed?
- Was the onset sudden or gradual?
- Did the onset appear to have been connected with another trauma or event?
- What situations present the most and least amount of difficulty?
- If the person does experience difficulty, is it accompanied by tinnitus (ringing in the ears), dizziness, headaches, or any other abnormal symptom?

- If a known hearing loss exists, does the person now use, or have they ever used, any form of hearing aid or assistive device? If so, the device should be checked for proper functioning. Is the device worn routinely? Does the patient (or family member) think that the device is meeting amplification needs at this time?

A thorough medical and occupational history may also be useful in establishing an etiology of the presenting condition. Clients are requested to provide a complete list of current and past medications with dosages, including any over-the-counter medications and herbal supplements. Any of these types of commonly consumed substances has the potential to adversely affect hearing and/or balance function. Changes in types of medication and dosages can also be contributory. Additionally, a synergistic effect may result from combinations of substances or a combination of a substance with another factor (such as noise exposure). Other causal and/or associated conditions include a history of diabetes, high cholesterol, hypertension, headaches, or dizziness; history of stroke, transient ischemic attack (TIA), accidents, or other trauma; a history of a serious health condition requiring ototoxic medication with long-term hospitalization; any cancer treatments; and past/present occupational or recreational history of noise exposure. Lastly, concerns of a family member or a familial history of late onset hearing loss may be contributory for the adult client as well.

Informal Observation

Another component that is critically important to the evaluation process is informal observation. Where children are concerned, observation and investigation of the child's auditory attentiveness, auditory response behaviors, and vocal quality may prove contributory. For the very young child, the quantity and quality of vocal play should be explored; deaf babies are not silent babies. What might distinguish the hearing baby from the deaf baby may not be the absence of vocal play, but rather the different characteristics that the deaf child's vocal play may take on. Also remember that hearing is not an all-or-nothing affair. Hearing loss can vary from slight to profound, and likewise, so can its impact. Thus, significance often lies in the particular character of a baby's utterance, rather than the presence or absence of it.

For the older child, adolescent, and adult as well, it is important to pay attention and take note of the person's speech and language skills. Are there unusual characteristics to their speech patterns? If, for example, a client's speech is characterized by distortions, substitutions, or omissions of high-frequency sounds or word endings, a high-frequency sensorineural hearing loss should be strongly suspected. Take note also of the vocal quality—is it very hypo- or hypernasal? How complex are their language patterns?

Informal observations can also assist in determining whether the information obtained thus far makes sense; that is, does the client's behavior and apparent communication ability match what they report on case history, as well as the results of testing? For example, does the client respond appropriately to the tester when the tester's face cannot be seen and no other contextual cues are available? If the client can respond appropriately under such circumstances, the likelihood of this person having sustained a severe to profound hearing loss is minimized. These are examples of ways in which the act of informally observing and making note of the client's behaviors can assist in establishing and/or supporting a differential diagnosis.

When the client is capable of appropriately responding to and answering questions while no visual information is available, and the test results you are shown seem to indicate a profound hearing loss, suspicion (a red flag) should immediately arise. The question one might explore in such a situation is whether the outcome of testing has a monetary or other tangible motivation. If it does, the astute clinician will be on guard for this and other red flags for pseudohypacusis. **Pseudohypacusis**, which is a term for false, exaggerated, or psychogenically motivated hearing loss, is sometimes accompanied by **telltale behaviors**. Some of these behaviors include fidgeting and vague answers during case history taking, leaning in and cupping one's ear toward a speaker, a report of sudden hearing loss with no logical medical history, excessively asking "Huh?" or "What?" and other such blatant overdramatizations of hearing loss. These behaviors are in stark contrast to what may have been obtained by pure tone testing or reported during the case history taking, and again may help the clinician in discerning a differential diagnosis.

Lastly, it is important to consider all test results in light of the behaviors observed. Are any discrepancies observed or suspected? Do these two sets of information match? There can be many reasons for such an occurrence, ranging from pseudohypacusis to a legitimate low incidence disorder to simple test inaccuracies. If there are discrepancies and the information does not match, then further assessment is a must, regardless of the assumed cause. Careful attention to a client's behaviors serves as an important and often informative and indispensible adjunct to the evaluation process.

Look, Play, Talk

The process of the clinician engaging in **"look, play, talk"** can be thought of as an additional, and child-specific, variation of the informal observation activity described previously. From the moment the child and parent(s) enter the test setting, the clinician should look at the child and take note of any and all nonverbal communication behaviors. For example, does the child make eye contact or use facial expression to display emotion? How and in what other types of actions does the child engage that show a communicative intent? Are any other significant nonverbal behaviors observed that may later prove useful in the assessment process?

Next, observe the child's play behavior. Provide the child with an age-appropriate toy/object and watch to see how the child plays with it. Is the child capable of manipulating the object? Does the child play appropriately with the toy? Can the clinician engage the child in a play activity with the toy/object? Then, talk to the child; can directions be followed? If you ask the child to take off his or her coat and get comfortable, does he or she understand and comply? Listen to the child as well; does the child speak or does she or he only point? As mentioned previously, if the child can speak, what does the speech sound like? Is it characterized by omissions, substitutions, and/or distortions of sounds or word endings? Talking and carefully listening frequently yields diagnostically significant information.

The process of "Look, play, talk" is an extremely important component of the evaluation process. Thus, it is incumbent on the clinician to take the time to establish a rapport with the parent(s), thus earning the trust of the child. The time it takes to do this will be time well spent, typically resulting in a smoother running test session and additional information regarding the child's developmental level and abilities.

The Process of Differential Diagnosis

If you have gone through the case history assessment as described, and done so meticulously, you will have collected a lot of information. This information plays a key role in establishing the differential diagnosis; the **differential diagnosis** is the method typically used to clinically distinguish or differentiate one disorder from another that presents with many of the same or similar symptoms and characteristics. The importance of establishing an accurate diagnosis cannot be overstated. Proper identification of hearing impairment and the concomitant difficulties is critical for establishing, preserving, and enhancing communication ability, as well as the quality of life, in all age populations across the life span. Unfortunately, erroneous and/or incomplete diagnoses are far too common, often resulting in a tragic loss in the ability to communicate and lead a healthy and productive life.

When considering the process of differential diagnosis, two key concerns are—as just suggested—the correct diagnosis of hearing loss as opposed to another similar, though erroneous, diagnosis, and the identification of possible additional comorbidly occurring conditions. A **comorbid** condition is one that occurs simultaneous to the hearing loss.

Numerous conditions present with many of the same or similar symptoms and characteristics as hearing loss. The concept of **look-alike** or imitator diseases is not restricted to hearing loss. In fact, when we hear about the great imitator diseases, some of the conditions that immediately come to mind may include syphilis, Lyme disease, and perhaps even multiple sclerosis or lupus. Less commonly do we hear hearing loss among the top contenders for this title. Despite this, the fact of the matter is that hearing loss *is* often mistaken for a number of different conditions. Misdiagnosis occurs all too often. Some of the hearing loss look-alike disorders include intellectual deficiencies, dementia, depression, behavior disorders, emotional disturbance, and attention deficit hyperactivity disorder; the list could go on. Clearly, the similarity of symptoms, and the possibility of these other disorders being simultaneously (comorbidly) present, causes some of the confusion and resulting errors.

It is absolutely essential that healthcare and other professionals (audiologists, SLPs, teachers, etc.) be aware of the possibility that hearing loss may be present, but obscured by other look-alike conditions, and also that two conditions may be comorbidly present. Appropriate intervention, whether that is medical or (re)habilitative, cannot be put into place if an accurate diagnosis is not established. What follows is a brief discussion of some of the conditions that have been observed to complicate the diagnosis of hearing loss or that occur simultaneously with it.

Autism Spectrum Disorder (ASD)

Multiple studies have documented the similarities between the presenting symptoms of autism spectrum disorder (ASD) and those of other sensory deficits (Hoevenaars-van den Boom, Antonissen, Knoors, & Vervloed, 2009; Myck-Wayne, Robinson, & Henson, 2011). For example, a child with severe to profound hearing loss will not respond when called and will also have difficulty developing speech and language skills without intervention. Similarly, the psychosocial characteristics of autism often include delays in language acquisition (Syzmanski, Brice, Lam, & Hotto, 2012). A very relevant question, as pointed out by Hoevenaars-van den Boom and colleagues, is that when it is hard to distinguish characteristics of autism and other sensory impairments in controlled studies, how much harder will it then be to do so in clinical practice (Hoevenaars-van den Boom et al., 2009)? To compound this situation further, the comorbidity of hearing loss with ASD appears to be increasing; the 2009–2010 Annual Survey of Deaf and Hard of Hearing Children and Youth (Gallaudet Research Institute, 2011) indicates that 1 in 59 eight-year-olds with hearing loss also received services for autism; this is considerably higher than the national estimate of 1 in 91 children with hearing loss (Kogan et al., 2009) and 1 in 110 with autism (Centers for Disease Control and Prevention, 2007). How, then, is the practicing clinician to distinguish between the two disorders, or ascertain if there is a case of dual diagnosis?

Let us first consider hearing loss. According to the National Institutes of Health (NIH, 1993), prior to universal hearing screening, the average age of identification of hearing loss in the United States was at close to 3 years of age, with lesser degrees of hearing loss going undetected for even longer. It's not surprising, then, that at the time of the NIH consensus statement it was reported that only 11 hospitals in the United States were screening more than 90% of their newborn infants prior to discharge. By the year 2005, as a result of universal newborn hearing screening (UNHS) programs, 95% of *all* infants in the United States were being screened prior to hospital discharge (Joint Commission on Infant Hearing, 2007). The age of identification of hearing loss dropped to an average of 3 to 6 months of age following the implementation of UNHS (Yoshinaga-Itano, 2004).

Based on this information, it would seem reasonable to assume that if a child presenting with delayed language development had a hearing loss, and the newborn hearing screening was completed and passed, then the risk of hearing impairment has been ruled out and the professional can move on to consider other possible etiologies. Under ideal circumstances this might actually prove to be the case; however, not only can genetic impairments occur

with late onset, but also numerous other risk factors can be responsible for causing late onset and/or progressive hearing loss. (Readers are again directed to Appendix 1 of the *Year 2007 Position Statement: Principles and Guidelines for Early Hearing Detection and Intervention Programs* [Joint Committee on Infant Hearing, 2007] for a more detailed listing of risk indicators associated with permanent congenital, delayed-onset, or progressive hearing loss in childhood.) It is important, therefore, that the speech-language pathologist refer any child who has any history of these risk factors for a complete audiologic evaluation, regardless of whether a newborn infant hearing screening has been passed.

Regarding ASD, Myck-Wayne and her colleagues (2011) reported that although the median age of identification of ASD has decreased over time (Shattuck et al., 2009), reliable identification does not occur until a child is approximately 24 months of age (Baron-Cohen, Allen, & Gillberg, 1992; Moore & Goodson, 2003). Some of the reasons for this include the apparent lack of a physical test that could conclusively identify the presence or absence of ASD, and that the symptoms of autism reportedly do not occur until approximately 24 months of age (Syzmanski et al., 2012). It would appear, then, that if a child has hearing loss and ASD, the hearing loss might be identified earlier; however, the reverse can't be ruled out either.

It is at this point that we can clearly recognize the essential role that the speech-language pathologist plays in the identification, treatment, planning, and interventions of individuals with communication disorders. Let us assume a child has been identified with a hearing loss and early intervention services have been provided, yet the child's development is not progressing at the anticipated rate. The speech-language pathologist is often the professional who spends the most time with the child (more than the audiologist, social worker, etc.), and thus, is in an ideal position to observe and document the lack of progress and make appropriate referrals. It is important to remember that delayed identification of one or the other disorder will confound efforts to provide early and appropriate intervention.

Finally, it is in the best interest of our patients (and families) that we all (speech-language pathologists, audiologists, and others) work together in collaboration. Accurate differential diagnoses, appropriate treatment planning, and individualized and comprehensive therapeutic interventions are facilitated, thus giving individuals with communication disorders the best possible chance of success.

Attention Deficit/Hyperactivity Disorder (AD/HD)

There is an abundance of information in the literature regarding the comorbidity trap among the three varieties of attention deficit/hyperactivity disorder (AD/HD), the broad category of hearing loss and auditory processing, and hearing loss specifically associated with otitis media. An entire textbook could be written addressing how each of these conditions may or may not be related to AD/HD. This section cannot hope to even scratch the surface of the broader topic and all its implications; instead, the intention of this section is merely to point out the similarity of symptoms between AD/HD and hearing loss for the purposes of differential diagnosis, and provide some general guidance for the speech-language pathologist who may encounter such a case.

Childhood AD/HD has been described as an educational disability that is thought to be due *not* to lack of skill, but to a problem of sustaining attention, effort, and motivation. Some deficits in specific skill areas (e.g., academic, social, organizational) are common among students with AD/HD. School-aged children with ADHD are reported to have more difficulty with the same academic work, and are generally 30% or more behind typical students in social skills and organization (Barkley, 2006). Other characteristics observed in children with AD/HD include an apparent inability to listen, and not following through with directions. Unfortunately for the professional attempting to diagnose and plan treatment interventions, the communication and educational challenges created by a hearing loss can sometimes cause students to behave in ways that may appear similar to those of the student with AD/HD (O'Connell & Casale, 2004).

The negative consequences of hearing loss can be seen in delayed and/or disordered speech-language development, social-emotional development, academic achievement, and vocational choices; the severity can range from slight to profound. As mentioned previously, many of the performance difficulties and problematic behaviors observed can potentially be the result of hearing loss or ADHD, or a combination of the two. In fact, the literature cites examples of AD/HD being examined as a condition that is secondary to hearing loss (O'Connell & Casale, 2004). It is not surprising, therefore, that a parent or teacher may be uncertain of whether a child's behaviors are the results of a hearing loss, ADHD, or even just plain willfulness.

For the professional who is faced with the situation of trying to determine whether a child has one or both disorders, a sensible solution may be to contact and refer to your local audiologist for a complete audiologic assessment and intervention. When an individual's access to sound and the environment has been remediated as appropriately and effectively as possible (with hearing aids, assistive devices, or the like), it may be possible to begin discerning how much of the behavior(s) observed relate to hearing ability versus another comorbid condition such as AD/HD.

Depression

The behavioral observations and case history reports for a new patient indicate that she is withdrawn and tends to isolate; has low self-esteem; does not engage with others in conversation in social, vocational, or academic settings; appears to have trouble concentrating and paying attention; and experiences headaches, dizziness, and nausea. What do you think the most likely etiology of these symptoms could be? Would you immediately think of a hearing loss as the most likely cause? Would you think, rather, that this person is depressed? How about a dual diagnosis of hearing loss and depression?

The fact of the matter is that the diagnosis for a patient with these behaviors and complaints could be either or both of these disorders. Symptoms such as headaches, dizziness, nausea, anxiety, withdrawal and isolation, trouble concentrating, not paying attention, and poor self-esteem are well documented in both the mental health and communication disorders literature as being potential indicators of depression as well as auditory system disorders (Anderson & Matkin, 1991; Dingle et al., 2011; Grover et al., 2012; Tarhan, Bastan, Aktas, Tarhan, & Safak, 2011).

The literature documents that these two disorders can and, indeed, do occur simultaneously in *all* age categories. It is well documented in the adult and geriatric populations (Lee, Tong, Yuen, & Hasselt, 2010). Although the risk of major depressive disorder in childhood is relatively small, it substantially increases with adolescence (Lewinsohn, Clarke, Seeley, & Rohde, 1994). In fact, hearing-impaired children are exceedingly vulnerable to poor psychosocial development, and are reported to experience a higher prevalence of depressive symptoms than normal hearing children (Theunissen et al., 2011). For the adult hard of hearing population, depression and anxiety are higher and quality of life is lower (Cetin, Uguz, Erdem, & Yildirim, 2010); in the older adult population, those with hearing loss appear more likely to experience emotional distress and social activity restrictions (Gopinath et al., 2012). Finally, it appears that none of the studies reviewed found any evidence to suggest that the coexistence of depression with hearing loss was dependent on any other variable, such as gender, age, level of hearing impairment, or educational background. This was true for both child and adult study data. Although we are not suggesting a direct causal relationship between hearing loss and depression, there certainly appears to be a link between the existence of hearing loss and general quality of life issues.

Given the significant number and variety of symptoms that are common indicators of both conditions, as well as the communicatively handicapping characteristics of hearing loss that are potentially remediable to varying degrees, it is important to either ascertain which disorder truly exists or confirm the presence of the comorbidly occurring conditions. The astute clinician will collaborate with and refer to other health professionals in order to clearly define the nature, severity, and characteristics of the individual's disorder(s). If a hearing loss can be identified and remediated, the patient's withdrawal, isolation, and other nonsocially interactive behaviors that are actually due to hearing loss can be remediated as effectively as possible. The patient and clinician are both, then, in a better position to identify other areas of concern. Planning and carrying out appropriate therapeutic interventions depends on accurate diagnoses.

Dementia

Dementia, one of several examples of age-associated conditions, has been described not as a disease, but as a syndrome that may have a negative impact on a variety of different functions such as memory, cognition, attention, problem solving, and language. Dementia can be caused by a variety of conditions, and has been documented as comorbidly occurring with, or presenting as a feature of, many other diseases as well. Presbycusis is a term that refers to age-related changes in hearing, or age-related hearing loss. This type of hearing loss can impact function, or at least appear to an observer as changes in the person's memory, cognition, language, and so on. If a person presents with these symptoms, which of these disorders is the cause—or is it both?

For many decades the literature has reflected the fact that dementia and hearing loss occur simultaneously. Weinstein (1986) found that 83% of institutionalized patients with a diagnosis of senile dementia also had some degree of hearing loss, and that the degree of hearing loss they experienced was more pronounced than in those without dementia. More recently, Lin and his colleagues (2011) concluded that hearing loss is independently associated with (incident all-cause) dementia. And finally, Lin (2012) found that individuals with mild, moderate, and severe hearing loss had a two-, three-, and five-fold risk of developing incident dementia, respectively, compared to normal hearing individuals, thus concluding that hearing loss is independently associated with incident dementia. How, then, does the clinician approach this individual?

With so many different potential reasons for decreased memory, cognition, impaired language, and even social isolation being observed in the older adult population, and the increased risk of comorbid conditions in the older adult population, it is prudent for the practicing clinician to ensure that, prior to any treatment planning and therapeutic intervention, a complete audiologic evaluation has been done and that the patient (or family) is complying with all recommendations (hearing aid fitting, etc.). Proper identification of hearing loss, with aural rehabilitative counseling and the use of hearing aids and assistive listening devices, has been found to reduce the adverse effects of hearing loss (Burkhalter, Allen, Skaar, Crittenden, & Burgio, 2009). Thus, once the individual is able to hear and communicate as effectively as possible, the clinician is in a better position to determine whether the behaviors being observed are truly a sign of dementia, or if the individual has inadequate access to sound.

Finally, there may be times that an older adult is referred for services as the result of a stroke or other traumatic event. It is important to remember that this type of insult can also create further damage to one's hearing. Therefore, even if your patient has a hearing aid that he or she has been using for a number of years, there is the possibility that following the traumatic event there has been further damage to the auditory system, and the device(s) may no longer be adequate. Do not assume that because an individual is wearing a hearing aid, that you need not concern yourself with their hearing status. Hearing loss can and does progress for any one of a number of reasons. The clinician must also consider that the patient's hearing aid may be malfunctioning. Whenever there is any cause for doubt or question, remember that auditory status can change, so contact your local audiologist. Collaboration with other professionals is in the best interest of your patients.

Summary

An initial and very important component of the diagnostic evaluation is the process of taking a thorough case history. Many different formats can be used for this purpose; there are commercially available case history forms, or the clinician may wish to derive his or her own. Each professional will make a judgment as to the best method for his or her own purposes—dependent, of course, on the population and setting in which they are working. The appendix to this chapter contains one commercially available form. We encourage the reader to review the information and forms available, and determine which will work best for his or her work environment.

The latter portion of this chapter addresses differential diagnosis, with a focus on comorbidly occurring conditions. We expect that you will find, as we have, that individuals with communication disorders frequently have other co-occurring conditions. In the process of making a differential diagnosis, it is beneficial to be organized and systematic in our thinking and approach to the diagnosis of hearing loss. As a guideline, the reader is reminded to use a collaborative approach; other speech-language pathologists as well as audiologists and other healthcare-related professionals are frequently indispensible in developing appropriate and individualized intervention services for the patients in our care.

Discussion Questions

1. Discuss the different components of a thorough case history.
2. What kinds of information can be gathered from informal observation of a client?
3. Describe some of the complications that may occur in the prenatal, perinatal, and postnatal period.
4. What are some of the childhood risk factors for hearing loss?
5. List and describe some of the red flag behaviors that may be informally observed during the evaluation process. What might some of these behaviors indicate?
6. Discuss the process of differential diagnosis.
7. Describe the similarity in symptoms between hearing loss and other possible comorbidities.

References

Anderson, K., & Matkin, N. (1991). *Relationship of long term hearing loss to psychosocial impact and educational needs, revised 2007.* Available from http://www.betterhearing.org/hearing_loss/children_hearing_loss/relationship_hearing_loss_learning.pdf.

Barkley, R. A. (2006). *Attention-deficit hyperactivity disorder: A handbook for diagnosis and treatment* (3rd ed.). New York: Guilford.

Baron-Cohen, S., Allen, J., & Gillberg, C. (1992). Can autism be detected at 18 months of age? The needle, the haystack and the CHAT. *British Journal of Psychiatry,* 161: 839–843.

Burkhalter, C. L., Allen, R. S., Skaar, D. C., Crittenden, J., & Burgio, L. D. (2009). Examining the effectiveness of traditional audiological assessments for nursing home residents with dementia-related behaviors. *Journal of the American Academy of Audiology,* 20: 529–538.

Centers for Disease Control and Prevention. (2007). Prevalence of autism spectrum disorder—Autism and developmental disability monitoring network, 14 sites. United States, 2002. In Surveillance summary. *Morbidity and Mortality Weekly Report,* 56: 12–27.

Cetin, B., Uguz, F., Erdem, M., & Yildirim, A. (2010). Relationship between quality of life, anxiety and depression in unilateral hearing loss. *Journal of International Advanced Otology,* 6 (2): 252–257.

Dingle, K., Clavarino, A., Williams, G. M., Bor, W., Najman, J. M., & Alati, R. (2011). Predicting depressive and anxiety disorders with YASR internalizing scales (empirical and DSM-oriented). *Social Psychiatry and Psychiatric Epidemiology,* 46: 1313–1324.

Elmorsy, S., Shabana, Y. K., Raouf, A. A., Naggar, M. E., Bedir, T., Taher, S., et al. (2010). The role of IL-8 in different types of otitis media and bacteriological correlation. *Journal of International Advanced Otology,* 6(2): 269–273.

Gallaudet Research Institute. (2011). *Regional and national summary report of data from the 2009–2010 annual survey of deaf and hard of hearing children and youth.* Washington, DC: GRI, Gallaudet University.

Ghonaim, M. M., El-Edel, R. H., Basiony, L. A., & Al-Zahrani, S. S. (2011). Risk factors and causative organisms of otitis media in children. *Ibnosina Journal of Medicine and Biomedical Sciences,* 3(5): 172–181.

Gopinath, B., Hickson, L., Schneider, J., McMahon, C. M., Burlutsky, G., Leeder, S. R., et al. (2012). Hearing-impaired adults are at increased risk of experiencing emotional distress and social engagement restrictions five years later. *Age and Ageing,* 41: 618–623.

Grover, S., Kumar, V., Chakrabarti, S., Hollikatti, P., Singh, P., Tyagi, S., et al. (2012). Prevalence and type of functional somatic complaints in patients with first-episode depression. *East Asian Archives of Psychiatry,* 22: 146–153.

Hoevenaars-van den Boom, M. A. A., Antonissen, A. C. F. M., Knoors, H., & Vervloed, M. P. J. (2009). Differentiating characteristics of deafblindness and autism in people with congenital deafblindness and profound intellectual disability. *Journal of Intellectual Disability Research,* 53(6): 548–558.

Joint Committee on Infant Hearing. (2007). Year 2007 position statement: Principles and guidelines for early hearing detection and intervention programs. *Pediatrics,* 120(4): 898–921.

Joint Committee on Infant Hearing. (2007). *Year 2007 Position Statement: Principles and Guidelines for Early Hearing Detection and Intervention.* Available from www.asha.org/policy.

Kogan, M. D., Blumberg, S., Schieve, L., Boyle, C., Perrin, J., Ghandour, R., et al. (2009). Prevalence of parent-reported diagnosis of autism spectrum disorder among children in the US, 2007. *Pediatrics,* 124(4): 1–8.

Lee, A. T. H., Tong, M. C. F., Yuen, P. S. O., & Hasselt, C. A. (2010). Hearing impairment and depressive symptoms in an older Chinese population. *Journal of Otolaryngology,* 39(5): 498–503.

Lewinsohn, P. M., Clarke, G. N., Seeley, J. R., Rohde, P. (1994). Major depression in community adolescents: age at onset, episode duration, and time to recurrence. *Journal of the American Academy of Child & Adolescent Psychiatry,* 33: 809– 818.

Lin, F. (2012). Implications of hearing loss for older adults. *Audiology and Neuro-Otology,* 17(Suppl.): 4–6.

Lin, F., Metter, J., O'Brien, R., Resnick, S., Zonderman, A., & Ferrucci, L. (2011). Hearing loss and incident dementia. *Archives of Neurology,* 68(2): 214–220.

Moore, V., & Goodson, S. (2003). How well does early diagnosis of autism stand the test of time? Follow-up study of children assessed for autism at age 2 and development of an early diagnosis service. *Autism,* 7(1): 47–63.

Morzaria, S., Westerberg, B. D., & Kozak, F. K. (2004). Systematic review of the etiology of bilateral sensorineural hearing loss in children. *International Journal of Pediatric Otorhinolaryngology,* 68: 1193–1198.

Myck-Wayne, J., Robinson, S., & Henson, E. (2011). Serving and supporting young children with a dual diagnosis of hearing loss and autism: The stories of four families. *American Annals of the Deaf,* 156(4): 379–390.

National Institutes of Health. (1993). Early identification of hearing impairment in infants and young children. NIH Consensus Statement Online, 11(1): 1–24.

O'Connell, J., & Casale, K. (2004). Attention deficits and hearing loss: Meeting the challenge. *Volta Review,* 104(4): 257–271.

Sack, K. E. (2012). Taking away the diagnosis. *Texax Heart Institute Journal,* 39(1) 1.

Shattuck, P., Durkin, M., Maenner, M., Newschaffer, C., Mandell, D., Wiggins, L., et al. (2009). Timing of identification of children with an autism spectrum disorder. Findings from a population-based surveillance study. *Journal of the American Academy of Child and Adolescent Psychiatry,* 48(5): 474–483.

Sheer, F. J., Swarts, J. D., & Ghadiali, S. N. (2012). Three-dimensional finite element analysis of Eustachian tube function under normal and pathological conditions. *Medical Engineering and Physics,* 34: 606–616.

Syzmanski, C. A., Brice, P., Lam, K. H., & Hotto, S. A. (2012). Deaf children with autism spectrum disorders. *Journal of Autism and Developmental Disorders,* 42: 2027–2037.

Tarhan, E., Bastan, B., Aktas, A. R., Tarhan, B., & Safak, M. A. (2011). Spontaneous intracranial hypotension syndrome with bilateral hearing loss and hyperacusis: A case report and review of the literature. *Journal of International Advanced Otology,* 7(2): 271–277.

Theunissen, S. C. P. M., Rieffe, C., Kouwenberg, M., Soede, W., Briaire, J. J., & Frijns, J. H. M. (2011). Depression in hearing-impaired children. *International Journal of Pediatric Otorhinolaryngology,* 75: 1313–1317.

Weinstein, B. (1986). Hearing loss and senile dementia in the institutionalized elderly. *Clinical Gerontologist,* 4(3): 3–15.

Yoshinaga-Itano, C. (2004). Levels of evidence: Universal newborn hearing screening (UNHS) and early detection and intervention systems (EHDI). *Journal of Communication Disorders,* 37: 451–465.

Appendix 4-A

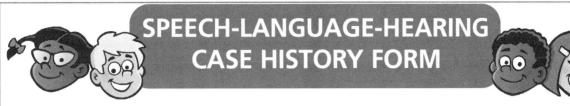

SPEECH-LANGUAGE-HEARING CASE HISTORY FORM

Identifying and Family Information:

Child's Name:_____ Birthdate:_____ Sex: ☐ M ☐ F

Father's Name:_____ Daytime Phone:_____

Address:_____ Cell Phone:_____

_____ E-mail:_____

_____

Mother's Name:_____ Daytime Phone:_____

Address:_____ Cell Phone:_____

_____ E-mail:_____

_____

Doctor's Name: _____ Doctor's Phone: _____

Child lives with (check one):

    ☐ Birth Parents   ☐ Foster Parents   ☐ One Parent

    ☐ Adoptive Parents   ☐ Parent and Step-Parent   ☐ Other _____

Other children in the family:

Name	Age	Sex	Grade	Speech/Hearing Problems

Child's race/ethnic group:

    ☐ Caucasian, Non-Hispanic   ☐ Hispanic   ☐ African-American

    ☐ Native American   ☐ Asian or Pacific Islander   ☐ Other _____

Is there a language other than English spoken in the home? ☐ Yes ☐ No

    If yes, which one?_____

    Does the child speak the language?   ☐ Yes ☐ No

    Does the child understand the language?   ☐ Yes ☐ No

    Who speaks the language? _____

    Which language does the child prefer to speak at home? _____

Speech-Language-Hearing

Do you feel your child has a speech problem? ☐ Yes ☐ No
If yes, please describe. _____
_____
_____

Do you feel your child has a hearing problem? ☐ Yes ☐ No
If yes, please describe. _____
_____
_____

Has he/she ever had a speech evaluation/screening? ☐ Yes ☐ No
If yes, where and when? _____
What were you told? _____
_____
_____

Has he/she ever had a hearing evaluation/screening? ☐ Yes ☐ No
If yes, where and when? _____
What were you told? _____
_____
_____

Has your child ever had speech therapy? ☐ Yes ☐ No
If yes, where and when? _____
What was he/she working on? _____
_____

Has your child received any other evaluation or therapy (physical therapy, counseling, occupational
therapy, vision, etc.)? ☐ Yes ☐ No
If yes, please describe._____
_____
_____
_____

Is your child aware of, or frustrated by, any speech/language difficulties?_____
_____

What do you see as your child's most difficult problem in the home? _____
_____

What do you see as your child's most difficult problem in school?_____
_____

Birth History

Was there anything unusual about the pregnancy or birth?   ❑ Yes   ❑ No

    If yes, please describe. _____

_____

_____

How old was the mother when the child was born? _____

Was the mother sick during the pregnancy?   ❑ Yes   ❑ No

    If yes, please describe. _____

_____

How many months was the pregnancy?_____

Did the child go home with his/her mother from the hospital?   ❑ Yes   ❑ No

    If child stayed at the hospital, please describe why and how long. _____

_____

_____

Medical History

Has your child had any of the following?

❑ adenoidectomy	❑ encephalitis	❑ seizures
❑ allergies	❑ flu	❑ sinusitis
❑ breathing difficulties	❑ head injury	❑ sleeping difficulties
❑ chicken pox	❑ high fevers	❑ thumb/finger sucking habit
❑ colds	❑ measles	❑ tonsillectomy
❑ ear infections	❑ meningitis	❑ tonsillitis
How often?_____	❑ mumps	❑ vision problems
❑ ear tubes	❑ scarlet fever	

  Other serious injury/surgery: _____

Is your child currently (or recently) under a physician's care?   ❑ Yes   ❑ No

    If yes, why?_____

_____

Please list any medications your child takes regularly: _____

_____

_____

Developmental History

Please tell the approximate age your child achieved the following developmental milestones:

_____ sat alone	_____ grasped crayon/pencil
_____ babbled	_____ said first words
_____ put two words together	_____ spoke in short sentences
_____ walked	_____ toilet trained

Does your child...
- ❑ choke on food or liquids?
- ❑ currently put toys/objects in his/her mouth?
- ❑ brush his/her teeth and/or allow brushing?

Current Speech-Language-Hearing

Does your child...
- ❑ repeat sounds, words or phrases over and over?
- ❑ understand what you are saying?
- ❑ retrieve/point to common objects upon request (ball, cup, shoe)?
- ❑ follow simple directions ("Shut the door" or "Get your shoes")?
- ❑ respond correctly to yes/no questions?
- ❑ respond correctly to who/what/where/when/why questions?

Your child currently communicates using...
- ❑ body language.
- ❑ sounds (vowels, grunting).
- ❑ words (shoe, doggy, up).
- ❑ 2 to 4 word sentences.
- ❑ sentences longer than four words.
- ❑ other _____.

Behavioral Characteristics:

❑ cooperative	❑ restless
❑ attentive	❑ poor eye contact
❑ willing to try new activities	❑ easily distracted/short attention
❑ plays alone for reasonable length of time	❑ destructive/aggressive
❑ separation difficulties	❑ withdrawn
❑ easily frustrated/impulsive	❑ inappropriate behavior
❑ stubborn	❑ self-abusive behavior

School History

If your child is in school, please answer the following:

Name of school and grade in school: _____

_____

Teacher's name: _____

_____

Has your child repeated a grade? _____

_____

What are your child's strengths and/or best subjects? _____

_____

Is your child having difficulty with any subjects? _____

_____

Is your child receiving help in any subjects? _____

_____

Additional Comments

_____

_____

_____

_____

_____

_____

_____

_____

_____

_____

_____

_____

_____

_____

_____

Chapter 5

Pure Tone Audiometry and Masking

Deborah R. Welling, AuD, CCC-A, FAAA
Associate Professor and Director of Clinical Education
Department of Speech-Language Pathology
Seton Hall University

Carol A. Ukstins, MS, CCC-A, FAAA
Educational Audiologist
Office of Special Education
Newark Public Schools

Key Terms

Air conduction
Auditory masking
Auditory threshold
Behavioral observation
    audiometry (BOA)
Bone conduction

Conditioned play
    audiometry (CPA)
Diagnostic
Interaural attenuation
Minimum response
    level (MRL)

Screening
Shadow curve
Visual reinforcement
    audiometry (VRA)

Objectives

- Understand the principles behind air and bone conduction testing, and the unique information that each contributes
- Understand the circumstances that necessitate masking to be performed
- Understand the similarities and differences between diagnostic and screening air conduction testing
- Discuss the different procedures employed during behavioral pediatric assessment and how they differ
- Understand the differences between the results of earphone and sound field testing

Introduction

"Raise your hand when you hear the sound." You probably heard this phrase at some point in your life when you had your hearing checked as a school-aged child. At that age, *pure tone audiometry* was a foreign term. However, as a speech-language pathologist, pure tone audiometry is a frequently used term that defines the most common behavioral procedure used to determine both the degree and etiology of hearing loss. Although not all techniques in this chapter will be performed by a speech-language pathologist, it is important to understand the process, principles and procedures, and clinical implications of air conduction audiometry.

Air Conduction Audiometry

What You Need to Know

Pure tone **air conduction** is an immensely practical measurement. Sound traveling through air conduction is the normal way an auditory stimulus reaches our ears during typical day-to-day activities. For example, when someone is speaking, their words reach our ears through the air. Sound reaches our outer ear and is then sent down the ear canal to the eardrum, through the middle ear, and further on to the inner ear where it reaches the organ of hearing. There it is converted to a neural signal that then travels up the auditory pathway to our brain for comprehension. Any break in this chain of hearing, at any point along the entire auditory pathway, can cause air conduction results to be abnormal. Abnormal results are a hearing loss. It is important to conclude from this that when we test hearing using air conduction audiometry, we are assessing the integrity of this entire auditory pathway; however, this determination is only part of the story. Air conduction's limitation is that the results tell us only that there *is* a problem; they do not give us the entire picture. If abnormal results are obtained, air conduction results cannot tell us *where* the hearing problem originates in the ear.

How It Works

Pure tone air conduction audiometry is the behavioral procedure used to establish the loudness or intensity threshold in decibels (dB) at which a person just begins to hear sound via this normal mode of sound transmission. Air conduction audiometry involves putting one of two styles of transducers, standard or insert earphones, on a person's ears and then having him or her raise a hand (or perform some other task) every time he or she hears a beeping sound. The air-conducted signal enters the ear and goes through the entire auditory system; hence, it represents the hearing sensitivity of the auditory system as a whole. This procedure can be done as either a screening or a diagnostic modality.

Technically Speaking

As previously stated, air conduction is the normal means of sound transmission in day-to-day situations. Pure tone air conduction audiometry is the behavioral procedure that is utilized for the purposes of establishing the loudness or intensity threshold in dB at which a person just begins to hear sound for this normal mode of sound transmission. The air-conducted signal is presented by a transducer; either supra-aural or inserts earphones, and can be performed as either a screening or diagnostic threshold procedure. As a **screening**, a pass/fail paradigm is employed in response to an agreed-upon intensity level (possibly 10, 15, or 20 dB, depending on the setting and population). As a **diagnostic** procedure, thresholds are established for individual frequencies. Regardless of whether it is done as a diagnostic or a screening procedure, air conduction testing evaluates the integrity of the entire auditory system (conductive, sensorineural, and central mechanisms), and results represent the degree of sensitivity of the entire auditory system; that is, if a hearing loss exists, we can make a statement regarding the degree of hearing loss only. As mentioned earlier, the findings cannot localize the site of damage (etiology of hearing loss). Further testing must be completed to make the determination between a conductive and a sensorineural pathology. In order to establish the etiology, bone conduction audiometry must be completed (see later in this chapter), and the results are used in conjunction with the air conduction findings.

Methodology

When you are ready to begin air conduction testing, you should first be aware that the way in which instructions are given can have an impact on the way in which the patient responds. For example, if you merely instruct the person to raise a hand (or some other task) when a sound is heard, you may not find the very softest (threshold) level that the person is capable of hearing. **Auditory threshold** is the lowest-decibel hearing level at which responses occur in at least one half of a series of ascending trials (American Speech-Language-Hearing Association [ASHA], 2005). Instructing the patient to "listen very carefully and respond, even if you only think you hear the sound" is likely to result in a much better (more sensitive) response from the patient. In addition,

ASHA's *Guidelines for Manual Pure-Tone Audiometry* (2005) recommends the following:

- Indicate that the purpose of the test is to find the faintest tone that can be heard
- Emphasize that it is necessary to sit quietly, without talking, during the test
- Indicate that the participant is to respond whenever the tone is heard, no matter how faint it may be
- Describe the need to respond overtly as soon as the tone comes on and to respond overtly immediately when the tone goes off
- Indicate that each ear is to be tested separately with tones of different pitches
- Describe inappropriate behaviors such as drinking, eating, smoking, chewing, or any additional behavior that may interfere with the test
- Provide an opportunity for questions that the listener may have

Proper placement of the supra-aural earphones (or insert earphones) during air conduction testing is the next critical step in the testing process. If you are using the standard (supra-aural) earphones, make sure that the small dime-sized hole (diaphragm) that the sound comes out of lines up with the opening to the ear canal. The same holds true if you are using insert earphones; make sure that you select an appropriately sized tip and that when it's inserted it fits flush in the ear canal, and does not stick out. Inappropriately placed earphones may adversely affect hearing test results, possibly suggesting a hearing loss when one does not, in fact, exist. It is particularly important to pay attention to earphone placement when testing small children or clients with cranial-facial abnormalities because it will be evident upon initial earphone placement that transducers are fitting loose or "sloppy" on the head. In cases like these, it is important to periodically recheck earphone placement throughout the test procedure because the earphones may slip or become displaced due to natural head movement.

Pure tone air conduction audiometry is considered a behavioral test of the auditory system. Therefore, the next consideration involved in air conduction testing is how the examiner will have the client indicate that she or he has heard the sound. For example, an adult may be asked to raise a hand, press a switch, or the like. Children under the age of 5 or 6 years (chronologically or developmentally) may be trained to drop a block or participate in some other game/play type activity each time a sound is heard. Additional details regarding the testing of children will be addressed later in this chapter. Regardless of the population

or the method used during testing, consistent and repeatable responses are the goal in order to obtain reliable results.

When performing diagnostic threshold testing, the frequencies of sound used typically include 250 Hz, 500 Hz, 1000 Hz, 2000 Hz, 4000 Hz, 8000 Hz, and occasionally 125 Hz as well. When there is a significant difference between the decibel levels of the responses at two adjacent frequencies, a threshold measurement will be made at additional interoctave frequencies (750 Hz, 1500 Hz, 3000 Hz, and 6000 Hz) as well.

Testing is completed one ear at a time and one frequency at a time. The clinician will typically start in the right ear (or the better ear if there is a difference) at 1000 Hz first; proceed to 2000 Hz, 4000 Hz, and 8000 Hz; repeat testing at 1000 Hz as a reliability check; and then go down to 500 Hz and 250 Hz before moving on to the left (or other) ear. At each frequency, the initial intensity of the sound will be presented at a decibel level that is assumed to be higher (louder) than the level at which the person just begins to hear. In this way, the patient is familiarized with the sound stimulus. Each time the listener responds that the sound has been heard, the intensity level is decreased by 10 dB; each time the person does not hear the sound it is increased by 5 dB. The intensity level of the sound is continually increased and decreased until the clinician finds the decibel level that the patient responds to one-half of the time, with the minimum number of responses needed to determine the threshold of hearing being two out of three responses at a single level (American National Standards Institute, 2004). The results obtained are recorded on an audiogram (see **Figure 5.1**).

When performing air conduction testing as a screening, as opposed to a diagnostic evaluation, many of the same considerations should be taken into account. In an audiometric screening, we are not usually testing as many frequencies and we are not searching for threshold; rather, we use a pass/fail paradigm. Frequencies used typically include 1000 Hz, 2000 Hz, 3000 Hz, and 4000 Hz. Due to the problems of background noise, 500 Hz is tested only when conditions permit. If the screening is not completed in a sound-treated room, the deleterious effects of background noise will influence the reliability of threshold testing at the lower frequencies. A typical screening technique starts with the right ear. The client is again familiarized with the sound at a level assumed to be sufficiently louder than the suspected threshold level. Then the sound is lowered directly to a predetermined decibel level (usually 15 dB HL or 20 dB HL, depending on the setting), and the person either hears the sound and passes the screening or does not hear the sound

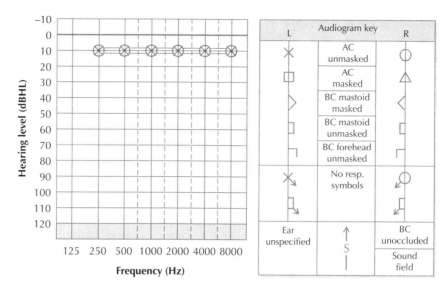

Figure 5.1 Typical audiogram demonstrating normal pure tone air conduction responses in both ears; the "O" markings represent the right ear, and the "X" markings represent the left ear.

and fails. The inability to hear and respond at any one frequency, in either ear, constitutes a failure and requires a referral for further evaluation.

Bone Conduction Audiometry
What You Need to Know

Bone conduction audiometry has more significance diagnostically than practically; that is to say that, unlike air conduction, bone conduction is not the normal way that we hear and communicate in day-to-day situations. To review, when a person speaks, the sound is transmitted through the air (air conduction), and it eventually reaches the listener at the outer ear before traveling further through the auditory system and reaching the organ of hearing (cochlea) in the inner ear. Bone conduction, on the other hand, is when sound is transmitted by vibrating the skull, a bone, and is conducted via that vibration to directly stimulate the cochlea (which is surrounded by bone) in the inner ear. We do not typically communicate with others by vibrating their skulls; at least, one would hope not. However, if you have ever experienced a car driving past with the bass control of its stereo turned up to maximum, you have experienced firsthand the vibration of sound via bone conduction. The results of this test are diagnostically significant because they can be used to help us determine the location or etiology of the hearing loss. When the results of air and bone conduction testing are used in combination, both the type

of hearing loss and the severity can be established. Neither test alone can give us both pieces of information.

How It Works

Bone conduction audiometry is also considered a behavioral audiometric measure. In bone conduction audiometry, a bone conduction oscillator is placed either behind the ear (called mastoid placement) or on the forehead (called forehead placement). The client is again asked to respond in the same fashion that was established for pure tone air conduction testing—either raise a hand or perform some other task every time she or he hears a beeping sound.

Unlike air conduction, the bone conduction oscillator vibrates the skull; as a result, the cochlea in the inner ear (sensorineural mechanism) is stimulated directly, thus bypassing the outer and middle ears (conductive mechanism). When, for example, a client is tested by air conduction and demonstrates a moderate degree of hearing loss, the next step is to test by bone conduction. The results of air conduction testing (using supra-aural or insert earphones) are then compared to the results of bone conduction (using the bone conduction oscillator); based on a comparison of these results, we can determine how much of the moderate hearing loss is due to conductive damage, how much is due to sensorineural damage, or if some combination of damage to the two pathways is involved. Thus, the results of this test in combination with the results of air conduction testing can help the audiologist determine the type of hearing loss (conductive, sensorineural, or mixed).

In summary, bone conduction alone cannot determine the severity of the hearing loss; it can only help us determine the type of hearing loss. Air conduction alone, on the other hand, cannot determine the type of hearing loss, but it does indicate the degree. Only the combined measurements of both air and bone conduction thresholds can lead us to determine both nature (type) and severity (degree) of a hearing loss.

Technically Speaking

Whereas air conduction testing transmits sound through the entire auditory system (outer, middle, inner ear and central auditory pathways) by using standard supra-aural or insert earphones, bone conduction testing stimulates the cochlea directly by vibrating the skull through the use of a bone conduction vibrator. This may be accomplished by placing the vibrator on either the mastoid bone (behind the ear) or on the forehead. Although there is evidence in the literature that the forehead is the preferred placement site for bone conduction testing (Fagelson and Martin, 1994; and others), it appears that many audiologists continue to prefer the mastoid process.

Upon stimulation, the bone-conducted signal goes directly to the cochlea in the inner ear and continues up the auditory pathway to the temporal lobe. Thus, the responses obtained reflect the integrity of the cochlea and/or retrocochlear structures. Based on a combination of these results and the air conduction findings, a determination of site of lesion and type of hearing loss can be gleaned.

If a difference between the ears exists (such as a sensorineural hearing loss with one ear significantly better than the other), the responses to unmasked bone conduction testing would reflect the better cochlea, because there is essentially no interaural attenuation by bone conduction. Alternately, in the case of a bilateral conductive hearing loss, the unmasked bone conduction responses will reflect the ear with the greatest conductive component (air–bone gap). Masking, interaural attenuation, and related concepts will be explained later in this chapter.

Methodology

In preparation for bone conduction audiometry, the clinician removes the earphones used for air conduction and places the bone conduction oscillator on the client, either on the forehead or, more frequently, on the mastoid bone behind the ear. It is noteworthy to mention that the mastoid selected for testing (right or left side) does not matter because regardless of placement, the clinician cannot be sure which cochlea is actually responding. The reason is because the bone oscillator is vibrating the entire skull, which will simultaneously stimulate both cochleas, unless masking is performed. Additional details regarding the concept of masking will be addressed in the next section.

The actual procedure for obtaining bone conduction thresholds is the same as for air conduction. The clinician uses either standard hand raising or a conditioning procedure for the response pattern and then does a threshold search, as described previously. The results are plotted on the audiogram form.

Masking

Generally speaking, speech-language pathologists do not need to know how to perform masking; in fact, it is likely that they never will need to do so. However, if speech-language pathologists are to provide the best possible services for their clients, proper interpretation of the audiogram often incorporates the interpretation of masked thresholds as well. Therefore, the purpose of this section is merely to help the speech-language pathologist understand how the process of masking is carried out in order to enhance understanding of audiometric test results and the implications those findings will have on therapeutic interventions.

What You Need to Know

One of the major objectives of the basic audiological evaluation is assessment of auditory function of each ear independently (Yacullo, 1999). Unfortunately, a potentially problematic situation occurs during a routine hearing test when the hearing sensitivity of one ear is significantly better or worse than the hearing sensitivity of the other ear. Let's consider a situation where a person has completely normal hearing in one ear and a profound hearing loss in the other ear. When we perform air conduction testing, using standard supra-aural earphones, testing results would reflect normal hearing in the "good" ear. However, when we switch to the "bad" ear, a complication arises. The amount of sound that will need to go into the earphone in order for the bad ear to respond will eventually become so loud that you run the risk of the good ear hearing and responding to the sound before the bad ear has a chance. In this scenario it becomes physiologically impossible for the client to listen with the bad ear and expect reliable test results. When the responses of the good ear are recorded falsely as responses of the bad ear, we call this a **shadow curve**. The term *cross over* (or *cross hearing*) is used when the evaluator identifies the existence of a shadow curve. When it is suspected that the stimulus used for testing is crossing over to the better hearing ear, masking is employed as a further diagnostic test procedure.

How It Works

Simply put, **auditory masking** is the process in which one sound is blocked out by another sound. Clinically, masking is used to prevent the test sound from being heard by the nontest ear. The process of masking can be observed in many everyday situations, such as when background noise prevents us from hearing what another person is saying. In the testing of auditory thresholds, when an asymmetrical hearing loss is suspected, the audiologist needs to perform clinical masking in order to determine how the poorer ear hears when not influenced by the better ear.

During this procedure, once a shadow curve is identified, the poorer ear is retested while, at the same time, masking noise is put into the better ear to prevent it from participating in the process. In this way it is possible to determine the hearing abilities of each ear independent from the other.

Technically Speaking

Attenuation, as it refers to hearing, is the reduction or lessening in the strength of a sound. **Interaural attenuation** is the difference, in decibels, between the intensity of sound that was presented to the poorer ear and the amount of sound that actually reached the good ear. The mathematical difference is the amount of sound that was "lost" and got absorbed by the skull, before it got loud enough to reach the other ear. This amount of sound, in decibels, is the interaural attenuation.

There is an abundance of available literature that documents the impact that interaural attenuation has on audiometric test results and provides normative data for the purposes of masking (Killion, Wilber, & Gudmundsen, 1985; Munro & Agnew, 1999; Munro & Contractor, 2010). These data are routinely taken into account to ensure the accuracy of the results.

Sound Field (SF) Testing
What You Need to Know

We most frequently envision a person receiving a hearing test while wearing either supra-aural or insert earphones; however, this is not the only way a hearing test can be performed. *Sound field* refers to a controlled acoustic environment. Previously, we have referenced a sound booth in which sound field testing takes place, and later we will discuss sound field assistive listening devices, which refers to instrumentation modifying an acoustic environment. *Sound field testing* is a term used to describe a test situation in which a client's hearing is assessed while he or she is seated in the sound-treated room or booth. The sound stimulus is delivered through speakers mounted in the booth instead of through earphones. Many of the same guidelines used for pure tone audiometry via earphones need to be considered for sound field testing as well, such as client instruction, choice of response mode, listening for the faintest sound, and so on. This type of test setup may be used for both unaided and aided behavioral hearing assessment procedures; the stimuli used may be warbled pure tones, narrow bands of noise, or speech stimuli. The type of stimulus used for testing should be specifically noted on the audiogram.

Sound field testing is frequently the methodology of choice when performing behavioral hearing assessment on very young and/or difficult to test populations. It is extremely useful, for example, when a tactilely defensive child refuses to wear the earphones. However, sound field testing can also be used for other types of assessments and clients. For example, a sound field testing setup is useful for follow-up procedures when behavioral performance with hearing aids, assessing cochlear implants, and/or testing with FM systems. Although the practice of performing some of these sound field functional assessments with hearing aids and/or other assistive devices may not be standard practice in all facilities, it is the expressed opinion of these authors that such functional evaluations can yield valuable information.

An important caveat must be addressed regarding sound field testing. Specifically, when audiologic assessments are performed in this manner, with the sound coming out of speakers instead of directed to individual ears through earphones, the results only represent the hearing status of the better ear, if there is a difference between the ears (that is, one ear being significantly better than the other). For example, if a baby with normal hearing in the right ear and a profound hearing loss in the left ear is being tested behaviorally in a sound field, the responses to the sounds presented through the speakers will be observed at normal levels because the right ear has normal hearing. It is only when we use earphones that we are able to test each ear individually and determine that the left ear has a profound loss of hearing. Any loss of hearing, even slight or unilateral, is cause for concern and intervention; therefore, even when a behavioral audiogram is performed in the sound field and shows responses in the normal range, a conclusion of normal hearing in both ears cannot be made. A follow-up evaluation must be performed in order to obtain ear-specific information and rule out the presence of a unilateral hearing loss.

In the sections that follow, you will find descriptions of various procedures that are frequently performed in a sound field, with pediatric and/or difficult to test populations. It should be noted, however, that these procedures and methods of obtaining behavioral results are not limited to the sound field; that is to say that whenever possible, they may also be performed with the use of earphones and/or a bone conduction oscillator, in order to obtain additional diagnostic and ear-specific data.

Behavioral Pediatric Assessment

A wealth of research is available supporting the use of objective procedures such as otoacoustic emission (OAE) testing and auditory brainstem response (ABR) testing in the newborn infant hearing screening process. In 2007, the Joint Committee on Infant Hearing (JCIH) of the American Speech-Language-Hearing Association (ASHA) published an updated consensus statement titled *Principles and Guidelines for Early Hearing Detection and Intervention (EHDI) Programs.* In this position statement, the JCIH endorses early detection of and intervention for hearing loss, with the ultimate goal to maximize linguistic and communicative competence and literacy development for children who are deaf or hard of hearing. In particular, the JCIH recommends that all infants have access to a hearing screening using physiologic measures by 1 month of age (ASHA, 2007). It further recommends, however, that following failure of either the initial screening or subsequent rescreening, an audiologic evaluation be performed and behavioral measures, as developmentally appropriate and feasible, be completed as a cross-check measure. It is imperative to understand that although the objective procedures such as OAE and ABR testing are clearly important, and even indispensable, in the identification, assessment, and intervention of a hearing impairment, only behavioral tests are true and direct measures of hearing (Hicks, Tharpe, & Ashmead, 2000; Madell, 2011). As such, behavioral measures of hearing sensitivity necessarily remain an integral part of the diagnosis and treatment of hearing loss.

With regard to behavioral pediatric assessment, whether of pediatric age chronologically or developmentally, it is important to understand that the responses observed may not actually be threshold levels for the given child. Recall

that a threshold-level sound is the very softest sound that a person is capable of hearing 50% of the time. The responses that are observed and reported on during pediatric assessments are often not the softest sounds that a child is actually capable of hearing; rather, they might merely be the softest sounds that the child was willing or able to respond to on a given date. This type of measurement is often referred to as a **minimum response level (MRL)**, in recognition of the fact that the child's true hearing ability might be better than the results would otherwise indicate. The developmentally younger the child is, the more likely the responses are MRLs instead of actual thresholds.

The following sections on behavioral observation audiometry (BOA), visual reinforcement audiometry (VRA), and conditioned play audiometry (CPA) describe the behavioral techniques that are frequently utilized in a sound field setting (often out of necessity for a variety of reasons) with pediatric and/or difficult to test populations. As noted in the preceding section, these procedures are not limited to the sound field setting. Whenever possible they can, and should, also be employed while using earphones and/or bone conduction oscillators in order to obtain ear-specific and diagnostically useful information.

Behavioral Observation Audiometry (BOA)
What You Need to Know

Behavioral observation audiometry (BOA) is a methodology used when attempting to subjectively test the hearing of a child with a developmental age of up to 6 or 7 months. Objective procedures (such as OAE and ABR) record physiologic activity; they do not require the active participation of the client and are measures of auditory function only. BOA is a behavioral technique that requires a subjective response from the child each time a sound is heard, and the results are a direct measure of hearing sensitivity.

Technically Speaking

During BOA the responses that children typically demonstrate are reflexive ones (eye blinks, startle responses, etc.), not conditioned responses, and they are generally assumed to be representative of gross responses to sound, as opposed to threshold (the softest possible) responses. As mentioned previously, these responses are not likely to be the softest sounds that a child is actually capable of hearing; rather, they might merely be the softest sounds that the child responds to on a given date. As such, it is imperative that the results of BOA testing be viewed in conjunction with all other test results available, including electrophysiologic measures, before arriving at any diagnostic conclusions. Additionally, when behavioral pediatric assessment is warranted, it is not uncommon for multiple test sessions to be required in order for sufficient behavioral audiologic information to be obtained.

Methodology

Hearing testing using BOA is typically accomplished in a sound field with different sounds being presented through calibrated speakers. Some of the auditory stimuli used might include warble pure tones, noise, and unfiltered and/or filtered speech and music stimuli. The child is typically seated in the test (sound-treated) room on the parent's lap; meanwhile, the audiologist presents the sounds through the speakers, and then observes the child's responses to those sounds. Some of the overt responses observed may include rudimentary head turn, eye widening, changes in sucking or breathing, startle, and changes in state of arousal.

Ideally, this type of testing would be performed by two audiologists working in tandem to ensure the accuracy of the results obtained. However, in many cases when a second audiologist is not available, an available speech-language pathologist working in the same department may be called on to assist. The audiologist (or assisting SLP) in the sound room is responsible for keeping the individual engaged and providing an extra set of eyes to help ensure validity and reliability. Simultaneously, the audiologist on the control side, in addition to observing the child's responses, manipulates the frequency, intensity, and variety of auditory stimuli being presented to the client through the calibrated speakers. If one of the examiners judges a behavior to be a response to sound while the other examiner does not, the behavior in question is not considered a response to the sound. Both examiners must be in agreement about each behavior observed as a response.

Visual Reinforcement Audiometry (VRA)/ Conditioned Orientation Reflex (COR)

What You Need to Know

When a child reaches approximately 6 to 7 months of age developmentally, conditioning them to respond to sound becomes increasingly successful. At this developmental stage, which lasts through about 24 months of age, accurate behavioral hearing test results are achievable using a conditioning procedure known as **visual reinforcement audiometry (VRA)**. The basic premise underlying the VRA procedure is not only that a child has a natural instinct to turn searchingly for an interesting sound when it's heard, but also that the child will continue to do this when "rewarded" with an appealing visual stimulus (such as lights, lighted animated toys, videos, etc.).

Technically Speaking

VRA is another procedure that is frequently performed in the sound field using two audiologists, or with the assistance of an available speech-language pathologist. This type of behavioral hearing testing can be easily accomplished by again having the child sit on his or her parent's lap. The visual reinforcers are situated on top of each of the speakers in the sound field. One audiologist (or assistant) is directly facing the child and will keep the child engaged during the test process. At the same time, the other audiologist on the control side of the test suite is operating the audiometer and presenting the test sounds through the speakers. These stimuli can be warbled tones, narrow bands of noise, or live or recorded speech. The child is intentionally situated between the two speakers, typically at a calibrated position (denoted on the ceiling of the sound booth), and at such an angle as to require a noticeable head turn in search of the sound, if and when the child hears the sound. This arrangement is displayed in **Figure 5.2**.

Methodology

The first step in the process is to condition the child to associate the sound (auditory) with the visual (animated toy). This is easily accomplished by sending a sound through the speakers that is assumed to be "clearly loud enough" for the child to hear; the child's attention is then directed toward the sound and the animated toy is activated. When the connection between the two has been clearly established, the audiologist (or assistant) keeps the child otherwise engaged while the audiologist on the control side systematically presents a combination of sounds. Some of the sounds used during this procedure may include warbled pure tones, narrow bands of noise, unfiltered and filtered speech and music, and the like. Both examiners watch for responses, and each time a response is observed the child is rewarded with the toy animation (or video, lights, or other visual stimulation) as reinforcement.

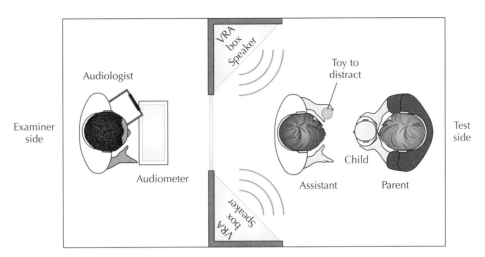

Figure 5.2   Typical audiometric test room arrangement when visual reinforcement techniques are utilized.

An ideal test session is when the child remains interested in this activity long enough to finish getting a complete audiogram. Unfortunately, it's all too common for the child's interest to wane before completing the hearing test, thus necessitating multiple test sessions to obtain results across all frequencies. Additionally, although this test is most often performed with speakers in the sound field, it may also be done with the use of earphones, for the purposes of getting ear-specific information for difficult to test populations.

Conditioned Play Audiometry (CPA)
What You Need to Know

When children reach 2 1/2 years of age through approximately 5 years of age, either developmentally or chronologically, they can typically be engaged in **conditioned play audiometry (CPA)** techniques. The older children in this age range are generally able to participate in almost any game, whereas the younger children in this category need the task to be modified into a simpler form. When a simpler task is utilized, this is sometimes referred to as *modified play techniques.*

Technically Speaking

CPA is designed to gain audiological test results by making the evaluation process into a game. The child is conditioned to play a game; for example, drop a block into a bucket, put a ring on a stick, and so on each time a sound is heard. Almost any game will suffice, so long as it produces responses that

are repeatable and consistent. A challenge that is frequently encountered during CPA is finding games that hold the child's interest throughout the evaluation process.

Methodology

CPA may be performed by one tester; however, two audiologists are useful with some of the younger children in this age range. Again, a speech-language pathologist is frequently called on to assist in this testing procedure, especially if the child being tested is on that specific speech-language pathologist's caseload. Again, familiarity with the younger child being tested is felt to be advantageous in obtaining reliable test results.

The clinician places the earphones on the child. Ideally, CPA is completed using earphones and a bone conduction oscillator, when possible, so that ear-specific information can be obtained. However, this technique may also be used in a sound field for situations where the child is unwilling or unable to accept earphones. Please refer to the previous section of this chapter regarding earphone placement on younger children.

In lieu of lengthy verbal instructions, these authors have had good success conditioning children to perform the desired task by simply demonstrating and engaging the child in the play activity. A good rule of thumb is the fewer words/directions, the better. Many children who are in this situation are being tested to rule out hearing loss as contributory to developmental language issues, so extensive verbal direction can result in the child being confused or simply shutting down to the task at hand.

The clinician selects a game that is developmentally appropriate for the child and begins to engage and condition the child to the activity. The diagnostic threshold search or screening then proceeds as described previously. Results are plotted on the audiogram form, along with notes regarding the method used to obtain them and the clinician's judgment as to the reliability of the information obtained.

Summary

Pure tone air and bone conduction audiometry are the backbone of the audiologist's behavioral testing measures. A clear understanding of the scientific basis of air conduction and bone conduction testing will aid the speech-language pathologist in thoroughly understanding not only threshold and MRL responses, but also how the responses were obtained. It is only with this clear understanding and the appropriate interpretation of air conduction and bone conduction results that a measure of both degree and type of hearing loss can be determined.

Discussion Questions

1. What type of information regarding hearing sensitivity is provided by air conduction testing?
2. What type of information regarding hearing sensitivity is provided by bone conduction testing?
3. What is the difference between an audiologic screening and an audiologic evaluation?
4. When would you expect masking to be performed in pure tone testing? Incorporate the term *interaural attenuation* into your answer.
5. What type of testing technique would be used with a 5-year-old child with normal cognitive functioning to get the most reliable test results possible? Why?

References

American National Standards Institute. (2004). *American National Standards method for manual pure-tone threshold audiometry.* ANSI S3.21-2004. New York: Author.

American Speech-Language-Hearing Association (ASHA). (2005). *Guidelines for manual pure-tone audiometry.* Available from http://www.asha.org/policy.

American Speech-Language-Hearing Association, Joint Committee on Infant Hearing. (2007). *Year 2007 position statement: Principles and guidelines for early hearing detection and intervention.* Available from http://www.asha.org/policy.

Fagelson, M., & Martin, F. N. (1994). Sound pressure in the external auditory canal during bone-conduction testing. *Journal of the American Academy of Audiology,* 5(6): 379–383.

Hicks, C. B., Tharpe, A. M., & Ashmead, D. H. (2000). Behavioral auditory assessment of young infants: Methodological limitations or lack of auditory responsiveness. *American Journal of Audiology,* 9: 124–130.

Killion, M. C., Wilbur, L. A., & Gudmundsen, G. I. (1985). Insert earphones for more interaural attenuation. *Hearing Instruments,* 36(2): 34–36.

Madell, J. R. (2011). Testing babies: You can do it! *Behavioral Observation Audiometry,* 21(2): 59–65.

Munro, K. J., & Agnew, N. (1999). A comparison of interaural attenuation with the etymotic ER-3A insert earphone and the telephonic TDH-39 supra-aural earphone. *British Journal of Audiology,* 33(4): 259–262.

Munro, K. J., & Contractor, A. (2010). Interaural attenuation with insert earphones. *International Journal of Audiology,* 49: 799–801.

Yacullo, W. S. (1999). Clinical masking in speech audiometry: A simplified approach. *American Journal of Audiology,* 8: 106–116.

Chapter 6

Speech Audiometry

Deborah R. Welling, AuD, CCC-A, FAAA
Associate Professor and Director of Clinical Education
Department of Speech-Language Pathology
Seton Hall University

Carol A. Ukstins, MS, CCC-A, FAAA
Educational Audiologist
Office of Special Education
Newark Public Schools

Key Terms

Binaural
Dynamic range (DR)
Masking
Monaural
Most comfortable
    listening level (MCL)
Phonemically
    balanced (PB)

Speech audiometry
Speech detection threshold
    (SDT)/Speech awareness
    threshold (SAT)
Speech reception threshold/
    Speech recognition
    threshold (SRT)
Spondee

Uncomfortable listening level
    (UCL)/Loudness discomfort
    level (LDL)/Threshold of
    discomfort (TD)
Word recognition testing/
    Speech discrimination
    testing/Word discrimi-
    nation testing (WDT)

Objectives

- Understand the variety of speech audiometry procedures and the type of information they can provide
- Understand how the results of speech audiometry relate to the pure tone findings and how they may be used as a check for response reliability
- Describe how speech audiometry may be performed on a variety of different developmental ages and populations
- Understand how to incorporate the results of speech audiometry to maximize effectiveness in the therapeutic setting

Introduction

Speech audiometry, along with pure tone audiometry, is a critical element of a comprehensive evaluation because our daily activity of listening is not composed merely of beeps, but is a complex neurological process called speech perception. At the forefront of this process is the detection and discrimination of a speech signal and comparing it with the levels of peripheral hearing determined through pure tone audiometry. When a hearing loss is identified, speech audiometry attempts to measure the impact the hearing loss has on the person's ability to understand and communicate using the aural/oral processes of speech and language. Speech audiometry should not be confused with the comprehensive evaluation of (central) auditory processing.

A Word About Terminology

Several of the tests in this chapter actually have several names that vary from state to state, facility to facility, or even audiologist to audiologist. This variation has its roots, in part, in regional preference, training facility (college/university), and age of the examiner (what year they graduated from school). Although the variation in terms for speech audiometry has been debated and discussed on many different levels, a single homogeneous term for each is rarely agreed upon by all. Every effort has been made to expose the reader to all terms currently in use, regardless of any underlying dispute, because the practicing speech-language pathologist will probably encounter most, if not all, of the testing terminology.

Derivation of Word Lists

Historically, the first speech tests were spoken or whispered messages presented at measured distances between the talker and the listener. These tests provided a gross estimate of an individual's ability to hear speech (American Speech-Language-Hearing Association [ASHA], 1988). Speech audiometry, as we know it today, is the result of efforts to formalize the measurement of this information.

As with many aspects of the field of audiology, the development of speech audiometry came from the U.S. military both during and after World War II. Not exempt from this part of audiology history, formal speech audiometry came from the development of articulation testing for military communication equipment. A desire to create a clear, intelligible speech signal for radio communication precipitated the development of methodologies by which spoken English could be assessed for both minimal audible thresholds (hearing threshold for speech) and intelligibility (discrimination), when transmitted through military communication technology of the day. This spurred the creation of spondaic word lists to determine hearing thresholds for speech, and phonemically balanced (PB) word lists to assess discrimination loss.

A **spondee** refers to a word that has two syllables with equal emphasis on both; some examples are hotdog, baseball, and toothbrush. **Phonemically balanced** refers to words that have been statistically analyzed for their phoneme content. This content is then compared to a sampling of spoken discourse and is again statistically analyzed for percentage of representation in that speech sample. Lists are then assembled of 25 and 50 words (referred to as half lists and full lists, respectively) that statistically represent each phoneme's occurrence in the English language using either a consonant-vowel-consonant (CVC) format or a consonant consonant-vowel-consonant consonant (CC-V-CC) format, using only monosyllabic words. The evaluation and determination of which words in the English language would be chosen for these lists is extensive, but may hold historical interest for some. Those individuals are directed to Hirsh and colleagues' article titled "Development of Materials for Speech Audiometry" (Hirsh et al., 1952).

Early recordings of these words were on vinyl disks (the type used in record players, not our CDs of today), but these were determined to have too much variability and distortion of the recoded signal. After a brief period of use, recordings were transferred onto a recordable tape format called reel-to-reel. In a continued effort to create a clearer signal, recordings later evolved to cassette format, decreasing the distortion even further. Today, word lists are recorded and reproduced onto compact discs, by all accounts our best technology of reproduction to date.

Speech Recognition Threshold (SRT)/Speech Reception Threshold (SRT)
What You Need to Know

A **speech reception (recognition) threshold (SRT)** provides a measure of a person's threshold for the recognition of speech stimuli, much in the same way as pure tone air and bone conduction testing provide thresholds for the reception of tones. The basic purpose of the SRT is to give an indication of how loud speech has to be for a person to *just barely* begin to hear it. Second, but no less important, the SRT serves as a reliability or cross-check for the accuracy of the pure tone findings.

How It Works

The SRT is defined as the softest level at which a person can recognize 50% of simple speech materials (ASHA, 1988). (See American National Standards Institute [ANSI] S3.6-1969 standard or subsequent superseding standards.) The decibel level of the SRT is not a level that would be sufficient to enable the person to carry on a conversation; rather, the SRT is merely the very softest level at which sound can be detected *and* recognized as a speech signal. The SRT is typically performed by air conduction (using supra-aural or insert earphones), and should be in agreement with the pure tone air conduction results at 500, 1000, and 2000 Hz (this is known as the pure tone average [PTA]). For example, if someone demonstrates a severe hearing loss by pure tone air conduction testing, the SRT results should also be obtained at similarly impaired decibel levels. Thus, the SRT is a good measure of the accuracy of test results.

Technically Speaking

The SRT is the minimum hearing level for speech (see ANSI S3.6-1969 standard or subsequent superseding standards) at which an individual can recognize 50% of the speech material (ASHA, 1988). The SRT is typically obtained using spondaic words (bisyllabic words with equal emphasis on the first and second syllables), but cold running speech or the identification of body parts using a pointing task are modifications that may also be used when necessary. When a procedural variation of this type occurs, there would typically be a notation on the audiogram. In addition, there are a variety of spondaic word lists available that are geared to meet the needs of different developmental ranges, as well as picture pointing tasks for those who, for a variety of reasons, may not be capable of orally repeating words.

The SRT provides a measure of the person's threshold for the recognition of speech much in the same way as pure tone air and bone conduction testing provide thresholds for the reception of simple sound. The SRT should be in agreement with the average PTA at 500, 1000, and 2000 Hz. Although some variability between the SRT and the pure tone responses can be expected (e.g., when a steeply sloping configuration of hearing loss exists), inappropriately large differences between the SRT and the pure tone results is suggestive of pseudohypocusis, otherwise known as false hearing loss.

Methodology

The SRT is tested one ear at a time, beginning with the better ear first. The patient is instructed to repeat the words they hear, even if the words are very faint. The words are

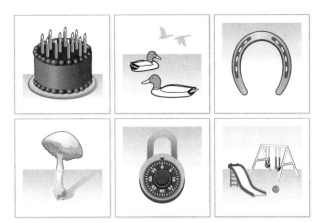

Figure 6.1   Spondee picture board for use with children.

then presented to the patient at a comfortably loud level in order to familiarize the listener with approximately 8 to 10 test word items that will be used for the test. The familiarization process ensures that the listener knows and is able to auditorily identify each of the words. In some cases, for instance, young children or nonverbal patients, familiarization can be done using a simple board of spondee pictures (see **Figure 6.1**). A closed set task of 6 or 10 pictures can be used without changing the validity of the thresholds obtained. Regardless of the response modality (picture pointing or verbal response), once finished with familiarizing, the clinician proceeds to search for the threshold by adjusting the volume of these same words (lowering by 10 dB each time the patient correctly identifies a word, and raising by 5 dB each time the response is incorrect), much in the same way that pure tone air conduction thresholds are tested. The softest decibel level at which the listener is able to correctly identify 50% of these simple words is the SRT for that ear. This procedure is then repeated for the other ear, and the results are reported accordingly.

Speech Detection Threshold (SDT)/Speech Awareness Threshold (SAT)
What You Need To Know

The **speech detection threshold (SDT)** is sometimes also referred to as the **speech awareness threshold (SAT)**. The SDT is very similar to the SRT in that it involves a patient's responses to the presence of speech; however, whereas the SRT requires that the person detect *and* recognize a sound as being a speech signal, the SDT simply requires that the person indicate they are aware of a speech sound without requiring that they know what the sound is (ASHA, 1988). As such, it is a simpler task and very useful in cases where, for whatever reason, a person is unable to repeat back words. Examples of this are when there is a significant language barrier, aphasia, or other cognitive or developmental impairment.

How It Works

The SDT can be performed using any speech sound (for example, the tester might say "ba, ba, ba" into the microphone); it does not require spondaic words as is the case for establishing the SRT. Additionally, because the SDT requires awareness as opposed to the recognition of a signal being a speech signal, the SDT response is generally obtained at a more sensitive (lower/better) decibel level. Again, as is the case with the SRT, the results should be in agreement with the pure tone responses and serve as a check of the accuracy of the audiogram.

Technically Speaking

The SDT, or SAT, is the minimum hearing level for speech at which an individual can just detect the presence of speech stimuli. The listener does not have to identify the material as speech, but must indicate awareness of the presence of sound (ASHA, 1988). The stimulus used for assessment of the SDT is not as important nor is it as prescribed as it is with the SRT; this is because the SDT is a detection only task and, therefore, the content of the speech signal used as a stimulus becomes less critical. Similarly to the SRT, the results of the SDT should be in relative agreement with the pure tone findings.

Methodology

The SDT is tested one ear at a time, beginning with the better ear first using traditional or insert earphones. The SDT is performed using words, connected discourse, or other such materials; the patient is simply required to raise a hand, drop a block, or use any other behavioral indication that the sound has been heard. It does not matter whether the patient knows, can identify, or understands what it is they have heard. This procedure is also performed in much the same way the air conduction thresholds are obtained; that is, the speech stimulus (this might be the spondaic word or it may also be vocalizations; such as, "ba, ba, ba") is presented at a level that is comfortably loud for the listener. The intensity is then lowered by 10 dB each time the patient detects the sound, and raised by 5 dB each time the sound has not been detected. Just as in pure tone air conduction testing, the intensity level of the sound

is continually increased and decreased until the clinician finds the decibel level that the patient responds to one-half of the time, with the minimum number of responses needed to determine the threshold of hearing being two out of three responses at a single level (ANSI, 2004).

Most Comfortable Listening Level (MCL)
What You Need To Know

The **most comfortable listening level (MCL)** is a speech audiometry measure audiologists have come to depend upon when assessing hearing and communication ability. The MCL is exactly as its name suggests—it is the decibel level that has been determined to be the most comfortable volume level at which the patient subjectively prefers to listen to speech.

How It Works

Subjectively, we each have a preferred level of loudness (or intensity) that we individually determine to be a comfortable level—neither too soft nor too loud for our preference. The stimulus of choice used for this test is typically cold running speech. Clinically, this level is often approximately 40 dB louder than the patient's SRT or SDT, although there is some variability from person to person. The MCL level is noted on the audiogram and may be used as the presentation level for a variety of other speech audiometry tests as well as hearing aid fitting and adjustment.

Technically Speaking

The most comfortable listening level (MCL) can be defined as the decibel level that is decided upon, by audiologist and patient together, as being the most comfortable level for the patient to listen to speech. It is neither too loud nor is it too soft, and the stimulus of choice used for this test is typically cold running speech. The purpose of obtaining this measure is not only to determine the level that the patient has the easiest time listening to speech, which typically results in the patient's best possible speech understanding ability, but also to use it for other speech audiometry procedures and other evaluations; particularly those involving the assessment and fitting of hearing aids. Large variations from a 40 dB reference to the SRT/SDT of the patient can be a clinically significant finding.

Methodology

The patient's MCL can be determined for each ear individually (**monaural** condition) or both ears together (**binaural** condition) using either earphones or the sound field via the speakers. Regardless of the condition (monaural or binaural), the process is the same. The audiologist carries on a conversation with the patient, all the while manipulating the intensity level of his or her voice with the audiometer, while getting the patient's input to determine the intensity level that is "most comfortable"; that is, the level that is neither too soft nor too loud. The audiologist might ask the listener to "pretend that you are listening to the television and let me know if you would raise the volume, lower it, or leave it the same." Ideally, the clinician will talk to the patient for several minutes so the patient will have the opportunity to listen to the way conversational speech varies over time, to help in determining an accurate MCL.

Uncomfortable Listening Level (UCL)/Loudness Discomfort Level (LDL)/Threshold of Discomfort (TD)
What You Need To Know

The **uncomfortable loudness level (UCL)**, also referred to as either the **loudness discomfort level (LDL)** or the **threshold of discomfort (TD)**, is the limit of the acceptable amount of sound in decibels, beyond which the patient would find sound to be unacceptably loud or even painful to listen to for any significant period of time. This measure is extremely important, particularly for the assessment and fitting of hearing aids and other such amplification devices.

How It Works

A large percentage of hard of hearing individuals experience the sensation of an abnormal growth in loudness. For example, instead of a slight increase in volume causing a slight increase in perceived loudness (as is the case with a normal hearing person), the hard of hearing person frequently experiences a sudden large increase in the perceived loudness of that sound with only that same slight increase in the volume control. Unfortunately, this usually results in the hard of hearing listener having a lowered tolerance for sound and a poor prognostic indicator for successful hearing aid use.

Technically Speaking

The uncomfortable loudness level (UCL) is the maximum sound intensity level in dB and it represents the upper limit of what the patient finds comfortable to listen to; beyond this level discomfort and/or pain may be experienced. This procedure should be done, carefully determining UCL levels (in dB) using both speech as well as pure tone stimuli (250 Hz through 4000 Hz inclusive).

Measurement of the UCL levels is particularly appropriate and vitally important during the evaluation process of the hard of hearing individual, as an evaluation of recruitment and /or a narrow dynamic range of hearing (see below). Should hearing aids be programmed without regard for the individual's UCLs, the patient may experience discomfort and as a result be unable or unwilling to routinely use their hearing aid(s).

Methodology

The procedure for assessing a patient's UCL is similar to that for assessing the MCL. It can be tested in both monaural and binaural conditions, and under earphones or in the sound field through the speakers. The speech material used is again ongoing conversation between the audiologist and the patient, and the intensity level is likewise adjusted. The patient is asked to listen to the tester's voice and indicate, in some way, when the intensity of the clinician's voice gets to a level at which any higher would become intolerable. This measure is then recorded and is extremely important in hearing aid evaluations, selection, and monitoring.

Dynamic Range (DR)
What You Need To Know

The **dynamic range (DR)** is the mathematical difference between the lowest level at which an individual begins to hear speech (the SRT) and the upper limit of comfort for speech (the UCL). This is sometimes also referred to as the range of comfort loudness (RCL) because it represents the range of loudness (from softest to loudest) that a person can hear without experiencing discomfort or pain.

How It Works

Normal listeners start to hear speech at a very faint (normal) level, and they do not start to experience discomfort or pain until sounds reach a very loud level. This is a very wide range of loudness within which the normal listener can comfortably experience sound. The hard of hearing listener is likely to experience an abnormal growth of loudness (discussed in the previous section), which results in an inability to tolerate loud sounds. In a hard of hearing individual, the sound stimulus must be louder before it can start to be heard; however, the threshold of discomfort may not be significantly louder than that of a normal hearing individual. Hence, the dynamic range of the hard of hearing individual is effectively reduced, and in some cases significantly so.

Technically Speaking

The dynamic range (DR) is a simple calculation of the mathematical difference between the SRT and the UCL. For example, a typical normal hearing person might have an SRT of 10 dB and a UCL of 110 dB, making the DR for this person 110 dB (UCL level) – 10 dB (SRT level), or 100 dB. Alternately, a hard of hearing person might have an SRT of 50 dB and a UCL of 90 dB, making the DR for this person 90 dB – 50 dB, or 40 dB. This narrowing of the DR is an extremely common scenario, and it presents a challenge to the audiologist who is fitting hearing aids. When working with clients pursuing hearing aid use, measures of SRT, MCL, UCL, and overall dynamic range, and the accuracy of these measures, can in many cases be the determining factor of successful hearing aid use.

Word Discrimination Testing (WDT), Speech Discrimination Testing, and Word Recognition Testing
What You Need To Know

Word discrimination testing (WDT), also referred to as **speech discrimination testing** or **word recognition testing**, is not an assessment of sensitivity; rather, it is an assessment of clarity. This procedure provides the audiologist with an estimate of how well a person is able to understand speech once it has been made comfortably loud for them. When the hard of hearing person demonstrates poor understanding of speech, even though the speech is being presented at the person's predetermined MCL, a distortional product of the hearing loss is identified. Typically, a patient with poor discrimination ability will have limited success with hearing aids. Alternately, if the person has very good discrimination ability when the signal has been made loud enough, he or she will likely be very successful with hearing aids.

In children, poor word discrimination scores may have a wide range of repercussions in educational planning, hearing aid use, and cochlear implant candidacy.

How It Works

Have you ever heard a person complain that they had no problems hearing you but just couldn't understand what you

had said? This phenomenon of hearing a speech signal, yet not understanding its content, describes a large portion of the hard of hearing population. It brings us to some basic facts about auditory pathology; that is, hearing loss not only impairs the loudness of sound that reaches the person's ear, but also may include a distortional element. These are two of the most basic characteristics of hearing loss—severity and clarity. Severity refers to how loud sound must be made for a person to just barely be able to hear it; clarity refers to how intelligible the signal is once it is presented at a comfortably loud level (MCL, for example). This explains why someone may "hear" something, but not necessarily be able to discriminate the content of what they have just heard. Word discrimination testing (WDT) attempts to quantify a person's ability to understand speech, once it has been made comfortably loud for the person.

Technically Speaking

Whereas pure tones (air and bone) allow us to establish the nature and quantify the severity of hearing impairment, and SRTs obtain threshold measures of hearing for speech, WDT focuses more on the impact the hearing loss has on communication ability by looking at a patient's ability to understand and discriminate the content of what she or he is hearing (Brandy, 2002). Testing is accomplished using any of several different variations of PB lists available. Word discrimination testing is generally performed at the level of a person's MCL and the results are categorized as excellent, very good, good, fair, poor and very poor. Generally speaking, the better one's WDT scores are, the less the hearing loss will impact their ability to communicate. The results obtained from the WDT are a necessary and integral part of the treatment and aural rehabilitation planning process.

Methodology

WDT is performed approximately 35–40 dB above the level of the SRT, or at the client's most comfortable listening level (MCL). For example, if a patient has an SRT of 20 dB HL, the presentation level of the speech stimuli used for WDT would be approximately 55–60 dB HL.

The most common speech stimuli used for WDT are phonemically balanced word lists, discussed previously. The basic procedure is to present a list of words at a comfortably loud presentation level, and instruct the patient to repeat what has been said. Again, how the instructions are presented to the patient will determine the accuracy of the measured outcome; for example, "Repeat what you have heard" vs. "Repeat what you have heard even if you just think you know the word" will affect patient performance on this task, yielding very different results. Once he or she has provided instructions, the examiner presents each test word item, one at a time, preceding each of the words with the phrase "say the word. . . ." Scoring is reported as a percentage based on 25 (half list) or 50 (full list) words, at the discretion of the examiner. For example, if a list of 25 words is presented and the listener correctly repeats back 22 out of 25 words, a WDT score of 88% would be recorded.

Modifications of this test procedure are often necessary when assessing the very young child, special populations, or anyone who either cannot or will not comply with the request for a verbal response. An example of such modifications is the Word Intelligibility by Picture Identification (WIPI) test developed by Ross and Lerman (1970). This tool allows the clinician to assess a young child's word recognition ability by presenting the child with a series of pictures; the words are presented to the child, one at a time, and the child is asked to "point to the. . . ." The score of these results, as indicated above, is a percentage of the words correctly identified. Similar materials are available that have been developed for use with nonverbal adults.

Masking for Speech

As a point of reference, if **masking** is needed for pure tone audiometry, it will probably need to be done for speech audiometry as well. The process of masking for SRT is similar to that for pure tone air conduction testing. The decibel level of the SRT in the poorer ear needs to be compared to the best (most sensitive) bone conduction threshold in the better ear; if a 40 dB or greater difference exists, the SRT needs to be retested using masking.

Similarly, if the SRT needed masking, the WDT will need masking as well. Generally speaking, the likelihood of needing masking is routinely greater for WDT than for threshold-level tests (pure tone air conduction and SRTs). This is due to the fact that the WDT is accomplished using a loudness level that is suprathreshold (louder than threshold) referencing the SRT (threshold).

Although speech-language pathologists are unlikely to be responsible for knowing how to perform effective masking, it is critically important that they understand the concept, what it represents, and the audiometric implications as well. Without accurately measuring and interpreting hearing test results, proper interventions and management strategies cannot be implemented accurately.

Summary

Although pure tone audiometry provides us with information regarding the degree and nature of the hearing loss, it is important to know that pure tone test results only provide part of the audiometric profile of a patient. Speech audiometry is equally important for the examiner to determine the communication status of the patient and the impact a hearing loss may or in some cases may not have on daily communication. Speech reception thresholds determined for each ear serve multiple purposes in testing—first, to determine a threshold for speech; second, to serve as a reliability check for the pure tone test results; and third, to serve as a reference for word discrimination testing. Word discrimination testing then allows the examiner to determine a person's ability to clearly distinguish one word from another. Performance on word discrimination testing is a prognostic indicator for successful hearing aid use in the patient with hearing loss.

Other tests of speech audiometry play a significant role in determining quality of life factors for a patient with hearing loss. MCL, UCL, and the computation of the dynamic range of hearing are important measures to consider when working with the hard of hearing patient.

Discussion Questions

1. Pure tone audiometry provides us with information regarding the degree and nature of the hearing loss. Why is speech audiometry also important?

2. What options for speech audiometry testing would you use when a child refuses to, or cannot, respond by repeating back a word?

3. Is it possible to apply the principle of masking to speech audiometry? If not, what principles preclude masking for speech? If yes, when would you expect to see masked thresholds for speech audiometry testing?

4. When would MCL and UCL be important information to have on a child? Incorporate the term *dynamic range* into your answer.

5. Mrs. Jones complains that her new hearing aids are "too loud" and she cannot hold a conversation with her grandson because she "does not understand a word he says." What are the two most likely reasons for Mrs. Jones's dissatisfaction with her new hearing aids? What measures of speech audiometry can you reference to check your suspicion? What would you recommend that Mrs. Jones do to remedy her complaints?

References

American National Standards Institute. (2004). *American National Standards method for manual pure-tone threshold audiometry.* ANSI S3.21-2004. New York: Author.

American Speech-Language-Hearing Association (ASHA). (1988). *Determining threshold level for speech.* Available from http://www.asha.org/policy.

Brandy, W. T. (2002). Speech audiometry. In J. Katz (Ed.), *Handbook of clinical audiology* (5th ed., pp. 96–110). Baltimore: Lippincott Williams & Wilkins.

Hirsh, I. J., Davis, H., Silverman, S. R., Reynolds, E. G., Eldert, E., & Benson, R. W. (1952). Development of materials for speech audiometry. *Journal of Speech and Hearing Disorders,* 17: 321–337.

Ross, M., & Lerman, J. (1970). A picture identification test for hearing-impaired children. *Journal of Speech, Language, and Hearing Research,* 13(1): 44.

Chapter 7

Otoscopy and the Middle Ear Test Battery

Deborah R. Welling, AuD, CCC-A, FAAA
Associate Professor and Director of Clinical Education
Department of Speech-Language Pathology
Seton Hall University

Carol A. Ukstins, MS, CCC-A, FAAA
Educational Audiologist
Office of Special Education
Newark Public Schools

Key Terms

Acoustic (stapedial) reflex
Acoustic reflex decay (ARD)
Acoustic reflex threshold
  (ART)
Atresia/microtia
Cerumen
Conductive hearing loss
Ear pit
Ear tag

Eustachian tube (ET)
External auditory canal
External auditory meatus
Keloids
Middle ear
Otitis media
Otoscope
Otoscopy
Outer ear

Pinna
Retrocochlear pathology
Tympanic membrane
Tympanometric compliance
Tympanometric pressure
Ear canal volume
Tympanometry
Universal precautions

Objectives

- Illustrate the principles and components of the middle ear test battery
- Understand the information the middle ear test battery provides and how it relates to audiometric results
- Understand and explain disorders that potentially impact the results of the middle ear test battery

Introduction

"Never stick anything smaller than your elbow in your ear!" is a common phrase that has been used by mothers, fathers, grandmothers, and grandfathers for years. Unfortunately, this warning goes unheeded by many, especially when faced with the annoying feeling that there is something in there. It is therefore the responsibility of the examiner to determine that sound has a clear pathway to channel itself through the peripheral auditory system. In practice, you will never cease to be surprised at what people put in their ears. Beyond the tympanic membrane (eardrum), sound can be further impeded in its journey to the cochlea by a host of middle ear pathologies as well.

The complete evaluation of the auditory system goes beyond measuring acuity. Using both otoscopy and the middle ear test battery, we can focus not only on in-depth evaluation of the auditory system, but also on the overall health of the ear. Otoscopy and tympanometry become an integral part of the evaluation as nonbehavioral measures used in the assessment process.

The figures referenced in this chapter are meant to provide the reader with an overview of the more common pathologies encountered in the daily practices of an audiologist or speech-language pathologist; however, they are in no way a comprehensive representation of all pathologies you may encounter. If something doesn't look right, find an audiologist with whom you can network and consult with regarding unknown or unidentified pathologies. A common clinical mistake is to think that because you are the only or perhaps first one to identify something as abnormal, that you are potentially working outside of your scope of practice. However, good clinical practice includes the willingness to question, question, question, and refer when necessary.

Visual Inspection

Most audiological procedures require highly calibrated technical tools or other equipment to evaluate. The visual inspection of the pinna and temporal area of the head requires only a trained eye, but is an integral part of the audiological evaluation that should not be overlooked. This visual inspection can yield important information used as a springboard to further diagnosis of auditory problems.

What You Need to Know

Many craniofacial abnormalities are strong indicators of hearing impairment. Simply stated, if there is a visible abnormality, there is probably a whole host of abnormalities that you can't see. It is therefore important to look at and touch the **pinna** in order to assess its size, shape, and relative placement as compared to the patient's other facial features. A portion of the **external auditory canal** (external ear canal) can also be seen without the use of any equipment. This portion of the canal should be examined for size, shape, and patency. Other aspects that should be evaluated are the presence or absence of drainage, distinct odor, **cerumen** (also known as ear wax), and foreign objects (American Speech-Language-Hearing Association [ASHA], 2004). This visual inspection of the ear should be performed prior to doing any tests of middle ear function and before any hearing test procedures (air conduction, bone conduction, speech audiometry, tests of otoacoustic emissions) as well. In the event that the visual inspection reveals any drainage, foul odor, and the like, tests of tympanometry should not be performed and immediate medical attention is indicated.

How It Works

Visual inspection is simply that—a visual inspection to identify any physical abnormalities that may exist. This chapter contains figures that will assist you in identifying the most common visual abnormalities of the ear; however, as previously mentioned, these should in no way be considered comprehensive. The speech-language pathologist should always consult with, or refer to, an audiologist or an otolaryngologist if an abnormality is observed or suspected.

Technically Speaking

Visual inspection of the pinna, surrounding temporal area of the ear, and facial feature symmetry is important to identify craniofacial abnormalities which may have a secondary characteristic of hearing loss. Structural integrity of the cranium can be both internal and external. Therefore visual inspection of the head is an integral part of the audiological evaluation as it can yield important information valuable in the diagnosis of the patient. Again, do not assume that if previous records do not indicate any craniofacial syndrome or other disorder that there has not been a missed diagnosis. Should any questions or concerns arise, you should immediately seek the opinion of others who work with the child.

Methodology

It is vitally important to take a comprehensive case history and create a bond with the patient prior to testing, because to visually inspect the pinna and surrounding area the examiner must touch the patient. Prior to making physical contact with a patient, it is important to adhere to policies of **universal precautions**. Hand washing and gloving are recommended as a precaution against transmission of pathogens.

First, the examiner should gently but firmly grasp the topmost portion of the pinna, evaluating for shape, thickness of ear cartilages, and the identification of pinna landmarks. An assessment of pain while touching the pinna should also be made at this time.

The area around the pinna should also be examined for abnormalities. **Figures 7.1** through **7.5** show common, but by no means comprehensive, typical and atypical findings.

Otoscopy

The process of examining the **external auditory meatus** (also known as the external ear canal), especially the eardrum, using an instrument that magnifies and lights the area (**otoscope**) is known as **otoscopy**. The examiner inspects the external ear canal using an otoscope to identify abnormalities as compared with the known norm. Although many speech-language pathologists shy away from otoscopy, it is cited in the scope of practice; with a small amount of training it can be completed easily and yield important results regarding your patient.

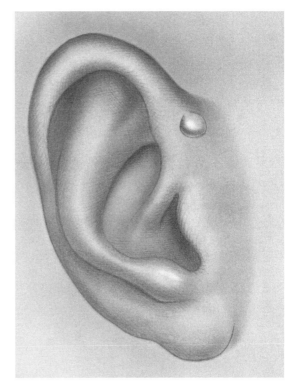

Figure 7.2   Ear tag.

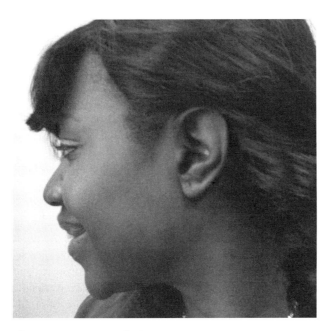

Figure 7.1   Normal pinna.

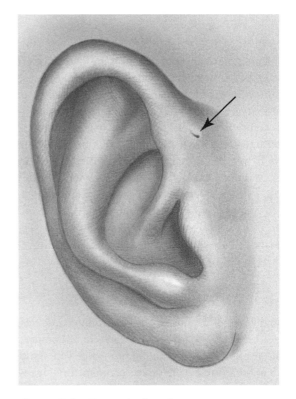

Figure 7.3   Preauricular pit.

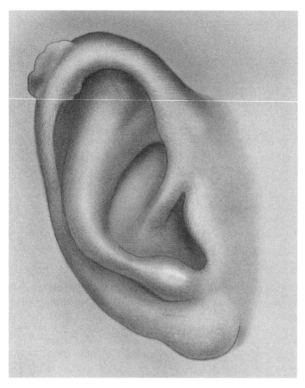

Figure 7.4   Keloid of the pinna.

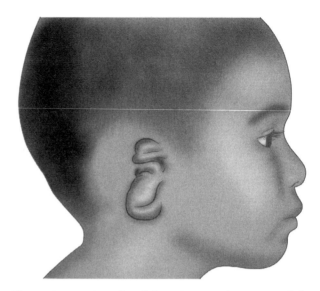

Figure 7.5   Microtia of the pinna with atresia of the external auditory ear canal.

What You Need to Know

Performing otoscopy on a patient is an important procedure in the audiological evaluation. Results of otoscopy will allow the examiner to identify several common problems that preclude sound from entering the ear. Two quite common abnormal findings are ear canal occlusion; by cerumen (ear wax) or foreign object, and the manifestation of middle ear pathology (**otitis media** or ear infection). It is important to point out that although abnormal findings on otoscopy can be identified and a patient can be referred to a physician for follow-up, it is outside the scope of practice for either an audiologist or a speech-language pathologist to diagnose a medical condition based on their findings.

How it Works

With the use of an otoscope, the examiner inspects the external ear canal to identify abnormalities as compared to the known norm. Below are figures which will assist you in identifying some of the most common findings when performing otoscopy. However, as previously mentioned,

otoscopy should in no way be considered comprehensive and the speech-language pathologist should always consult with, or refer to, an audiologist or an otolaryngologist if an abnormality is observed or suspected.

Technically Speaking

The normal pathway of sound gathered from our environment is via air conduction. In order for this sound to be gathered and channeled into the ear for the processing of what has been heard, the physical structures of the ear must be in working order. The identification of abnormalities in the **external auditory canal** (external ear canal) should be the precursor to any other testing completed by the examiner. Common abnormal findings are excessive cerumen (or ear wax), foreign objects, drainage from otitis media, infection of the ear canal wall, and abnormal tympanic membrane (ear drum) landmarks. The identification of such physical problems can result in the identification of a hearing loss as well. When a hearing loss is caused by a problem in the external ear canal, it is known as a hearing loss involving the conduction of sound into the ear or a **conductive hearing loss**. Again, it should be stressed that while the audiologist or speech-language pathologist is within their scope of practice to identify the presence of an abnormality upon otoscopic inspection of the external ear canal, a diagnosis of physical abnormality is outside of their scope of practice.

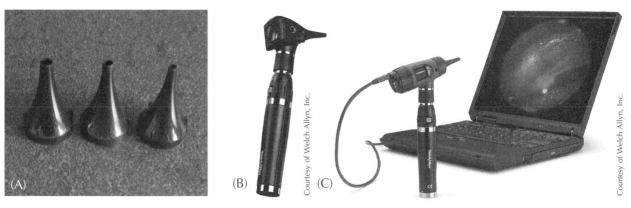

Figure 7.6   (A) Otoscope specula. (B) Otoscope. (C) Digital otoscope.

Methodology

As with visual inspection of the pinna, the examiner should exercise the principles of universal precautions while performing this procedure, because it involves direct physical contact with the patient. Otoscopic inspection of the external ear canal involves using an otoscope with a speculum (see **Figure 7.6**) chosen based on its aperture (or size of opening) as it compares to the relative size of the patient's ear canal on visual inspection by the examiner.

The external ear canal is normally a curvy *S* shape; therefore, in order to obtain a clear view of the entire canal straight down to the **tympanic membrane** (eardrum), the examiner must straighten the canal. This is accomplished by gently pulling up and back on the pinna (the specific direction may vary from person to person) and then inserting the otoscope speculum into the ear. The examiner looks for the normal landmarks of the tympanic membrane (see **Figure 7.7**) as well as physical abnormality (see **Figures 7.8** through **7.12**), such as perforations of the eardrum, drainage, redness, excessive wax, or the presence of pressure equalization tubes for the remediation of otitis media. Any observed abnormality should be formally documented and the patient should be referred to a physician for follow-up. It should be noted that the patient's form of medical insurance will determine whether this referral will be to the patient's primary care physician under a managed healthcare plan or directly to an otolaryngologist (ENT specialist). Regardless of specialty or qualifications, the need for medical follow-up should most definitely be stressed.

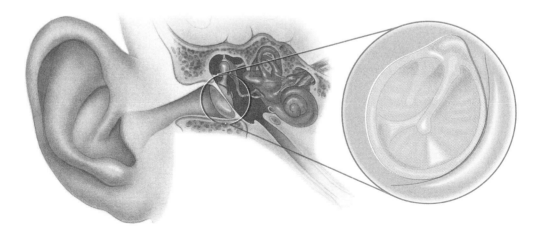

Figure 7.7   Normal tympanic membrane.

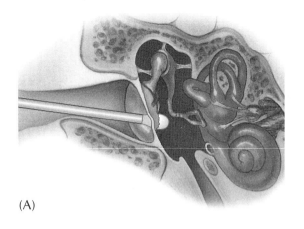

(A)

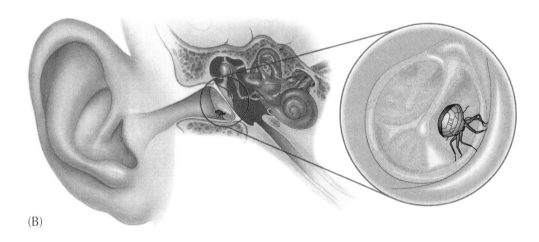

(B)

Figure 7.8 (A) Foreign body in the ear (cotton swab). (B) Bug in the ear.

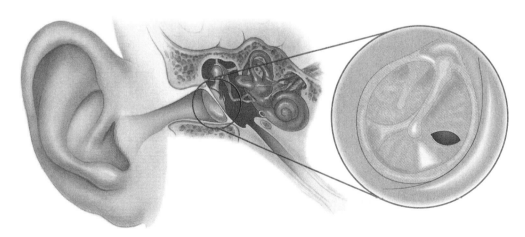

Figure 7.9 Perforated eardrum.

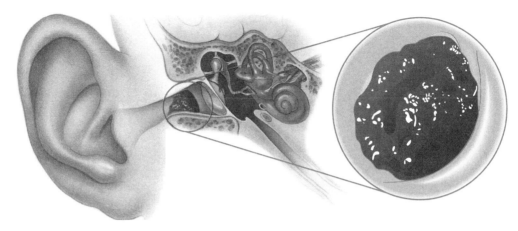

Figure 7.10   Excessive wax in the external ear canal.

Middle Ear Test Battery

Tests of **middle ear** function play another important role in the audiological evaluation. In addition to being objective measures of the auditory system, these tests yield important results regarding the health of the patient's ear and also can serve to support and/or further qualify the audiometric results. Many pathologies of the ear occur in the middle ear

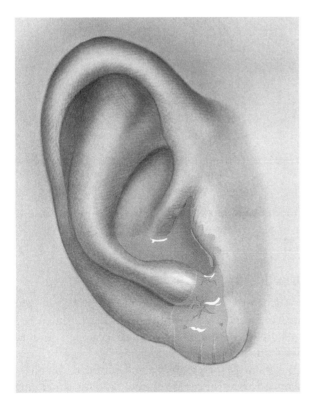

Figure 7.11   Drainage from the external ear canal.

system. Information obtained during tests of middle ear function can assist in the medical diagnosis of these pathologies by a physician. The accurate evaluation of the middle ear plays an important role in the diagnosis of conductive hearing loss as well.

Tympanometry

Visual inspection of both the external anatomy of the ear and structures of the external ear canal including the tympanic membrane are a vital part of the audiological evaluation as a whole. However, just as pure tone audiometry without speech audiometry provides us with only part of a picture, otoscopy and visual inspection of the ear provide us with only part of our assessment of a physical ear structure. In order to examine what we cannot see, tympanometry provides us with information regarding the health and functioning of the middle ear system.

What You Need to Know

Tympanometry is a procedure that allows us to examine the functioning of the middle ear system indirectly, by using measures of pressure and movement of the outer and middle ears as they work together as complementary systems. The results can provide an indication of any type of pathology that may prevent the efficient movement of sound from the **outer ear** (external ear canal) to the inner ear (cochlea). Tympanometry is also a useful procedure because it does not require a person to actively participate. Pure tone audiometry and speech audiometry procedures are considered behavioral audiological measures, whereas tympanometry is an objective measure and can

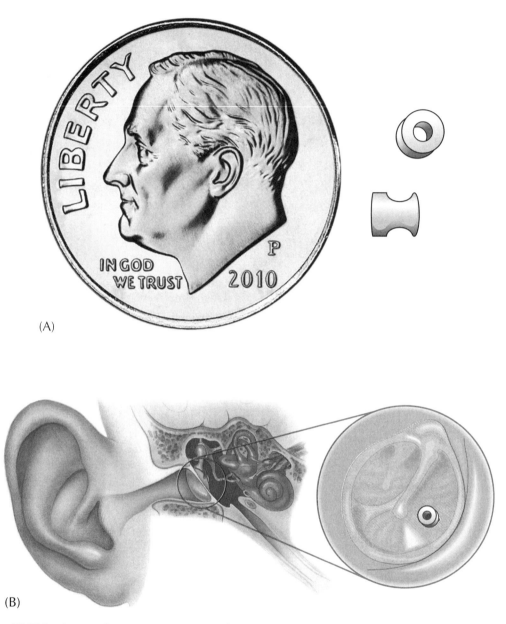

(A)

(B)

Figure 7.12 (A) This picture shows a pressure equalization (PE) tube next to a dime in order to illustrate the size. (B) An illustration of a pressure equalization (PE) tube in place in the eardrum.

be performed even if a patient cannot or refuses to participate in the process. It should be noted, however, that tympanometry does not tell us about hearing sensitivity per se, but only about potential physical abnormalities of the outer and/or middle ear that may be contributory in the diagnosis of a hearing loss. As with outer ear pathologies, when a hearing loss is caused by an abnormal condition in the middle ear, it's referred to as a conductive hearing loss.

How It Works

Tympanometry is based on three physical principles—pressure, compliance, and volume. Using a tympanometer, a probe tip is inserted into the external ear canal and data are collected from each ear individually. The actual readings obtained (corresponding pressure and compliance values as well as **ear canal volume**) are plotted on a graph known as the tympanogram, and are then classified based on established normative data. The resulting tympanogram(s) are printed out and are then interpreted by the examiner.

The tympanometer does not give us a measure of hearing; rather, it measures the mobility (compliance) of the ear drum as pressure is systematically varied in the external ear canal. Specifically, the measurements obtained indicate how the eardrum moves back and forth as pressure is first pushed in, and then pulled out of the ear.

Technically Speaking

Tympanometry works on the principles of pressure, compliance and volume. Mathematical data points are then collected and analyzed for their content. The speech-language pathologist does not need to master these mathematical principles as they relate to taking tympanometric readings; however, a brief description of each is important as background information of how these three principles articulate to generate tympanograms.

Pressure

Tympanometric pressure values are indicative of the amount of pressure in the middle ear cavity. These values are plotted on the horizontal (*x*) axis of the tympanogram. Pressure measurements are made in either decaPascals (daPa) or millimeters of water (mmH$_2$O) (these units are essentially equivalent), with 0 daPa representing normal atmospheric pressure.

The normal middle ear cavity maintains a pressure that approximates normal atmospheric pressure; this is accomplished through the opening and closing of the Eustachian tube. Abnormal tympanogram pressure may be suggestive of Eustachian tube dysfunction.

Compliance

Tympanometric compliance values are indicative of the amount of mobility (movement or compliance) of the tympanic membrane; these values are plotted on the vertical (*y*) axis of the tympanogram. Compliance can be measured in cubic centimeters (cc/cm³) or milliliters (ml) (these units are identical).

Tympanogram compliance that is significantly lower than normal may be suggestive of tympanosclerosis (scarring of the tympanic membrane) or otosclerosis (fixation of the stapes bone in the oval window). Compliance that is much higher than normal may suggest a disarticulation of the

bones of the ossicular chain or a hypermobile tympanic membrane. Either scenario requires a medical referral.

Ear Canal Volume (ECV)

The ear canal volume (ECV), also known as equivalent ear canal volume (EECV) or physical volume test (PVT), is a middle ear test battery measure that represents the estimated volume of the external ear canal from the probe tip at the opening of the ear canal to the tympanic membrane.

The range of normal varies depending on client age and gender. Excessively large ear canal volumes may be indicative of either a perforation of the tympanic membrane or an improperly functioning pressure equalization (PE) tube, thus representing a measure of the entire outer and middle ear volumes, instead of just the canal. Alternately, an abnormally small volume measure may be indicative of excessive wax buildup in the ear canal.

Figure 7.13 shows a standard tympanogram form. The middle ear pressure is plotted on the *x*-axis and the compliance (eardrum mobility) is plotted along the *y*-axis. Note that the ECV value is typically provided clearly on the tympanogram form.

Methodology

To prepare the patient for tympanometry as well as the other subtests in the middle ear test battery, the examiner must ensure that the patient is not talking, chewing, moving

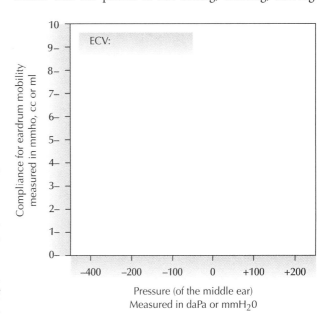

Figure 7.13 Standard tympanogram form used for the recording of results.

excessively, or doing anything else that will negatively impact the results. Again, as with visual inspection and otoscopy, the examiner should exercise the principles of universal precautions prior to making physical contact with the patient.

Based on a visual approximation of ear canal size and shape, a soft probe tip is selected from an assortment of sizes of tips and placed on the test probe of the tympanometer. Similarly to otoscopy, the pinna is pulled up and back, and the test probe, which is covered with the soft tip selected, is carefully positioned at the outside opening of the external ear canal (see **Figure 7.14**). Air pressure is then systematically varied in the ear canal while the pressure response of the tympanic membrane is monitored. The patient needs only to sit still; that is, no subjective behavioral response is required of the person. The process of obtaining the tympanogram readings of pressure, compliance, and ear canal volume takes a mere 3–5 seconds to complete; however, the reliability of these results is dependent on the motionlessness of the patient while the procedure is being performed. It may therefore become necessary, especially when testing young children or patients who are tactilely sensitive to objects or people in or about their ear, to otherwise distract the patient during testing.

Most tympanometers have a digital readout for the examiner to review the results and make a determination of their reliability (readability). The actual readings obtained (corresponding pressure and compliance values as well as ear canal volume) are plotted on the tympanogram, and are then classified based on established normative data. The resulting tympanogram(s) are printed out and interpreted by the examiner.

Acoustic Reflexes

Acoustic (stapedial) reflexes are involuntary contractions of the middle ear muscles—the stapedius muscle and the tensor tympani—that occur in response to high intensity sound. Testing for the presence of acoustic reflexes is another part of the middle ear test battery. The normally

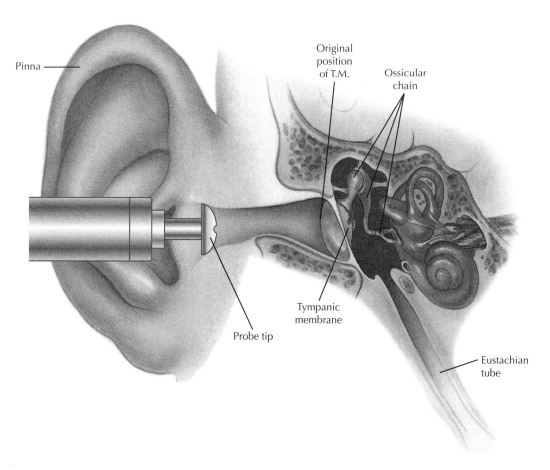

Figure 7.14   Side view of the placement of a probe tip into the ear.

functioning auditory system is expected to have reflexes present at specified levels. Similarly, there are normative acoustic reflex data for the variety of different types of hearing loss and conditions as well. As is the case with other components of the middle ear test battery, acoustic reflex testing should be viewed only in the context of the results of the complete evaluation. The results of acoustic reflex testing can potentially provide information to support, confirm, or rule out the hearing loss demonstrated by pure tones (Emanuel, Henson, & Knapp, 2012).

What You Need to Know

Acoustic reflex threshold (ART) testing would not be performed by a speech-language pathologist (SLP) because it is outside of their scope of practice. However, it is important for the SLP to understand what it is and what it represents in order to better understand and interpret the results they will find in a report from an audiologist.

How It Works

In a normally functioning auditory system, the muscles of the middle ear will contract in response to high intensity sound. This involuntary contraction occurs when "too much sound" is presented to the ear (when sound becomes too intense). However, *how much sound* is too much sound depends on the patient's hearing acuity. A normal hearing ear will react to a loud sound long before an impaired ear perceives the sound as being loud. Regardless, this muscle contraction can be measured and recorded.

The results of acoustic reflex testing have a number of potential uses. For example, if a patient is trying to fake a hearing loss, acoustic reflex testing may provide the objective data necessary to disprove such a claim. If a patient cannot or refuses to participate in behavioral testing, the presence or absence of a hearing loss might be gleaned, at least in part, from the results of acoustic reflex testing.

Technically Speaking

Acoustic reflex testing involves measuring the threshold at which the muscles of the middle ear contract. This is not a threshold of hearing sensitivity as is the case when we test pure tone air conduction thresholds. Rather, acoustic reflex threshold testing provides the threshold of when a sound becomes too intense for the person; as a result, it may serve as an indirect measure of hearing. That is to say, measurement of an acoustic reflex threshold can be a predictor of the presence or absence of a hearing loss, but the examiner should not base a diagnosis of normal hearing or hearing loss on the results of acoustic reflex thresholds alone, but on the cumulative results of the entire evaluation.

For the normal auditory system, an acoustic reflex threshold typically occurs at a level that is much louder than the level at which the person just starts to hear. Anticipated results vary, depending on the nature and severity of hearing loss, as well as the presence of recruitment or decruitment. The results of acoustic reflex testing can (potentially) provide information to support, confirm or rule out the hearing loss demonstrated by pure tones (Emanuel, Henson, & Knapp, 2012).

Methodology

The measurement of acoustic reflexes can be done while the probe tip is still in the person's ear canal from performing tympanometry. Either by manual manipulation or using an automatic sequence that most tympanometers are capable of performing, sound is presented to the ear while the examiner looks for a contraction response. Again, as with the tympanogram, the contraction response required is automatic and does not require the active participation of the patient to respond in any way. The tester then searches for the acoustic reflex threshold, which represents the decibel level that is too intense (loud) for the listener; it is typically performed at 500 Hz, 1000 Hz, 2000 Hz, and 4000 Hz.

Acoustic Reflex Decay Testing

Acoustic reflexes have a second property that can be evaluated and clinically useful. As we have just discussed, the ear produces contractions of the middle ear muscles in response to loud sounds at predictable intensity levels. This contraction should be maintained as the loud sound is continuously presented. When the acoustic reflex is unable to appropriately sustain itself, **acoustic reflex decay (ARD)** has occurred. The identification of a decaying acoustic reflex is suggestive of an abnormality of the auditory system and should be followed up with further diagnostic testing.

What You Need To Know

Acoustic reflex decay testing would not be performed by a speech-language pathologist (SLP) because it is outside of their scope of practice; however, as with acoustic reflex threshold testing, it is important for the SLP to understand what it is and what it represents in order to better understand and interpret the results they will find in a report from an audiologist.

How It Works

Acoustic reflex decay testing measures how long and how well the acoustic reflex is capable of sustaining itself. In the normal auditory system, the acoustic reflex should be able to maintain its contraction for a period of time before it drops off. Alternately, the auditory system whose reflex falls off too quickly is thought to be abnormal, and is in need of additional diagnostic testing.

Technically Speaking

Acoustic reflex decay is a test that measures the decrease in magnitude over time of the contraction of the acoustic reflex, when the patient is subjected to continuous high-intensity sound stimulation. Specifically, the reflex amplitude is expected to maintain half of the original measurement for a minimum of 10 seconds of continuous tone presentation. An auditory system in which the acoustic reflex decays to half or less of the original amplitude is demonstrating ARD, and is typically deemed in need of further diagnostic testing.

Historically, the presence of acoustic reflex decay has been associated with **retrocochlear pathology**, a pathological condition that occurs beyond (retro) the level of the cochlea. An example of a retrocochlear abnormality is an acoustic neuroma (tumor on the eighth cranial nerve) or a vestibular schwannoma (vestibular tumor). It should be noted, however, that in a recent study that surveyed middle ear practices for the diagnosis of retrocochlear pathology, Emanuel and her colleagues (2012) found that acoustic reflex decay testing has been on a downward trend over the past 25 years, presumably related to the availability of more sensitive measures such as magnetic resonance imaging (MRIs).

Methodology

Once acoustic reflex thresholds have been established, the examiner can check for acoustic reflex decay, if desired. With the probe tip still in the patient's ear from tympanometry, the examiner now measures reflex decay by raising the intensity of sound by 10 dB above the level of the acoustic reflex threshold and leaving the sound on continuously for 10 seconds. If the reflex is functioning normally it will sustain itself (within certain limits) for the 10-second period of time; if not, it will decay or decrease over time. This test can be performed either manually or as part of an automatic test sequence, and is typically performed at 500 Hz and 1000 Hz, assuming, of course, that an acoustic reflex threshold has been obtained at those frequencies in the first place.

Eustachian Tube Function

Eustachian tube function testing is another subtest of the middle ear test battery. The **Eustachian tube (ET)** is part of the middle ear anatomy that connects the middle ear space and the back of the throat. Normal opening and closing of the Eustachian tube equalizes the pressure of the middle ear space with the environment (normal atmospheric pressure). The persistence of otitis media is primarily due to a dysfunctional Eustachian tube (Sheer, Swarts, & Ghadiali, 2012); thus, the ET function assessment is a useful component of the middle ear test battery. A common example of Eustachian tube dysfunction is that plugged feeling one experiences when ascending or descending in an airplane.

What You Need To Know

Like the acoustic reflex threshold testing and acoustic reflex decay testing, the Eustachian tube function test is not a procedure that a speech-language pathologist would be expected to perform, because it is outside of their scope of practice. However, as with the other tests within the middle ear test battery, it is important for the SLP to understand what it is and what it represents in order to better understand and interpret the results from an audiological evaluation.

How It Works

A properly functioning Eustachian tube serves to equalize pressure between the middle ear space and normal atmospheric pressure. As previously discussed, tympanometry is based on three principles—pressure, compliance, and volume. By using a diagnostic tympanometer, pressure (in daPa) can be manually manipulated by the examiner. During this manipulation, if the middle ear system is able to equalize the pressure manually imposed in the external ear canal, the Eustachian tube is found to be functioning appropriately. If the pressure cannot be equalized, the Eustachian tube is not functioning as it should be.

Technically Speaking

The secondary function of the Eustachian tube is to clear away and protect the middle ear space from harmful secretions from the nasopharynx. Otitis media is one of the most common infectious diseases of childhood, and the most significant causative factor is dysfunction of the Eustachian tube (Elmorsy et al., 2010), so the Eustachian tube function test provides useful information, particularly when assessing the pediatric population.

Methodology

If the results of tympanometry are abnormal, and there is a suspicion of Eustachian tube dysfunction, Eustachian tube function testing can be accomplished while the probe used for tympanometry is still in the ear canal. The examiner manually introduces pressure into the patient's ear. During this manual manipulation of pressure, the patient is asked to swallow and yawn. If the pressure is equalized in the middle ear during this process, the Eustachian tube is functioning appropriately. In contrast, if pressure cannot be equalized, the Eustachian tube is determined to be functioning abnormally. Results are recorded appropriately.

Summary

The conductive hearing mechanism, which consists anatomically of the outer and middle ears, begins with the pinna, which collects auditory information from an individual's environment, connects to the external auditory canal, which in turn connects to the tympanic membrane and then the middle ear cavity. Visual inspection of the outer ear, otoscopic inspection of the external auditory canal, and the middle ear test battery all play a vital role in determining the overall health of a patient's ear. Throughout these portions of the ear, any pathology that results in hearing loss is considered conductive.

Middle ear anomalies (such as the common ear infection with fluid, ruptured eardrum, and the like) are of common and significant concern, particularly in the pediatric population. These conditions not only negatively affect health, but also can have an adverse impact on hearing ability. Irregular findings can be determined by completing a battery of tests of middle ear function, which may include tympanometry, acoustic reflex thresholds, acoustic reflex decay testing, and Eustachian tube function. Tests of middle ear function are considered nonbehavioral or objective measures of the audiological evaluation. As with visual inspection and otoscopy, the middle ear test battery yields important results pertaining to the health of the ear itself, but portions can also provide information that, when used in conjunction with pure tone results, can support and/or further qualify the audiometric findings.

Although the speech-language pathologist may never perform some tests of middle ear function clinically, comprehensive understanding of these test procedures will aid the professional in wholly understanding the pathologies that can affect auditory sensitivity and result in hearing loss.

Discussion Questions

1. Pure tone audiometry and speech audiometry are direct measures of hearing sensitivity. Why would we also need information regarding the outer and middle ear systems?
2. What three physical principles make up tympanometry?
3. A pediatric patient comes in for his weekly speech and language therapy session. He is complaining that he has not been able to hear out of his left ear since he was playing with beads with his younger brother on Saturday. What problem might you suspect? How can you evaluate your suspicion?
4. The Eustachian tube is part of which system of the ear? What function does it perform? Why is this important?

References

American Speech-Language-Hearing Association (ASHA). (2004). *Guidelines for the audiologic assessment of children from birth to 5 years of age.* Available from http://www.asha.org/policy.

Elmorsy, S., Shabana, Y. K., Raouf, A. A., Naggar, M. E., Bedir, T., Taher, S., et al. (2010). The role of IL-8 in different types of otitis media and bacteriological correlation. *Journal of International Advanced Otology,* 6(2): 269–273.

Emanuel, D. C., Henson, O. E. C., & Knapp, R. R. (2012). Survey of audiological immittance practices. *American Journal of Audiology,* 21: 60–75.

Sheer, F. J., Swarts, J. D., & Ghadiali, S. N. (2012). Three-dimensional finite element analysis of Eustachian tube function under normal and pathological conditions. *Medical Engineering and Physics,* 34: 605–616.

Chapter 8

Beyond the Basics

Deborah R. Welling, AuD, CCC-A, FAAA
Associate Professor and Director of Clinical Education
Department of Speech-Language Pathology
Seton Hall University

Carol A. Ukstins, MS, CCC-A, FAAA
Educational Audiologist
Office of Special Education
Newark Public Schools

Key Terms

Auditory brainstem
  response (ABR) study
Auditory steady state
  response (ASSR) study
Distortion product
  otoacoustic emissions
  (DPOAEs)

Electroacoustic measures
Electronystagmography
  (ENG)
Electrophysiologic measures
Evoked otoacoustic
  emissions
Otoacoustic emissions

Spontaneous otoacoustic
  emissions
Transient evoked
  otoacoustic emissions
  (TEOAEs)
Videonystagmography
  (VNG)

Objectives

- Compare and contrast the differences between behavioral and nonbehavioral testing techniques
- Understand which portion of the auditory system the otoacoustic emissions, auditory brainstem response, auditory steady state response, and electronystagmography/videonystagmography are assessing
- Explain the differences between the auditory brainstem response and auditory steady state response tests

- Discuss the type and significance of information that can be obtained from these measures
- Explain how the information from nonbehavioral tests can augment the results of behavioral audiometric tests results

Introduction

Behavioral hearing test procedures provide information regarding the individual's actual functional auditory abilities; clearly these procedures are necessary. Unfortunately, there are individuals who, for any of a number of reasons, are incapable of complying with the demands of this type of testing. What's more, these procedures are simply not designed to provide us with additional data regarding the structural/functional integrity of various parts of the auditory system.

The development of the physiologic procedures (electroacoustic and electrophysiologic) that will be discussed in this chapter has allowed for objective assessment of the auditory system. These procedures aid in the diagnoses, treatments, and outcomes of a variety of auditory-related conditions. Some examples of the utility of these procedures include universal newborn hearing screening (UNHS) programs, diagnosis of peripheral hearing loss versus an auditory neuropathy syndrome disorder (ANSD), auditory processing disorders, balance disorders, and many others.

Although these "beyond the basics" procedures are diagnostically outside of the speech-language pathologist's (SLP's) scope of practice, the SLP needs to have a solid understanding of the basic underlying concepts and significance that the results of these tests add to the overall diagnostic picture and the therapeutic interventions planning process. However, before you breathe a sigh of relief, tests of otoacoustic emissions are becoming increasingly popular as a screening method of choice with the young and/or difficult to test populations, and this *is* within the scope of practice for the speech-language pathologist.

Electroacoustic Measures

The term *electroacoustic* refers to the interaction or conversion of electric and acoustic energy. As it applies to the field of audiology, **electroacoustic measures** are, quite plainly, acoustic measurements that provide us objective information about how portions of the peripheral auditory system functions. This information, in turn, helps us in establishing and/or confirming the characteristics of some forms of auditory dysfunction. The very earliest electroacoustic

measurements to be used diagnostically in the field of audiology are tympanometry and acoustic reflexes (Hall & Swanepoel, 2010); however, in the following section we will address the electroacoustic measures known as otoacoustic emissions.

Otoacoustic Emissions
What You Need To Know

The normal healthy cochlea is not only able to hear sound, but also can produce sound. The sounds that the cochlea produces are known as otoacoustic emissions (OAEs). There are two types of otoacoustic emissions—spontaneous and evoked.

With an **evoked OAE**, a sound is sent into the ear, and in response the ear produces a sound and sends it back. By contrast, **spontaneous OAEs**, as the name suggests, are spontaneously present without any sound stimulation. However, because spontaneous emissions are present in only approximately 70% of the normal hearing population (Hall, 2000), no clinical significance can be attached to them. The evoked types of emissions, on the other hand, can be recorded in nearly 100% of normal hearing ears (Chan, 2001; Kemp, 1978; Probst, 1990), and therefore have immense clinical significance and utility.

As with a limited number of tests in the basic audiological evaluation, tests of evoked otoacoustic emissions are objectively measured, requiring no active participation on the part of the patient. Normal evoked otoacoustic emissions are typically present in only the healthy cochlea with essentially normal to near normal hearing. There are other forms of otoacoustic emissions in addition to what will be presented here for discussion. However, given the focus of this textbook, we will limit the following discussion to two types of evoked otoacoustic emissions (OAEs), i.e., transient evoked otoacoustic emissions (TEOAEs) and distortion product otoacoustic emissions (DPOAEs).

Otoacoustic emission screenings are used as a nonbehavioral method of screening hearing in populations when a traditional pure tone screening (the kind using response patterns such as hand raising or play audiometry technique) would not yield reliable results. As such, the speech-language pathologist must know the principles of otoacoustic emission screening, as it falls within scope of practice.

How It Works

The cochlea is a complex organ of hearing that houses both outer hair cells and inner hair cells. There have been many theories over the past century and a half to explain the workings of the cochlea and how we hear (Babbs, 2011). Although the controversy and research continue, it was documented as early as the 1940s that the ear can be more than a passive listener (Gold & Pumphrey, 1948). In fact, as later researchers have discovered (Davis, 1983; Kemp, 1978), the ear is capable of producing low intensity sound called otoacoustic emissions. Current research supports the theory that these emissions are produced, most likely, by the cochlear outer hair cells as they expand and contract (see Hall, 2000). Advances in technology during the 1970s saw the creation of microphone equipment capable of measuring these responses. Thus the clinical application of measuring otoacoustic emissions as an indirect assessment of hearing ability began.

Technically Speaking

To evoke an otoacoustic emission, a sound is sent into the ear, and in response the ear produces a sound and sends it back; this response can be recorded. By contrast, the spontaneous OAEs, as the name suggests, are spontaneously present without external stimulation. However, an important caveat must be noted at this juncture. Technically speaking, otoacoustic emissions are a physical sign that the auditory system is functioning normally or near normal, up through the level of the cochlea. Because we are measuring a physical property of the ear, otoacoustic emissions are not a direct measure of hearing sensitivity, and thus do not replace behavioral hearing testing methods. The literature provides abundant data demonstrating that evoked OAEs are not present in the damaged cochlea; therefore, the presence of an evoked OAE speaks to the health of the cochlea and auditory system up to this point. However, although perhaps occurring infrequently, damage may occur to the auditory system at points beyond the level of the cochlea and still cause hearing loss. It is possible, therefore, for a patient with retrocochlear pathology to produce evoked otoacoustic emissions and still have a hearing problem.

There are other forms of otoacoustic emissions in addition to those that will be presented here for discussion. However, given the focus of this text, we will limit our discussion to two types of evoked OAEs—**transient evoked otoacoustic emissions (TEOAEs)** and **distortion product otoacoustic emissions (DPOAEs)**.

Transient Evoked Otoacoustic Emissions (TEOAEs)

In the case of TEOAEs, the sound used to elicit or evoke a response is a transient stimulus of brief duration, such as a click or a tone burst. Generally speaking, normal TEOAE responses are associated with hearing threshold levels better than or equal to the level of a mild hearing loss of approximately 30 dB HL (Beringer & Westling, 2011).

Distortion Product Otoacoustic Emissions (DPOAEs)

The second type of otoacoustic emission that has clinical utility is DPOAEs, which are obtained when the ear is simultaneously presented with two separate pure tone frequencies. A DPOAE response may be obtained with slightly more hearing loss (e.g., research suggests that DPOAEs are not diminished in ears with a mild to moderate hearing loss of up to approximately 50 to 60 dB HL [Dille et al., 2010]).

Methodology

Preparation for the otoacoustic emissions test is similar to the preparation for tympanometry; however, in addition to making sure that the patient is still, the tester must be sure to limit other sounds in the room, due to the potential negative impact ambient noise will have on obtaining reliable results. First, the clinician inspects the pinna and external ear canal to ensure that the canal is patent and unobstructed; any blockage such as wax, foreign body, etc. will interfere with the recording of OAEs. Then, the examiner pulls up and back on the patient's pinna while gently placing the probe tip into the outer opening to the external auditory ear canal. The probe tip in reference is the same type of soft tip that is used for tympanometry, acoustic reflex testing, and the like (refer to Figures 8.1 and 8.2). Ideally, tympanometry will be performed either before or after the OAE procedure.

Regardless of which type of otoacoustic emission testing is being used, the probe introduces a sound stimulus into the ear canal, and the resulting cochlear emissions, if present, are picked up and recorded automatically by the equipment. No behavioral response of any type is required of the patient.

Test time for performing an OAE is very short—approximately 10 seconds for each ear for the screening procedure, and

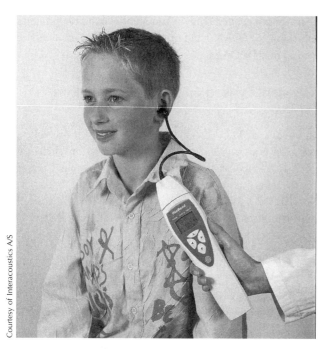

Figure 8.1 The Interacoustics OtoRead portable otoacoustic emissions (OAE) equipment.

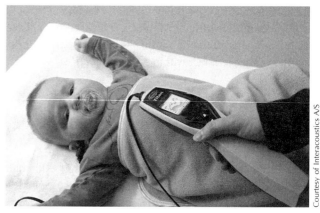

Figure 8.2 The Interacoustics Titan distortion product otoacoustic emission (DPOAE) equipment.

perhaps up to 1 minute for each ear for the diagnostic test. For this reason, performing hearing screenings using otoacoustic emissions—particularly when using the transient stimulus—is a quick and effective way of ruling out significantly handicapping hearing loss, especially in the very young and special needs populations. Otoacoustic emission testing is also the current choice for newborn hearing screenings in many hospitals.

Again, it must be stressed that otoacoustic emission testing is not a direct measure of hearing sensitivity, and thus does not replace behavioral hearing testing methods. Upon completion of otoacoustic emission testing, follow-up behavioral hearing evaluation should always be recommended.

Electrophysiologic Measures

The previous procedures have been measures of the auditory system up through and including the cochlea. **Electrophysiologic measures** evaluate the functional integrity of various structures along the auditory pathways beyond the cochlea, at the level of the eighth cranial nerve and brain stem. These test procedures are outside of the speech language pathologist's scope of practice. This section should be appropriately categorized as informational, but should not be disregarded, because the interpretation of electrophysiological measures will be necessary for a

comprehensive understanding of audiometric test results by the speech-language pathologist.

In this section we will limit our discussion to auditory brainstem response audiometry (ABR), auditory steady state response (ASSR), and electronystagmography/videonystagmography (ENG/VNG). All three procedures are objective assessments of various parts of the auditory and/or vestibular (balance) system.

Auditory Brainstem Response (ABR) Study

The **auditory brainstem response (ABR) study** is an indirect evaluation of hearing sensitivity that measures physiologic activity at the level of the eighth cranial nerve in response to an auditory stimulus. The ABR can be completed regardless of age, cognitive level of function, or state of consciousness. In some cases, pharmacological sedation is used to make sure that myogenic activity or other behaviors (crying, fidgeting, etc.) do not contaminate the test results (Sauter, Beck, & Speidel, 2012).

What You Need To Know

The auditory brainstem response measures the neurological response to an auditory stimulus at the level of the brainstem. As sound travels up the eighth cranial nerve, auditory nerve fibers bundle at certain points along the way. Each time the nerve fibers bundle, a waveform can be recorded as a response to the sound. This measured activity along the auditory nerve (eighth cranial nerve) in response to sound is a useful addition to other testing methods and procedures. In a normally functioning ear, assuming no other neural complications exist, the softest intensity at which the auditory nerve responds roughly corresponds to the softest level at which the person starts to hear. Hence, an estimation of hearing sensitivity can be made.

How It Works

As with any other test of neurological functioning, a neural response is elicited from stimulation specific to the anatomical function. As you may have experienced, physicians frequently use a reflex hammer, also called a percussion hammer, against an elbow or a knee to check deep tendon reflexes. We cannot stop our knees from flying into the air once hit. Similarly, we cannot stop our ears from responding neurologically once stimulated with sound. Although our ears do not fly up in the air as do our knees, we can measure their neural activity using electrodes placed at specific sites on the head. The waveforms or tracings elicited using a broadband click or tonal stimulus are then compared to the norm, and results are interpreted accordingly. See **Figure 8.3** for an example of an ABR tracing.

Technically Speaking

The purposeful stimulation of the eighth cranial nerve responsible for audition yields nonbehavioral (objective) results, which, although not a direct measure of hearing sensitivity, is a valuable clinical procedure. The auditory brainstem response study can also be a useful augmentation to behavioral hearing test results in the pursuit of etiological information. In terms of hearing loss, the ABR is most sensitive in distinguishing hearing levels in the normal through moderately or moderately severe range than in the profound range (Vander Werff, Brown, Gienapp, & Clay, 2002). As stated previously, it is outside of the scope of practice for the speech-language pathologist to perform ABR studies. Therefore, the technical basis behind such testing need not be extensive either.

Methodology

As discussed previously, it may be necessary to first consider the use of sedation in some patients prior to an auditory brainstem response study. The ABR test procedure then begins by having the patient sit or lie down comfortably. After careful cleansing of the skin, surface (noninvasive) electrodes are placed at various locations around the ears and head for monitoring and recording the neurological responses.

Testing is completed on each ear individually, using either clicks or tonal stimuli. Sound is then delivered to the test ear by either an insert earphone or a standard earphone, and the electrodes monitor and record the patient's response. The ABR procedure can be done as either a screening or a diagnostic assessment. A diagnostic ABR is

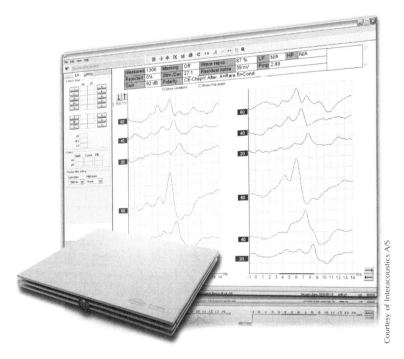

Courtesy of Interacoustics A/S

Figure 8.3   An illustration of the Interacoustics Eclipse auditory brainstem response (ABR) equipment.

typically a more elaborate procedure than an ABR screening and allows the audiologist to manipulate the variety of different test parameters, such as stimulus used, intensity presented, and so on. When performed as a screening, an automated ABR is completed more quickly and produces either a pass or fail/refer response.

Auditory Steady State Response (ASSR)

The **auditory steady state response (ASSR)** is very similar to the ABR just described. Like the ABR, it is an indirect assessment of hearing sensitivity measuring the neurological response to an auditory stimulus. ASSR differs from the ABR in that it can provide frequency-specific information and can help to differentiate between a severe and profound hearing loss.

What You Need to Know

The populations that benefit most from ASSR studies include the young and/or difficult to test. As such, sedation is again a consideration for those who are unable to be calm, quiet, and still for a period of time. Like the ABR, the ASSR is particularly useful as a supplement to other behaviorally obtained hearing test results in the pursuit of an accurate diagnosis. Specifically, the ASSR is useful when a severe or profound hearing loss is suspected—a distinction that is clearly meaningful and significant with regard to aural (re)habilitation and the selection of hearing aids versus cochlear implants (Beck, Speidel, & Gordon-Craig, 2009).

How It Works

As in the case of the ABR, the ASSR can measure the neural activity of the eighth cranial nerve using electrodes placed at specific sites on the head. ASSR differs from the ABR, however, because it uses a variety of stimuli that are more frequency specific as opposed to the "click" stimulus utilized by the ABR. The resulting waveforms or tracings are then compared to the norm and results are interpreted accordingly.

Technically Speaking

The ASSR study is an objective measure that evaluates the health of the structures along the auditory nerve and the brainstem and demonstrates how the brain "follows" certain characteristics of sound (Hall & Swanepoel, 2010); and, although not being a direct measure of hearing

sensitivity, estimations of hearing can be made based on the results. The ASSR differs from the ABR in several ways; for example, determining an ABR response becomes increasingly difficult as the stimuli approach a person's threshold—which is when the decision (response or no response) is most important. ASSR, on the other hand, uses an objective, sophisticated, statistics-based mathematical detection algorithm to detect and define hearing thresholds (Beck, Speidel, & Petrak, 2007). Additionally, the ASSR is more sensitive in distinguishing hearing levels in the profound range of hearing loss than in the normal through moderate or moderately severe range (Vander Werff et al., 2002), and thus it may be the more appropriate choice when assessing an individual suspected of having a significant hearing loss.

Methodology

Many children who fail the automated ABR screening are referred for an ASSR test. The procedures involved in the measurement of the ASSR are very much the same as those described for the ABR procedure. Specific protocols vary; however, the general test setup again includes the placement of surface electrodes at various locations around the ears and head, following careful cleansing of the skin. Testing is accomplished one ear at a time. The earphones deliver the sound stimulus to the ear(s), and the electrodes objectively monitor and record the electrical activity. The actual test parameters may include various frequencies and intensities of tonal stimuli for the purposes of obtaining an accurate, frequency-specific estimate of hearing sensitivity.

Electronystagmography/ Videonystagmography (ENG/VNG)

The semicircular canals are anatomically a portion of the inner ear. As such, the evaluation of the proper function of the inner ear balance system falls within the scope of practice for the clinical audiologist. Again, however, it is outside the scope of practice for the speech-language pathologist. Therefore, this section provides only a brief overview of electrophysiological evaluation of the vestibular system.

The electrophysiological assessment of vestibular function (whether using **electronystagmography [ENG]** or **videonystagmography [VNG]**) records a symptom known as nystagmus, which is an involuntary rhythmic oscillating movement of the eyes, either horizontally, vertically, or torsional (rotary). The eyes work in connection with the organs of the vestibular system within the inner ear and proprioception to establish our sense of balance and position in space. The measurement of nystagmus is important because it can be a symptom of pathology of the peripheral and/or central auditory mechanism. Both ENG and VNG consist of a series of procedures that allow us to measure the nystagmus, which in turns gives an indication of the health of the vestibular system. The difference between the ENG and the VNG is, quite simply, the means by which the eye movements are recorded. The ENG records the eye movements with the placement of surface (noninvasive) electrodes near and around the eyes, whereas the VNG uses video goggles (see Figure 8.4) that incorporate a camera to record and measure the person's eye movements. Results are then compared to the norm and interpreted for significant abnormalities, which may result in higher order testing like magnetic resonance imaging (MRI).

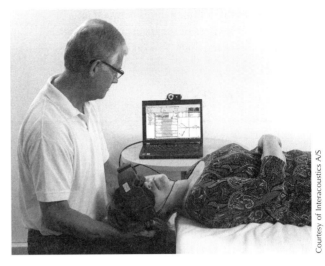

Figure 8.4 Videonystagmography (VNG) testing being performed on a patient, using Interacoustics VNG equipment.

Courtesy of Interacoustics A/S

Summary

Beyond the basic principles of behavioral audiometry and tympanometry are several tests based on the physical principles of the auditory system. Although not considered true tests of hearing, the conclusions that can be drawn from their accurate interpretation provide us insight into a patient's auditory abilities that may not be readily obtainable by conventional behavioral measures.

Distortion product otoacoustic emissions (DPOAEs) and transient evoked otoacoustic emissions (TEOAEs) provide information regarding the physical health of the ear that allows conclusions to be drawn about auditory sensitivity. Likewise, auditory brainstem response (ABR) studies and auditory steady state response (ASSR) studies yield electrophysiologic results from the eighth cranial nerve regarding the auditory pathways. Results of these tests also provide an indirect assessment of hearing, valuable for the course of (re)habilitation in those patients otherwise unavailable for other behavioral measures of auditory sensitivity. However,

with each of these tests, behavioral testing must be completed in order to substantiate the objective results.

Electronystagmography/videonystagmography (ENG/VNG) evaluate the balance system located within the semicircular canals of the inner ear. Measuring the eyes' involuntary response to changes imposed on the semicircular canals can provide valuable information regarding the cochlea's role in the balance system.

In practice, the speech-language pathologist will find that the screening measures of otoacoustic emissions will be useful under many circumstances. We hope to have made some sense of the alphabet soup of these nonbehavioral tests. ENGs, VNGs, ABRs, ASSRs, DPOAEs, and TEOAEs performed as diagnostic measures are outside the scope of practice for the speech-language pathologist, but should now be familiar terms, allowing for a more thorough understanding of results provided to you by the clinical audiologist.

Discussion Questions

1. Why must we interpret otoacoustic emission testing with caution?

2. What external factors may result in inaccurate or invalid results of otoacoustic emission testing?

3. What are the commonalities between tests of otoacoustic emissions and electrophysiological measures of hearing? How do they differ?

4. Which of the procedures discussed in this chapter are within the scope of practice for the speech-language pathologist?

References

Babbs, C. F. (2011). Quantitative reappraisal of the Helmholtz-Guyton resonance theory of frequency tuning in the cochlea. *Journal of Biophysics,* 11: 1–16.

Beck, D. L., Speidel, D. P., & Gordon-Craig, J. (2009, August). Developments in auditory steady-state responses (ASSR). *Hearing Review,* 16(8): 20–27.

Beck, D. L., Speidel, D. P., & Petrak, M. (2007, September). Auditory steady-state response: A beginner's guide. *Hearing Review,* 14(12): 34–37.

Beringer, E., & Westling, B. (2011). Outcome of a universal newborn hearing screening programme based on multiple transient evoked otoacoustic emissions and clinical brainstem response audiometry. *Acta Otolaryngologica,* 131(7): 728–739.

Chan, J. C. (2001). Spontaneous and transient evoked otoacoustic emission: A racial comparison. *Journal of Audiological Medicine,* 10(1): 20–32.

Davis, H. (1983). An active process in cochlear mechanics. *Hearing Research,* 9: 79–90.

Dille, M. F., McMillan, G. P., Reavis, K. M., Jacobs, P., Fausti, S. A., & Konrad-Martin, D. (2010). Ototoxicity risk assessment combining distortion product otoacoustic emissions with a cisplatin dose model. *Journal of the Acoustical Society of America,* 128(3): 1163–1174.

Gold, T. and Pumphrey, R. J. (1948). Hearing. 1. The cochlea as a frequency analyzer. *Proceedings of the Royal Society of London. Series B. Biological Sciences,* 135(881): 462–491.

Hall, J. W., III. (2000). *Handbook of otoacoustic emissions.* San Diego: Singular.

Hall, J. W., & Swanepoel, D. (2010). *Objective assessment of hearing.* San Diego: Plural.

Kemp, D. T. (1978). Stimulated acoustic emissions from within the human auditory system. *Journal of the Acoustical Society of America,* 64: 1386–1391.

Probst, R. (1990). Otoacoustic emissions: An overview. In Pfaltz, C. R. (ed.), *Advances in otorhinolaryngology* (Vol. 44, pp. 1–91). Basel: Karger.

Sauter, B. T., Beck, D. L., & Speidel, P. D. (2012). ABR and ASSR: Challenges and solutions, 2012. *Hearing Review,* 19(6): 20–25.

Vander Werff, K. R., Brown, C. J., Gienapp, B. A., & Clay, K. M. S. (2002). Comparison of the auditory steady state response and the auditory brainstem response thresholds in children. *Journal of the American Academy of Audiology,* 13: 227–235.

Chapter 9

Interpretation of Audiometric Results

Deborah R. Welling, AuD, CCC-A, FAAA
Associate Professor and Director of Clinical Education
Department of Speech-Language Pathology
Seton Hall University

Carol A. Ukstins, MS, CCC-A, FAAA
Educational Audiologist
Office of Special Education
Newark Public Schools

Key Terms

Asymmetrical hearing loss
Audiogram
Audiometric zero
Aural atresia
Conductive hearing loss
Familiar sounds audiogram

High frequency sensorineural hearing loss (HF SNHL)
Interaural attenuation
Mixed hearing loss
Ossicular discontinuity
Otitis externa

Otitis media
Otosclerosis
Pseudohypacusis
Sensorineural hearing loss
Speech banana audiogram
Tympanogram

Objectives

- Interpret the various components of the audiometric test battery, and understand how each plays a role in the diagnosis of hearing loss
- Critically assess an audiogram for consistency and validity
- Understand how the various degrees and types of hearing impairment impact communication development and skills
- Understand how the results of audiometric tests will impact the planning of speech-language therapeutic intervention
- Illustrate various ways of explaining audiometric test results to patients and their families

Introduction

The previous chapters introduced some of the basics of audiological equipment, terminology, procedure definitions, and methodologies. With this understanding, it will now be possible to look at the results that you will have in front of you, what they mean, and how to, in some cases critically, interpret the results for the purpose of therapeutic interventions. We emphasize again that the reader use Chapters 3 through 9 together as a cohesive unit.

A secure understanding of terminology, equipment used, patient expectations, and procedures employed will greatly enhance the reader's understanding of audiological test results and their implications. Our journey of interpretation will begin with how to read the audiogram.

Reading the Audiogram

A typical **audiogram** form is shown in **Figure 9.1**. An audiogram is a graphic depiction of a person's hearing sensitivity; when pure tone thresholds are obtained, they are charted on this grid. You will notice that frequency in Hertz (Hz) is represented along the *x*-axis, and intensity in the decibels hearing level (dB HL) is represented along the *y*-axis. Directing our attention first to the *x*-axis, labeled *Frequency in Hertz (Hz)*, the solid lines are marked with frequencies in full octaves ranging from 125 Hz through 8000 Hz; the broken lines in between mark the interoctave frequencies (750 Hz, 1500 Hz, 3000 Hz, and 6000 Hz). When a patient's threshold at two adjacent frequencies varies by 20 dB or greater, standard practice requires the audiologist

to test the frequency in between (the interoctave frequency) as well. Looking now to the intensity on the *y*-axis, labeled *Hearing level in decibels (dB HL)*, we see that it is broken down into 10-dB segments and spans the range from –10 dB HL through 120 dB HL. The solid black line corresponding to 0 dB HL across the entire frequency range is also known as **audiometric zero**, which represents the lowest level at which normal hearing people begin to detect sound. You may recall that 0 dB on the HL scale corresponds to a different amount of dB on the sound pressure level scale (dB SPL), and does not mean "no sound," which explains how we can have negative decibels. Negative dB on the HL scale simply means that the listener can hear sound at more sensitive levels than the average normal hearing person.

It is important to note that because we are working on a scale of –10 to +120 dB to describe the hearing sensitivity of a person, hearing loss should never be described in percentages. That being said, you will frequently hear hearing losses interpreted as a percentage. Mathematically, this is typically an incorrect interpretation unless the person is basing the percentage on a 130% scale rather than a 100% scale. The prudent professional should discourage this type of interpretation or report of hearing loss by either related health professionals or by the patient and encourage correct interpretation of mild-to-profound degrees.

Audiogram Symbols

The symbols used for recording the results are shown in **Table 9.1**. Although the exact symbols used might vary from clinic to clinic, the symbols presented in Table 9.1 are the ones most commonly used and are those recommended by the American Speech-Language-Hearing Association (ASHA) in 1990 and 1999. When unmasked pure tone air conduction (using standard or insert earphones) is done, the results for the right ear are represented with an O and for the left ear with an X. When masking is applied, based on the guidelines previously discussed, the symbols used are Δ for the right ear and □ for the left ear. The coding of right ear responses in red ink and left ear responses in blue, although sometimes still seen, is no longer as popular as it once was, because photocopying and electronic transmission (computer-generated audiograms and scanning of documents) often means this color coding is lost. When air conduction testing is done in the sound field through the speakers, the response is marked with an S on the audiogram.

The symbols used to record bone conduction vary depending on whether the bone conduction oscillator is placed on

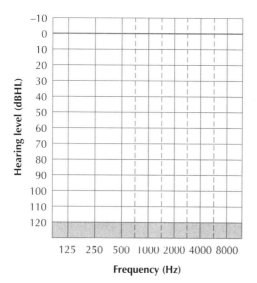

Figure 9.1 An example of the typical audiogram form used for recording audiometric results.

Table 9.1   Audiometric Response Symbols Key Recommended for Use by ASHA (1990 and 1999)

	Right Ear	Unspecified	Left Ear
AC unmasked	O		X
AC masked	Δ		□
BC unmasked (mastoid)	<		>
BC masked (masked)	[		]
BC unmasked (forehead)		V	
BC masked (forehead)	⌐		⌐
Sound field		S	

Data from American Speech-Language-Hearing Association. (1990). Guidelines for audiometric symbols. *ASHA*, 32(Suppl. 2), 25–30.; American Speech-Language-Hearing Association. (1999). Joint audiology committee clinical practice statements and algorithms [Guidelines]. Available from www.asha.org/policy

the forehead or the mastoid process behind the ear. When unmasked forehead placement is employed, the symbol used is a V. With unmasked bone conduction using mastoid placement, the < symbol is used on the left side of the line to represent the right ear, and the > symbol is used on the right side of the line to represent the left ear. (Refer back to Table 9.1.) This may seem a bit confusing, at least at first glance; but if you think of looking at someone face to face, that person's right ear is on your left and their left ear is on your right. If you look at the audiogram as though you are looking directly at the person's head, picture the symbols as the right and left ears, respectively; the symbols then make more pictorial sense.

When masking is applied for bone conduction testing, the [symbol is used on the left side of the line to represent the right ear, and the] symbol is used on the right side of the line to represent the left ear. (Refer again to Table 9.1). When masked bone conduction testing using forehead placement is performed, the ⌐ symbol is used on the left side of the line for the right ear and ⌐ is used on the right side of the line for

the left ear. Again, picture these symbols as ears as you are looking at a person, and little confusion will remain.

The process of bone conduction testing and recording, and thus reading the results, is often more complicated than for air conduction. Recall that when the bone conduction oscillator is used, the skull is stimulated fairly uniformly, and whichever cochlea is better is the one that will respond, regardless of the side of the head (mastoid process) the oscillator is actually placed on. Furthermore, if there is no simultaneous use of masking noise to separate out and distinguish the hearing ability of one cochlea from that of the other, the audiologist may not be sure which cochlea is responding. Therefore, if an audiogram is marked with an unmasked bone conduction response and the ears are different according to the air conduction responses, we will not know which cochlea the bone conduction response belongs to until the masking procedure is completed and noted as well.

Referring to Table 9.1, as well as to Table 9.2, you will notice that ASHA's guidelines for audiometric symbols do

Table 9.2   Audiometric No-Response Symbols Key Recommended for Use by ASHA (1990 and 1999)

	Right Ear	Unspecified	Left Ear
AC unmasked	ₒO		X↘
AC masked	Δ		⌐↘
BC unmasked (mastoid)	⩽		⩾
BC masked (masked)	⌐↙		⌐↘
BC unmasked (forehead)		V↓	
BC masked (forehead)	⌐↙		⌐↘
Sound field		S↓	

Data from American Speech-Language-Hearing Association. (1990). Guidelines for audiometric symbols. *ASHA*, 32(Suppl. 2), 25–30.; American Speech-Language-Hearing Association. (1999). Joint audiology committee clinical practice statements and algorithms [Guidelines]. Available from www.asha.org/policy

AUDIOMETRIC RESULTS

AIR CONDUCTION

			RIGHT EAR									LEFT EAR						
	250	500	1000	1500	2000	3000	4000	6000	8000	250	500	1000	1500	2000	3000	4000	6000	8000
Unmasked																		
Masked																		
Noise level																		

BONE CONDUCTION

			RIGHT EAR						FOREHEAD						LEFT EAR			
	250	500	1000	2000	3000	4000	250	500	1000	2000	3000	4000	250	500	1000	2000	3000	4000
Unmasked																		
Masked																		
Noise level																		

Figure 9.2   Audiometric results recorded numerically in bar graph format as opposed to being plotted on an audiogram (as seen in Figure 9.1)

not include any recommendations for recording the responses while a patient is wearing a hearing aid, cochlear implant, or other assistive device. Although each facility is free to use any symbol they choose, they should include a key to assist those who will be reading and interpreting their aided audiogram. The symbols used to denote such responses might include A to indicate the response with a hearing aid, AR for aided in the right ear, AL for aided in the left ear, and CI to indicate a response with a cochlear implant. Similarly, measures of speech audiometry may also be performed; specifically, speech recognition threshold/speech reception threshold (SRT), word discrimination test scores (WDT), and thresholds of discomfort (TDs) for both tones and speech. Examples of aided audiograms will be provided and discussed in the section on "Other Audiometric Data" that appears later in this chapter.

When there is no response to a particular sound stimulus in a particular condition, regardless of whether it is masked or unmasked air conduction, bone conduction, sound field, or aided conditions, the corresponding symbol is marked on the audiogram with a downward arrow attached to it, to indicate that the patient did not hear the sound at the maximum limit of the equipment. Refer to Table 9.2 for some of the ASHA-recommended no response symbols.

Another method of recording audiometric results is by using what is referred to as a "bar graph," which records the numbers, as opposed to an audiogram, which charts them. **Figure 9.2** provides an example of this type of format. Although the use of a standard audiogram seems to be

more popular, the method may vary from center to center and is a matter of preference.

Audiogram Interpretation
Degree of Hearing Loss

Hearing is not an all or nothing affair; people do not simply hear everything or hear nothing. An individual can have perfectly normal hearing, profoundly impaired hearing, or any degree of hearing loss between the two. **Figure 9.3** presents an audiogram depicting various degrees of hearing loss suggested by Clark (1981), as reported and endorsed by ASHA. In the following sections we will continue the journey of interpretation with descriptions of the categories appearing on the audiogram as depicted in Figure 9.3 and the corresponding Table 9.3. It is important to point out that it is always the air conduction thresholds (sometimes collectively referred to as the *air line*) that we look at to determine the degree (severity) of hearing loss, not the bone conduction results (or *bone line*).

An important caveat to remember when reading this section is that someone's hearing loss rarely falls neatly into only one category; that is, it is very common to see hearing loss that might be mild in degree at 250 Hz and then slopes to a profound degree by the time it gets to 8000 Hz. Hence, you may often come across an audiogram and/or evaluation report that describes a "mild sloping to severe" hearing loss. In such cases, the handicap experienced might be more severe as opposed to mild, depending on the specific pattern demonstrated. For example, if the more severely

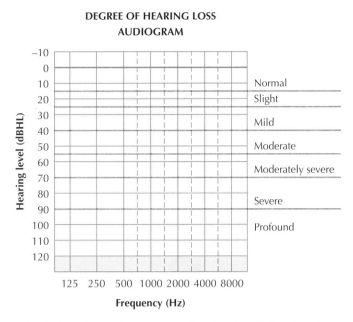

DEGREE OF HEARING LOSS
AUDIOGRAM

Figure 9.3   An audiogram depicting the various categories for classifying the degree of hearing loss.

Table 9.3   Categories of Degree of Hearing Loss

Decibels in Hearing Level (dB HL)	Degree Category
–10 to 15	Normal
16 to 25	Slight
26 to 40	Mild
41 to 55	Moderate
56 to 70	Moderately severe
71 to 90	Severe
91 and above	Profound

impaired responses are in the higher frequencies, the impact will definitely be more severe than mild, because the consonants carry the bulk of the meaning.

Normal Hearing

Normal hearing sensitivity, at one time considered to be –10 dB HL through 25 dB HL, is generally accepted to be in the range of –10 dB HL through 15 dB HL (refer to Figure 9.3), particularly where children are concerned. One of many reasons for this shift may be related to more current research about incidental learning. Incidental learning takes place naturally and spontaneously as a result

of a child being aware of and interacting in his or her environment, without the use of any formal direction or structure. Research clearly indicates that this is one of the ways children learn. In fact, although word learning in infancy may begin as a slow laborious task, during the second year of life the nature of word learning changes. Most typically developing 18- to 24-month-olds learn new words incidentally, without direct adult instruction and with only limited exposures to the words' labels and referents (Brackenbury, Ryan, & Messenheimer, 2005). Hearing sensitivity that exceeds the limits of 15 dB HL may not be sensitive enough for optimal incidental learning. In addition to concerns about children, there is also evidence in the literature that adults continue to learn by informal incidental means (Jubas, 2011), and sensitive thresholds of no poorer than 15 dB HL are important for this population as well.

Other circumstances necessitate, or at the very least would benefit from, hearing being within the limits of –10 dB HL to 15 dB HL. Some of these conditions include, for example, excessively noisy settings, poor (reverberant) acoustical environments, and when a speaker's face is not visible. Although these authors acknowledge that there are some populations for whom an upper normal limit of 25 dB HL is sufficient, such as a geriatric individual with limited mobility or restricted to a nursing home facility.

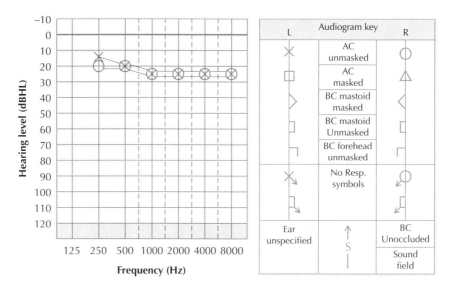

Figure 9.4   An audiogram illustrating a "slight" degree of hearing loss (between 16 dB HL and 25 dB HL). The type of hearing loss is unknown without the addition of bone conduction results.

Minimal/Slight Hearing Loss

Air conduction thresholds that fall within the range 16 dB HL through 25 dB HL are within the range of a minimal/slight hearing loss. Refer to Figure 9.4 for an example of a minimal/slight audiogram. Hearing threshold levels consistently within this range, particularly where children are concerned, can have an adverse effect on communication development and performance, the degree of which can potentially be significantly greater than the terms *minimal* or *slight* would seem to suggest. The literature supports that the presence of a minimal/slight hearing loss in a child can negatively impact speech and language understanding, academic achievement, and social interactions. Although not every child suffers consequences as a result of these minimal decrements in hearing sensitivity, for a significant portion of this population, a loss of any degree appears sufficient to interrupt the normal continuum of communication development and academic skills (Yoshinaga-Itano, 2008).

One example of the potential effects of minimal hearing loss is not hearing the endings of words, which in turn can cause difficulty with the concepts of possession or plurality (missing the /s/ ending), or past tense (missing the /ed/ ending). Acoustically, these individuals may not be able to hear whispered, soft levels or distant speech; they also may have difficulty understanding the message when a speaker's face is not visible or when in the presence of background noise or reverberant conditions. Someone who experiences any of these conditions in a classroom setting is at risk for academic difficulties and possible failure as a result.

In addition to the speech, language, and academic effects, this degree of hearing decrement may hamper social and emotional growth for several reasons. A person with this hearing loss may be viewed as confused, immature, or even aloof as a result of missing out on hearing soft-level conversation, or generally being unaware of subtle conversational cues. These children may act out, or they may become fatigued more easily than other children, due to the extra effort they must expend during the day to listen, hear, and learn. The fact that there is a hearing loss is often not apparent. As a result, these children are sometimes erroneously believed to have behavioral problems, and they often do not receive the appropriate intervention that they so desperately need.

Hopefully it will be apparent to the reader that all individuals, regardless of age, must be seen for an audiologic screening and/or evaluation in a timely manner, to either rule out or accurately diagnose a hearing loss. Additionally, making educators and other professionals aware of the need for proper diagnoses and management strategies is crucial for the achievement of effective educational outcomes for these children (Goldberg & Richburg, 2004) as well as for adults. The determination of intervention needs and recommendations is best provided on a case by case basis.

Mild Hearing Loss

A mild hearing loss (refer to Figure 9.5) is one in which air conduction thresholds fall within the 26 dB HL to 40 dB HL range. You can simulate and experience the effects of a mild hearing impairment by blocking off your ear canals, either

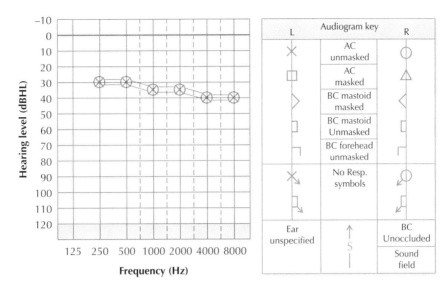

Figure 9.5   An audiogram illustrating a "mild" degree of hearing loss (between 26 dB HL and 40 dB HL). The type of hearing loss is unknown without the addition of bone conduction results.

with your fingers or with ear plugs. Some of the physical and emotional reactions you may experience include surprise at the level of difficulty a "mild" loss creates, and frustration when the speaker's face cannot be seen. Either of these experiences could understandably cause you to stop paying attention. Clearly, the term *mild* does not accurately imply the resulting consequences and level of difficulty perceived. Hence, like the minimal hearing loss category, the degree terminology can be very misleading to those who are uneducated about hearing loss and the concomitant effects.

Research on the effects of mild hearing loss indicate that although not all children with mild bilateral hearing loss (and unilateral hearing loss) have significantly delayed development compared with their peers with normal hearing, approximately one-third evidence significant difficulties in their language, academic, and social-emotional development (Yoshinaga-Itano, 2008). The potential impact this degree of hearing loss can have on understanding speech and language includes missing anywhere from 25% to 40% of the speech signal with a hearing loss of 30 dB HL and as much as 50% of discussion with a hearing loss of 40 dB HL (Anderson & Matkin, 2007). For a youngster, this can translate to missing half of class instruction and dialogue. Further hampering the understanding of speech-language communication is the presence of background noise, reverberation, and distance from the speaker. Academically, it is not uncommon for delays to arise in early foundational reading skills such as the ability to associate a sound with its corresponding letter (phoneme–grapheme correspondence). For the adult population, this degree of

hearing loss and the attendant loss of speech-language understanding (word discrimination ability) will have a variety of negative consequences, whether the individual is in the higher education arena or in a work setting.

The social and emotional impact that mild hearing loss can have on children includes the tendency for the child to be seen as off in his or her own world, hearing only when it is something she or he wants to hear, daydreaming, and the like, especially because the existence of a mild hearing loss is not always apparent. As a result, feelings of low self-esteem may begin to set in, and there may be a tendency for the child to isolate. The adult population suffers the social effects of mild hearing loss as well, sometimes demonstrating depression and social isolation in addition to the functional disability experienced. Regardless of age, whether adult or child, it is common for those who suffer from mild hearing loss to experience physical symptoms such as fatigue, headaches, or other behaviors as a result of the increased amount of energy expended in an effort to hear.

Moderate Hearing Loss

A moderate hearing loss is one in which the air conduction thresholds fall within 41 dB HL through 55 dB HL on the audiogram (refer to Figure 9.6). Regardless of age and life circumstances, this degree of hearing loss can have a significant negative impact on all aspects of communication and development. The literature suggests that the amount of speech signal that an individual can miss out on can range from 50% with a hearing loss of 40 dB HL to as much as 80% or more with a hearing loss of 50 dB HL (Anderson & Matkin, 2007).

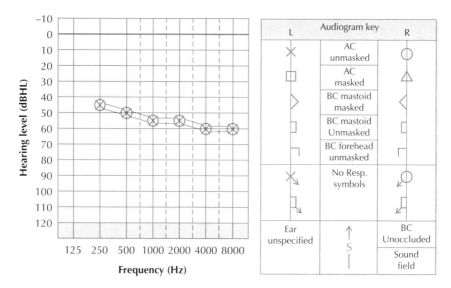

Figure 9.6 An audiogram illustrating a "moderate" degree of hearing loss (between 41 dB HL and 55 dB HL). The type of hearing loss is unknown without the addition of bone conduction results.

Full auditory access is a critical factor if a child is to have the best possible chance for normal speech and language development. A moderate hearing loss is a barrier to the necessary opportunities. Without appropriate identification and intervention strategies in place, there is a likelihood that the child will sustain delayed or disordered syntax, limited vocabulary, imperfect speech production, and flat voice quality (Anderson & Matkin, 2007). Without the appropriate opportunities to learn language, these children will fall behind their hearing peers in communication, cognition, reading, and social-emotional development (Joint Committee on Infant Hearing, 2007). Recall that the presence of background noise, reverberant conditions, distance from the speaker, and the speaker's face not being visible can all have further negative effects on communication. Without the use of hearing aids or some other assistive device or technology, a youngster with a moderate hearing loss will encounter tremendous difficulty, even if their particular classroom happens to be a relatively quiet space. Even with appropriate amplification, a child is at a considerable disadvantage in most listening environments, especially the average noisy classroom. It is well documented that hearing aids alone in a classroom setting do not allow the hard of hearing student to overcome the deleterious effects of poor classroom acoustics. Children also may not become involved in extracurricular activities, sports, or other socially interactive events; instead, they may isolate.

An adult with a moderate hearing loss will encounter similar difficulties. Without the use of amplification, they are also likely to miss 50% to 80% of the content of speech with a hearing loss of 40 dB HL to 50 dB HL, respectively, even if they are in quiet (good) listening conditions (Anderson & Matkin, 2007). As indicated previously, even when hearing aids are worn the presence of background noise and reverberant conditions will continue to cause difficulties; group settings, distance from a speaker, and/or not being able to see the speaker's face will be problematic as well. It is noteworthy that an adult with moderate hearing loss, in general, has an advantage over a youngster with the same degree of loss. An adult is more likely to be able to figure out pieces of a conversation when only part is heard; on the other hand, a child will not have had the life and language experience and exposure to fill in the missing bits of information.

In the adult population, the social effects might include no longer being able to enjoy going to restaurants, the theater, and other such large and/or noisy group settings because of their high degree of difficulty. They may cause them to avoid family gatherings, which may lead to strained relationships and even depression, a symptom that is not uncommon in the elderly population.

Moderately Severe Hearing Loss

Air conduction thresholds that fall within the 56 dB HL to 70 dB HL range on the audiogram (refer to **Figure 9.7**) are

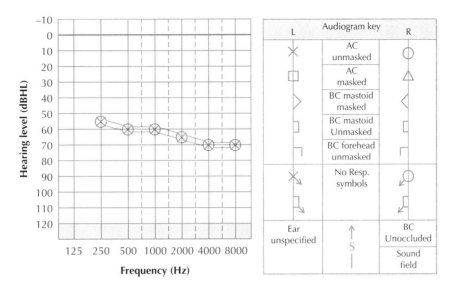

Figure 9.7   An audiogram illustrating a "moderate to severe" degree of hearing loss (between 56 dB HL and 70 dB HL). The type of hearing loss is unknown without the addition of bone conduction results.

categorized as a moderately severe hearing impairment. A hearing loss that falls within this range can be extremely handicapping; the individual with a loss at 55 dB HL can literally miss out on as much as 100% of average-level conversation. When we consider that the decibel level of average conversational speech is generally considered to be in the range of 45 dB HL to 50 dB HL (Martin & Clark, 2012), it is apparent that someone who is not aware of sound until 55 dB HL will be altogether unaware of average conversational speech if they are not using a hearing aid or other device. Whether it's an infant developing speech and language skills, a school-aged child trying to function academically in a classroom, or an adult attempting to function and communicate in a variety of settings, intervention strategies (hearing aids, aural rehabilitation, speech-language intervention, etc.) must be routinely in place.

Early hearing detection and intervention is critical for the young child with this degree of hearing impairment, for without it delayed and/or disordered speech-language skills can be expected. Some of the areas that are impacted, in varying degrees depending on the child, include disorders of syntax, morphology, vocabulary, and semantics, as well as speech intelligibility. For example, a child with hearing loss in this range typically has speech production errors comparable to those of normal-hearing children with articulation or phonological delays (Schow & Nerbonne, 2007). Additionally, there will be a well-documented difference in language development between the hard of hearing child

and his or her normal-hearing peers within the educational setting. However, this difference is not always apparent to all individuals who work with children. From child care centers, early childhood education programs, and even as late as kindergarten and first grade, the speech-language pathologist is often the first professional called upon to examine the child's apparent unintelligible speech patterns.

In the average classroom setting and without hearing aids, the moderately severe hearing-impaired child will be unable to understand and follow instruction and conversation, and is likely to be unaware of much of the conversation that is going on around him or her. Frequently, these children can be identified as always receiving guidance from another student in the classroom, which draws the attention away from the child with hearing loss toward the "little classroom helper" who recognizes the need to assist the "slower" student.

Adults will experience difficulties in similar situations as well. Even with the use of hearing aids (and/or other devices), the presence of background noise or reverberation, the speaker's face not being visible, and distance from the speaker may all prove to be especially problematic situations that greatly reduce the adult's ability to hear and understand. In such settings, recommendations may include full-time use of hearing aids and other prescribed devices, as well as ancillary support services as needed.

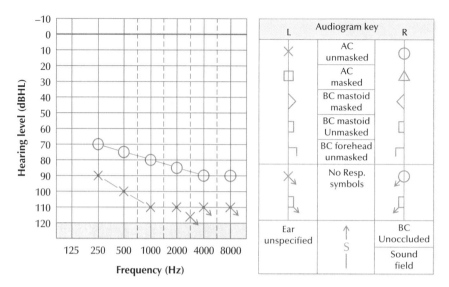

Figure 9.8 An audiogram illustrating a "severe" degree of hearing loss (between 71 dB HL and 90 dB HL) in the right ear and a "profound" degree of hearing loss (91 dB HL and greater) in the left ear. The type of hearing loss is unknown without the addition of bone conduction results.

Severe and Profound Hearing Loss

A hearing loss that falls within 71 dB HL to 90 dB HL is categorized as a severe hearing loss; when it falls at 91 dB HL and greater it is known as a profound hearing loss. Refer to the audiogram in **Figure 9.8** for an example of a severe and profound hearing loss. When we consider that a hearing loss at 56 dB HL to 70 dB HL can result in missing as much as 100% of speech, how much greater then is the impact of a hearing loss of this magnitude on speech-language development and overall communication skills?

Bearing in mind the discussion in the previous section regarding the impact of a moderately severe hearing loss, early intervention for the child with severe and profound hearing loss is that much more critical. For these youngsters, the earlier the child wears amplification consistently with concentrated efforts by parents and caregivers to provide rich language opportunities throughout everyday activities and/or provision of intensive language intervention (sign or verbal), the greater the probability that speech, language, and learning will develop at a relatively normal rate (Anderson & Matkin, 2007).

At the other end of the age spectrum, advancing age is the single most important (and nonmodifiable) risk factor for hearing loss in older adults (George, Farrell, & Griswold, 2012). However, adults may also sustain a hearing loss since birth (congenitally and prelingually), or it may be of later or progressive onset as a result of other causes. Therefore, the potential impact on speech, language, and range of overall communication skills is quite varied.

In terms of accessibility of sound, without hearing aids or other devices, individuals with severe and profound hearing loss (adults as well as children) are unaware of average-level conversational speech, and are most likely not even aware of loud-level speech. Additionally, often (although perhaps not always) there may be no access to even the loudest of environmental sounds. With appropriate amplification (or cochlear implantation) these individuals may be aware of average-level speech; however, the amount of speech that is actually understood is extremely variable and can range from reasonably good to none at all. This depends, at least in part, on the nature as well as the severity of the hearing loss. In addition to the age of onset of the hearing loss and whether it was incurred pre- or postlingually, other possible variables include age at time of identification, age at time of intervention, and the possible presence of comorbidities.

The speech-language pathologists may find themselves providing therapy to clients with profound hearing loss who may have relocated from other countries or from areas where early intervention services for children are not readily available or accessible. In such cases, even the procurement of hearing aids may be difficult. Because there is such

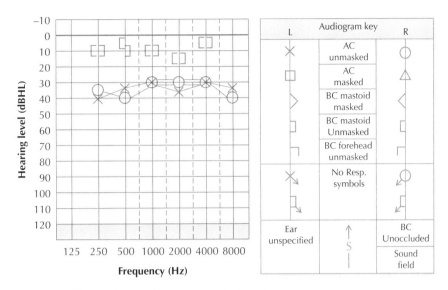

Figure 9.9 An audiogram illustrating a bilateral conductive hearing loss.

a wide range of variables, the reader is encouraged to network with local audiologists who may have prior experience in working with these and other such challenging cases.

Type of Hearing Loss (Reading the Bone Line)

If you are to interpret the audiogram and understand its implications, knowing the type of hearing loss is essential. Although determining the degree of hearing loss is based on the air conduction thresholds, determining the type of hearing loss is based on the bone conduction thresholds (sometimes collectively referred to as the *bone line*). In the following sections we will review the three main types of hearing loss (conductive, sensorineural, and mixed) along with some causes and characteristics of each.

Conductive Hearing Loss

You can determine what type of hearing loss a person has by looking at the relationship of the bone conduction thresholds with the air conduction thresholds. When the air conduction thresholds are outside of the normal range but the bone conduction thresholds are completely within normal limits, a **conductive hearing loss** is present. **Figure 9.9** shows an audiogram with a conductive hearing loss. Notice that the air conduction thresholds are at approximately 30 dB HL to 40 dB HL across all frequencies in both ears. The masked bone conduction thresholds, however, appear at 0 dB HL across all frequencies in both ears. This difference

between the air conduction thresholds and the bone conduction thresholds is known as an air–bone gap. This means that the hearing loss is mild in degree as determined by the air conduction thresholds being at 30 dB HL to 40 dB HL, and it is conductive in nature as determined by the bone conduction thresholds being completely within normal limits at 0 dB HL. Hence, this is a mild conductive hearing loss.

A conductive hearing loss occurs as a result of damage to or pathology of the conductive mechanism. The conductive mechanism is made up of the outer and middle ears. Any physical damage, structural abnormality, or obstruction that occurs in this portion of the auditory system can prevent sound from being transported into the inner ear. The primary characteristic of this type of loss is typically a reduction in sensitivity, and not a loss of the clarity of speech. Therefore, when sound is made loud enough, the person's ability to discern the content is usually intact, as demonstrated by the person's characteristically excellent word discrimination scores.

A variety of different pathologies can cause conductive hearing loss; they may be either congenital (present at birth) or acquired (not present at time of birth, onset sometime afterward). In contrast to sensorineural hearing loss (see the next section), the conductive type of hearing loss is typically medically and/or surgically treatable. An example of a medically treatable conductive hearing loss is antibiotic therapy for **otitis media**.

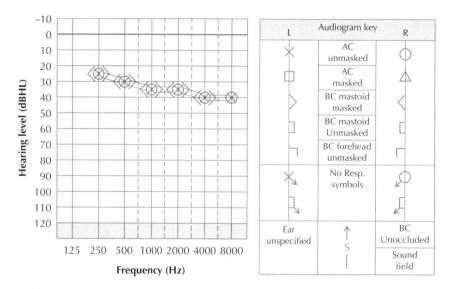

Figure 9.10 An audiogram illustrating a bilateral sensorineural hearing loss.

Some other examples of conductive pathology include impacted cerumen (wax); foreign bodies in the external ear canal; congenital **aural atresia** (complete absence of the ear canal opening); **otitis externa** (inflammation of the outer ear); **ossicular discontinuity** (disruption of the ossicles); cholesteatoma; and perforation of the tympanic membrane (eardrum). There are some types of conductive pathologies that are nonresponsive to medical and/or surgical treatment, or medical and/or surgical intervention may be contraindicated or unsuccessful. A patient—if appropriate and given the choice—may opt for a hearing aid in lieu of medical or surgical treatment. An example of this situation might occur with **otosclerosis**, (fixation of the stapes bone), ossification of the middle ear, or ossicular discontinuity, all of which result in a conductive hearing loss. Specifically in the case of otosclerosis, the literature reports that surgery is unsuccessful in up to 28% of individuals seeking surgical remediation for their hearing loss (Felix-Trujillo, Valdez-Martinez, Ramirez, & Lozano-Morales, 2009). A patient in this situation might understandably opt for rehabilitation with a hearing aid as opposed to undergoing the surgery. Alternately, there may be situations involving a chronic condition that may benefit from the use of hearing aids or assistive technology, in addition to medical and/or surgical services; for example, as might be the case with chronic otitis media.

A closing comment regarding conductive pathology, regardless of etiology, it is prudent for the speech-language pathologist to regularly review files and determine how long the patient's conductive condition has been present.

Monitoring and follow-up medical and audiologic services are important to ensure that the patient's healthcare and communication needs are routinely being met.

Sensorineural Hearing Loss

Again, you can determine the type of hearing loss by looking at the bone conduction thresholds in relation to the air conduction thresholds. When air conduction thresholds are abnormal and bone conduction thresholds are equally abnormal, a **sensorineural hearing loss** is present. Figure 9.10 shows an audiogram with a sensorineural hearing loss. Notice that the air conduction thresholds are at approximately 30 dB HL to 40 dB HL across all frequencies in each ear, and the bone conduction thresholds appear at the same levels as the air conduction thresholds at each frequency. When air and bone conduction thresholds are at the same levels at each frequency, this is known as a sensorineural hearing loss.

A sensorineural hearing loss occurs as a result of damage to the sensorineural mechanism, which is made up of the inner ear and auditory nerve. In the case of sensorineural hearing loss, sound is transmitted through the outer and middle ear unobstructed; the problem arises in either the inner ear or auditory nerve. Most sensorineural hearing loss is permanent. Sensorineural hearing loss is often remediated with the use of hearing aids, or cochlear implants if the nature and severity are sufficiently severe.

There are numerous etiologies of sensorineural hearing loss; here we can name but a few. Sensorineural hearing loss

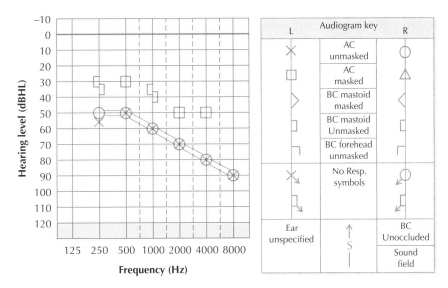

Figure 9.11   An audiogram illustrating a bilateral mixed hearing loss.

may be congenital or acquired, genetic or nongenetic, and syndromic or nonsyndromic. Common congenital causes of sensorineural hearing loss include premature birth, maternal diabetes, lack of oxygen, hyperbilirubinemia, maternal infection, or alcohol and drug abuse. Causes of acquired sensorineural hearing loss may include measles, mumps, meningitis, head trauma, noise exposure, ototoxic drug intake, and aging (known as presbycusis).

A common characteristic of sensorineural hearing loss is being able to hear low frequencies (many vowel sounds as well as background noise) better than the higher frequencies (many consonant sounds). This can lead to the frequent perception that the person with this type of hearing loss can hear, but they do not seem to understand, or that they may be choosing to ignore you. In fact, sensorineural hearing loss combines a loss of sensitivity with a diminished ability to understand speech, even when it is made louder. This characteristic of sensorineural hearing loss is why someone who suffers from it may turn the television up extremely loud, yet still not be able to understand what is being said. Other symptoms these individuals may experience include tinnitus (ringing or buzzing), an abnormal (inappropriately rapid) growth of loudness (recruitment) once they hear the sound, and vertigo (dizziness and loss of balance).

Mixed Hearing Loss

A **mixed hearing loss** is merely a hearing loss that is a combination (or mix) of a conductive component plus a sensorineural component. The audiometric pattern in a mixed hearing loss is one in which bone conduction thresholds are outside of normal (indicating the sensorineural component) and the air conduction thresholds are even further impaired (indicating the addition of the conductive component). This difference between the air and the bone conduction thresholds is another example of an air–bone gap. Looking at the mixed hearing loss in **Figure 9.11** note that the air and bone conduction thresholds are outside of the normal range, and are also separated by an air–bone gap.

A common example of a mixed hearing loss is when someone who has a preexisting sensorineural hearing loss (perhaps as a result of maternal in utero infection) then acquires otitis media (the common ear infection). There are numerous other possible causes of mixed hearing loss, all of them having one thing in common—they are a combination of a sensorineural component and a conductive component. Treatment and remediation for a mixed hearing loss varies depending on the specific etiologies involved.

Given the vast number of possible etiologies of sensorineural and conductive hearing loss combined, it is difficult to give the functional characteristics of a typical mixed hearing loss. Generally speaking, the symptoms that any given individual demonstrates will depend on the specific etiologies of the two separate components that make up the mixed loss. For instance, if we use the previous example of a congenital sensorineural hearing loss combined with the acquired ear infection, the air conduction results would tell

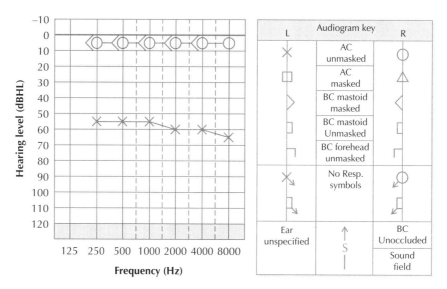

Figure 9.12   An audiogram with all unmasked responses.

us how much sensitivity loss there is while the characteristics of the sensorineural component will impact the word discrimination ability. A common complaint that may alert the speech-language pathologist to this type of condition may be the report of a sudden significant decrease in the person's ability to hear or that his or her hearing aids are suddenly not working to overcome the degree of hearing loss.

Configuration of Hearing Loss

At this juncture, degree and type of hearing loss have been established; now you must consider the configuration, or shape, of the hearing loss. In the following sections, two common configurations of hearing loss will be described.

Asymmetrical Hearing Loss

An **asymmetrical hearing loss** is, quite simply, when a person's hearing sensitivity is significantly different in one ear versus the other. This might involve an audiogram in which one ear is completely within normal limits and the other ear has a sensorineural hearing loss. (This would also be referred to as a unilateral hearing loss.) Alternately, you might see an audiogram with hearing loss in both ears, but the degree of loss is significantly different in one ear than the other. We will first discuss interpreting the validity of such an audiogram.

Let us take the example of a unilateral type of asymmetrical hearing loss. We will assume our patient has normal hearing

in the right ear and a profound sensorineural hearing loss in the left ear. If masking is not used when this person is tested for pure tones, the unmasked audiogram will not be accurate. **Figure 9.12** demonstrates unmasked hearing test results for this hypothetical case. Referring to Figure 9.12, notice that the air conduction thresholds for the right ear are completely normal, whereas the air conduction thresholds for the left ear are at approximately 55 dB HL to 65 dB HL. These unmasked air conduction thresholds in the left ear are actually a shadow curve of the right ear, and they are due to the phenomenon of cross-over. In our example, cross-over and cross-hearing occurred because the intensity of the sound in the left earphone became so great that the sound exceeded the interaural attenuation. **Interaural attenuation** can be thought of as the reduction (in decibels) caused by the skull as sound travels from the test ear to the nontest ear (Brannstrom & Lantz, 2010). These unmasked thresholds in the left ear are erroneous; that is, they don't actually represent the hearing in the left ear at all. Rather, they simply indicate how loud the test sound was in the left earphone for the sound to cross over to the right (better) ear to respond. When this occurs, the audiologist must mask.

Our audiologist in this example employs the masking process, which involves putting noise into the better (right) ear to "keep it busy" while at the same time retesting the poorer (left) ear. When this is done, the new thresholds for the pure tones that are obtained for the left ear (now without the help of the right good ear) are known as the *masked thresholds*. The result of this process is a masked

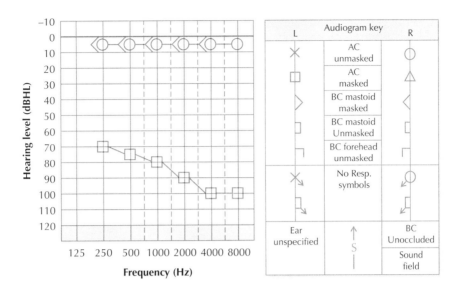

Figure 9.13   An audiogram for the same patient as the one in Figure 9.12, but masking for the left ear air conduction has now been completed. The left ear now shows a severe to profound degree of hearing loss; the type of hearing loss is still undetermined.

audiogram, much like the one shown in Figure 9.13. In contrast to the unmasked results for this patient (Figure 9.12), the masked audiogram provides a true indication of the severity of hearing loss in the left ear.

It's noteworthy to mention that although speech-language pathologists (SLPs) are unlikely to be responsible for knowing how to perform effective masking, it is critically important that they understand the concepts, what they represent, and the audiometric implications. An important caveat for the SLP to keep in mind is that if the audiogram in front of you looks like the unmasked one in Figure 9.12, showing large gaps between the ears and no masking, the appropriate course of action is to contact the audiologist as soon as possible to request more information or clarification of your patient's hearing status. The speech-language pathologist must be able to accurately interpret the hearing test results provided, in order for proper interventions and management strategies to be routinely in place.

In terms of the communication impact of such a hearing loss, it is first important to recognize that having "one normal ear" is not sufficient. Regardless of patient age or life situation, unilateral sensorineural hearing loss can result in significant and sometimes severe difficulty. Most commonly, there are difficulties with discrimination in background noise and reduced ability to localize sounds (Pennings, Gulliver, & Morris, 2011). Individuals with this type of impairment experiences difficulty understanding the message when their bad ear is directed toward the speaker, because their head—physically—interferes with the sound reaching the better ear. This is known as the *head shadow effect*, and accounts for why noisy settings can be particularly problematic and wearisome. Moreover, this becomes an especially troublesome and challenging situation for children, whose speech-in-noise listening skills do not reach full development until the adolescent/teenage years (Finitzo-Hieber & Tillman, 1978; Neuman, Wroblewski, & Rubinstein, 2010; Rothpletz, Wightman, & Kistler, 2012). Young children who have this asymmetrical unilateral configuration of hearing loss are at an even further disadvantage, because children with unilateral hearing impairment require a more advantageous listening condition to perform equally as well as their normally hearing counterparts (Pennings et al., 2011; Ruscetta, Arjmand, & Pratt, 2005).

Although different age categories and life circumstances may necessitate different considerations and interventions for individuals with unilateral hearing loss, an important take-away message is that a hearing loss of any degree appears sufficient to interrupt the normal continuum of communication development and academic skills (Yoshinaga-Itano, 2008). Do not assume that one normal ear can do the job of two.

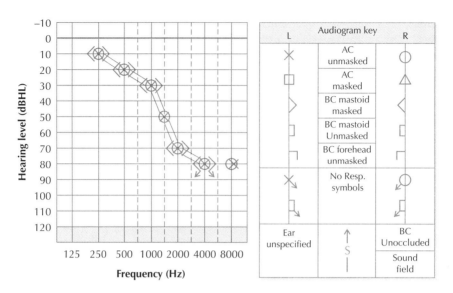

Figure 9.14   An audiogram illustrating a high frequency sensorineural hearing loss bilaterally.

High Frequency Sensorineural Hearing Loss

The two most common causes of sensorineural hearing loss in adults are presbycusis (hearing loss due to aging) and noise-induced hearing loss (NIHL) (National Institute on Deafness and Other Communication Disorders, 1997, 2002). Furthermore, the American Academy of Audiology (AAA, 2008) estimates that about one in eight children (more than 5 million) suffers from NIHL as well. The configuration of hearing loss frequently associated with both of these etiologies is a high frequency hearing loss pattern.

The precise definition of a **high frequency sensorineural hearing loss (HF SNHL)** seems to vary from source to source. Some researchers define HF SNHL as occurring above 2000 Hz (Roup & Noe, 2009), some define it as occurring above 3000 Hz (Hornsby & Ricketts, 2005), and still others use 4000 Hz through 8000 Hz (Robinson, Baer, & Moore, 2007). For our purposes, we will simply define it as a sensorineural hearing loss of greater severity in the higher frequencies than in the lower frequencies, where thresholds may be in the normal to near-normal range. What this means is that there may be normal or relatively normal hearing up to approximately 2000 Hz, and then a sloping sensorineural hearing loss at frequencies of 3000 Hz and above. Refer to **Figure 9.14** for an audiogram showing a high frequency sensorineural hearing loss, again, bearing in mind the variability.

Regardless of the etiology, the consequences of HF SNHL can be quite significant. Low frequency information includes speech sounds such as the vowels and the /n/, /m/, /l/, and /r/

(in addition to background noise); the higher frequency range typically includes the consonant sounds. The contribution of high frequency consonant sounds to our ability to understand speech and language is well documented in the literature as well as routinely observed; unfortunately for individuals with this type of loss, consonants tend to carry most of the meaning of speech. Imagine that you are hearing only the vowel sounds of a speech message; it is unlikely that you would understand the content. Now imagine that you are hearing only the consonant sounds; you would have a much better idea of what the person was trying to say.

You can visualize the effect of a HF SNHL. If you compare the "speech banana" audiogram (depicted in the "Speech Banana Audiogram" section later in this chapter) to the hearing loss shown in Figure 9.14 (or better yet, use your own client's audiogram), you will be able to approximate the sounds that will be most problematic for this individual. Furthermore, you will be able to see why, as has been repeatedly reported in the literature, the discrimination of consonants (such as fricatives) will be especially difficult for individuals with HF SNHL (Robinson et al., 2007). The speech audiometry results (discussed further in the next section of this chapter) may also provide additional insight into the degree of difficulty your client may experience.

Another difficulty associated with HF SNHL is having the impaired word discrimination even further degraded by the presence of background noise. Remember, a person with HF SNHL classically has much better (perhaps even normal) hearing sensitivity for low frequencies. The frequency characteristics of background noise (low frequency sound) will have a masking effect and physically block out the high frequency consonant sounds. This is known as the "upward spread of masking."

For youngsters who have high-frequency sensorineural hearing loss, even a small amount of hearing loss can have profound negative effects on speech, language comprehension, communication, classroom learning, and social development (Centers for Disease Control and Prevention, 2013). NIHL renders sound as distorted or muffled, and may lead to an uncertain grasp of many of the grammatical aspects of spoken language, including weak consonants such as fricatives (/f/, /s/, /sh/, and /h/) and stops (/p/, /t/, and /k/), along with morphemes that mark verb tense, possessives, and plurals (-ed, 's, and –s) (Levey et al., 2012).

One last issue about HF SNHL and its consequences should be pointed out. The audiometric results are expected to provide a guideline as to the degree and types of difficulties that a given individual may experience as a result of the hearing loss. However, there is evidence to suggest that some individuals in this category (high-frequency hearing loss above 2000 Hz) may experience listening difficulties not readily apparent from their word discrimination score results (Roup & Noe, 2009). For example, during the evaluation the individual may demonstrate very good-to-excellent word discrimination ability in a controlled acoustic environment; however, in real-life listening situations they may have noticeable difficulties communicating.

Speech Audiometry

So far in this chapter we have covered the characteristics of degree, type, and configuration of hearing impairment; however, any audiometric picture that does not include the results of speech audiometry is incomplete. It is important to understand that although there are certain general characteristics to each type of hearing loss—such as a person with conductive loss typically having very good understanding ability and a person's sensorineural loss often being accompanied by a loss of speech discrimination ability—a lot of variability is observed from etiology to etiology and from person to person. Speech audiometry measures attempt to quantify a person's ability to recognize and understand the content of the speech signal they are hearing; the speech-language pathologist must have a secure understanding of these measures and what they mean, in order to design effective outcomes for their clients.

Speech Recognition Threshold/Speech Reception Threshold (SRT)

The speech recognition (sometimes called reception) threshold (SRT), a procedure that attempts to measure a person's threshold for speech, serves as a validity check for the results of pure tone results. Because the SRT is normally done by air conduction (using earphones), it is expected to corroborate the pure tone air conduction results. Specifically, the SRT should be in agreement with the pure tone average (PTA), which is the average of the thresholds at 500 Hz, 1000 Hz, and 2000 Hz. To calculate the PTA you simply add together the three thresholds at those frequencies, and then divide by three. For example, if a person has thresholds of 40 dB at 500 Hz, 50 dB at 1000 Hz, and 60 dB at 2000 Hz, the PTA would be 40 + 50 + 60 = 150 and then 150/3 = 50. Therefore, the expected SRT for this individual should be perhaps 50 dB HL, with an acceptable variability of 5 dB. Exceptions to this may occur when there is a very steeply (precipitously) sloping hearing loss; in those instances the SRT might be closer to an average of the two better PTA frequency thresholds, typically, being the average of 500 Hz and 1000 Hz.

What does it mean if an SRT does not fall within these guidelines? Very simply, disagreement between the SRT and the PTA is an indication of inconsistency in test results. This inconsistency may provide an early indication of **pseudohypacusis** (false or exaggerated hearing loss). It may also be due to test variables such as equipment malfunction or misunderstanding of the instructions by the patient (ASHA, 1988), language or cognitive impairments, or an indication of developmental stage. If your patient's audiogram shows an inconsistency between the SRT and the PTA, you should look for explanatory notes either on the audiogram or within the evaluation report, providing rationale.

Speech Detection Threshold (SDT)/ Speech Awareness Threshold (SAT)

The speech detection threshold (SDT) is another threshold measure for speech, but unlike the SRT in which the person identifies the sound as being a speech signal, with the SDT the person only needs to be aware that sound is present. As such, the SDT is an easier task and is generally slightly better (lower dB level) than the SRT, typically by approximately 5 to 10 dB. Like the SRT, the SDT serves as a validity check of pure tone findings, but is more closely related to the best air conduction threshold as opposed to the three PTA frequencies (500 Hz, 1000 Hz, and 2000 Hz). In fact, if a person has a very steeply sloping hearing loss, the SDT is likely to be a great deal better than the PTA.

What does it mean if the SDT is not consistent with the pure tone air conduction findings? Similar to the previous section, if there is an unexplained discrepancy between the SDT and the pure tone findings, there is a distinct possibility of there being a case of pseudohypacusis. It is also possible, however, that an equipment malfunction or a cognitive, language, or development delay or disorder exists. These possibilities need to be explored in such cases where inconsistencies exist. You should consult the written report or your local audiologist for additional clarification.

Word Discrimination Testing

The results of word discrimination testing (WDT), whether referred to as speech recognition scores or speech discrimination scores, are a fundamental part of the audiologic evaluation. These scores represent an approximation of the person's ability to understand what has been said when speech has been made loud enough for them to hear it. The type of speech used is typically phonetically balanced word lists, such as CID W-22's and NU-6 lists. In terms of the results, conductive hearing loss, generally speaking, is frequently associated with very good discrimination scores. A sensorineural loss, on the other hand, is typically accompanied by somewhat poorer and variable scores, as has been noted in the literature (Brandy, 2002; Penrod, 1994) as well as observed by these authors during clinical practice. However, there are cases of sensorineural hearing loss with uncharacteristically good WDT scores relative to the audiogram, and the reverse is possible as well. Therefore, it bears repeating that any report that reflects only the nature and severity is incomplete. It is critically important for the SLP to have available *all* information for the purpose of speech-language assessment, intervention, and remediation planning processes for all patients.

The audiogram in front of you should include, at minimum, WDT scores in the quiet condition (no competing noise) in each ear separately; sometimes the audiogram also will have WDT scores in the presence of background noise. Perhaps you may have an audiogram in front of you that includes a person's WDT scores both with and without visual (lip reading) cues. The categorizing of the results generally follows a scale of excellent (100%) through very poor (less than 50%); Table 9.4 provides the general scoring guidelines. It is important to recognize that these are *suggested guidelines only and should be interpreted with*

Table 9.4 General Guide for the Interpretation of Word Discrimination Test (WDT) Scores

WDT Score (%)	General Interpretation
92 to 100%	Excellent
84 to 90%	Very good
78 to 82%	Good
70 to 76%	Fair
60 to 68%	Poor
Less than 60%	Very poor

caution; as already suggested, WDT score variability may occur within hearing loss categories as well as in an individual from day to day or one test session to the next.

A noteworthy consideration is that standard WDT is completed in an ideal "laboratory" type setting; that is, the sound treated booth, a quiet environment with no noise or distractions and the patient's attention focused—at all times—on the task at hand. Real-life listening conditions are not as ideal as this setting. Even when the WDT is done with background noise, the person is still in a somewhat ideal laboratory type of setting, with focused attention and without distraction. So again, these results need to be interpreted cautiously because they are only a "snapshot" of a person's true word discrimination ability.

Lastly, if the results of WDT do not make sense or do not seem possible, you should contact your local audiologist. For example, if the WDT scores in front of you indicate that a person repeats back 100% of words correctly at a decibel level that is softer (better) than any of the pure tone air conduction thresholds, a case of pseudohypacusis should be suspected. Refer to the "Pseudohypacusis" section later in this chapter.

Other Audiometric Data
Sound Field Unaided

Often the audiogram in front of you will have unaided sound field data; there are several reasons why this may be the case. For example, if the patient is a young child or one who has multiple or developmental disabilities (see Figure 9.15), the individual may not have been capable of or amenable to accepting the earphones, thus necessitating the sound field test condition (refer to Figure 9.16; also, refer back to Table 9.1 for the ASHA symbols key). An instance of when sound field unaided hearing testing might specifically be desirable

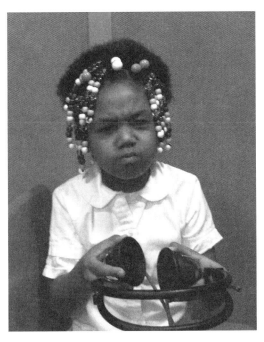

Figure 9.15 A picture of an "unhappy" child who does not want to wear the earphones.

is for comparison purposes, as might be the case when anticipating that a patient will soon be fit with hearing aids or cochlear implants and needing those results to document device benefit.

When reviewing and interpreting the results of unaided sound field testing, for whatever reason it was performed, it is important to keep in mind that these data represent the hearing of the better ear, if there is a difference between the ears. For example, if a patient has one ear that hears normally and one ear that is profoundly impaired, the better (normal) ear will pick up sound at normal levels. Thus, in the sound field condition we cannot rule out the possibility that someone has a unilateral hearing loss. If unaided sound field testing was performed out of necessity, as might be the case with a very young child, follow-up testing to obtain ear-specific information is always necessary and recommended, even when the results appear to be within normal limits.

Sound Field, Aided (Hearing Aid or Cochlear Implant)

A routine part of an audiologic assessment on a hearing-impaired patient should be the aided audiogram. Although we recognize that in some facilities the aided audiogram may have gone by the wayside in favor of some of the objective hearing aid verification options, it is the expressed opinion of these authors that aided functional data can provide very useful information. Very simply, the aided audiogram is a graph that contains a person's responses to speech and tones while they are wearing some device meant to improve hearing sensitivity. These devices may include hearing aids, cochlear implants, or some combination of both. The aided audiogram provides an estimation of the amount of benefit the person is receiving while they are using their device(s), and determines if the patient's needs

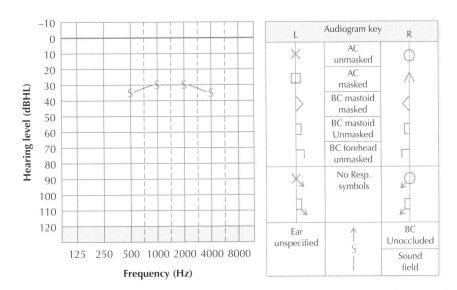

Figure 9.16 An audiogram showing the results of unaided sound field testing. With sound field audiometric results, we cannot be sure which ear is responding.

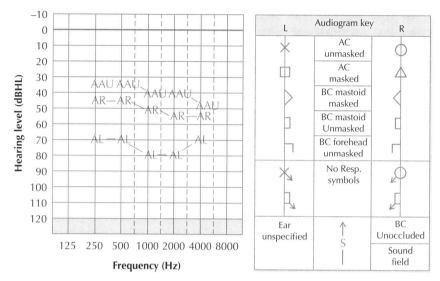

Figure 9.17 An example of an "aided audiogram." The symbol "AR" represents how the individual hears with a hearing aid on the right ear only. The symbol "AL" represents how the individual hears with a hearing aid in the left ear only. The symbol "A-Au" represents how the individual is hearing with both ears simultaneously aided.

are being met as effectively as possible, or if a different solution should be explored. The aided audiogram is also an excellent counseling tool for those individuals who may be resistant to or fail to see the benefit of amplification.

Although ASHA does not have a specific symbol to indicate the response with either a hearing aid or cochlear implant, hearing aid results are frequently noted using the symbol A

(see Figure 9.17), and a cochlear implant is often noted using the symbol CI (see Figure 9.18). The aided audiogram in front of you should clearly indicate what types of devices your patient is using, and which symbols denote specific responses.

The aided audiogram might even have symbols that indicate your patient uses a hearing aid in one ear while using a

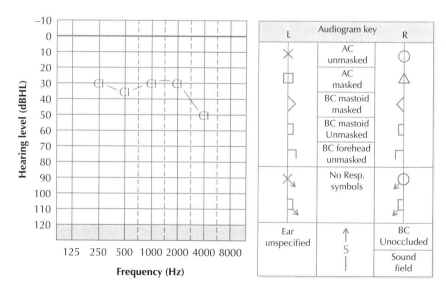

Figure 9.18 An aided audiogram with the symbol "CI" being used to illustrate how a person responds while using a cochlear implant.

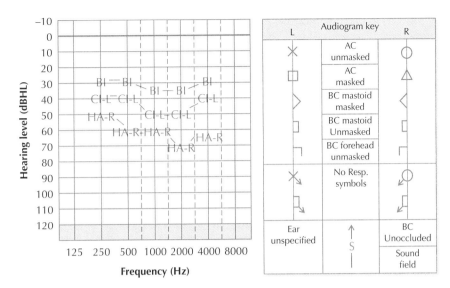

Figure 9.19 An aided audiogram comparing performance of a hearing aid on the right ear (HA-R); cochlear implant on the left (CI-L); or simultaneously using a hearing aid on the right ear and the cochlear implant on the left. This simultaneous condition is referred to as a bimodal listening condition.

cochlear implant in the other ear. This scenario is not uncommon, particularly where a child is concerned. When this occurs, for example, the audiogram might be noted with HA-R to indicate the condition of only the hearing aid on the right ear, CI-L to indicate the cochlear implant on the left ear, and perhaps AU to indicate the simultaneous use of the HA on the right ear and the CI on the left ear. See Figure 9.19 for an example of an aided audiogram of this type. Again, symbols may vary, but the symbols key will be indicated on the specific audiogram.

Regardless of the specific fitting strategy used for your patient, the audiogram and/or audiologic evaluation report should include information regarding device settings and details (for example, optimal volume setting or schedule of how and when the devices are to be worn) of which you should be aware. Remember, as the SLP providing services for this individual, you must familiarize yourself with this information in order to be as effective as possible with your therapeutic interventions.

Some of the types of information you might find on an aided audiogram include the person's responses to sound at different frequencies (either warbled pure tones or narrow bands of noise). You may also see SRT and WDT in quiet and in noise, and with or without visual (speech reading) cues. Sometimes results are obtained and reported for a variety of conditions, such as right ear aided only, left ear aided only, cochlear implant right, cochlear implant right

with hearing aid left, and so on. Quite simply, the aided responses to specific frequencies can show the audiometric benefit when the devices are worn. Aided speech audiometry gives a guideline as to how well a person can understand speech when it has been made audible to them through the hearing aids or cochlear implants. Remember, however, that these are merely approximations; actual performance in real-life situations may (and should be expected to) vary.

Clearly, just knowing the patient's type and degree of hearing loss with SRT and WDT ability is not enough. Again, it is incumbent upon the SLP to seek out and incorporate the aided data in order to gain a better understanding of the patient's performance with amplification. This information is vitally important in the evaluation and treatment planning process for all of their hearing-impaired patients. A hearing-impaired individual can only function as well as their devices. It is critical to success that the hearing aids are routinely utilized (as recommended) and that they remain in good working condition.

Tympanogram Interpretation

Tympanometry is not a hearing test, and so cannot tell us whether a person has normal or impaired hearing; rather, this test gives us an objective indication of how the conductive mechanism is physically functioning. The results of tympanometry should be used in conjunction with the hearing test results; they can provide evidence to help distinguish between sensorineural and conductive causes. Also, tympanometry can provide data supporting the existence of fluid in the middle ear, a common childhood disease that requires immediate medical referral. The Liden-Jerger system is commonly used for the classification of **tympanograms** (Liden, 1969; Jerger 1970); it breaks the results into the following categories: type A, type As, type Ad, type B, and type C. We will address each of these tympanometric types. Refer to **Figure 9.20** for an example of each tympanogram type.

Tympanometric results reflect measurements of middle ear compliance and pressure along with the volume of the external auditory ear canal. It is worth pointing out that the precise separation between normal and abnormal pressure and compliance values differs very slightly, from researcher to researcher. Regardless, the Liden-Jerger classification remains the benchmark for reporting data. Although tympanometry screening is part of the SLP's scope of practice, most of today's tympanometry screening equipment not only runs automatically, but also displays the results against a shaded background that visually defines the normal range, thus making interpretation that much easier.

Ear Canal Volume (ECV)

The ECV measure is also known as equivalent ear canal volume (EECV) or physical volume test (PVT). A normal healthy ear canal ranges in size from 0.3 ml to 1.0 ml in children and from 0.65 ml to 1.75 ml in adults (Alencar, Iorio, & Morales, 2005). This value can simply be read off the tympanogram printout; no calculation is needed. Refer to Figures 9.20A through 9.20E; the ECV can be seen on each of the tympanograms in these figures. The ECV, although providing valuable information, should be interpreted along with the tympanogram and not in isolation.

The significance of seeing a reduced ECV is that there is a likelihood of excessive wax being in the ear canal. A second scenario related to an exceptionally small ECV is that of a young child with craniofacial abnormalities. These may be a result of an underlying genetic syndrome (for example in the case of Down's syndrome) or other contributing condition such as hydrocephaly.

If results reflect an excessively large ECV, the measurement may not only reflect the volume of the external ear canal, but the middle ear cavity as well. Scenarios that may be responsible for such a finding may be either a perforation (hole) in the eardrum or a properly functioning pressure equalization tube (PE tube) in the eardrum. (To know the

difference, one should either reference the case history narrative for the presence/absence of PE tubes or the Otoscopy section of the test results narrative where the visualization of a PE tube should be noted if seen by the evaluating audiologist.) The significance of the ECV in relation to tympanogram type will be noted in each of the following sections.

Type A Tympanogram

The type A tympanogram is displayed in Figure 9.20A and is a pattern suggesting normal conductive system (outer and middle ear) functioning. The type A tympanogram is characterized by a peak pressure (as noted by the horizontal axis) between +50 daPa/mm H_2O and –100 daPa/mm H_2O to be considered within the normal pressure range, and between −100 and −200 to be considered borderline range; normal peak compliance (as noted by the vertical axis) reaches a height between 0.25 mmho/cc/ml and 1.05 mmho/cc/ml for children and between 0.3 and 1.7 for adults (Margolis & Hunter, 2000). The value of the ECV in a type A tympanogram is typically normal (from 0.3 ml to 1.0 ml in children and from 0.65 to 1.75 ml in adults [Alencar et al., 2005]). Although the numerical data are important to establish "the normal range," most devices include some type of reference, typically a box on the equipment read-out, denoting these normal parameters. The SLP needs only to judge if the results fall within this predetermined range on the

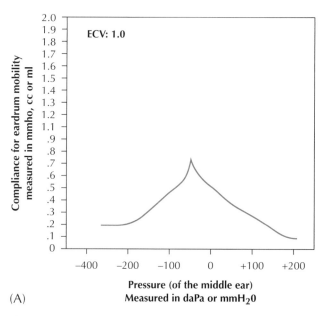

(A)

Figure 9.20A   A normal type A tympanogram, which is consistent with normal middle ear function.

digital readout. The significance of this pattern is that there is no evidence of pathology in the outer or middle ear; this is not to say that there is no hearing loss. Rather, it is saying that if the audiogram shows a hearing loss (in all likelihood, possibly as much as 99% of the time), it is not conductive in nature. A sensorineural loss can have a normal type A tympanogram because this type of loss arises from a problem in either the inner ear or the auditory nerve, not the outer or middle ear (the conductive system).

Type As Tympanogram

The subscript *s* in the classification of a tympanogram as As is a reference to the fact that the compliance of the pattern is **shallow**. A pattern of this type is characterized with a pressure value within normal limits (between $+50$ daPa/mm H_2O and -100 daPa/mm H_2O to be considered within the normal pressure range [Margolis & Hunter, 2000]), but the compliance value is very low or shallow. The compliance value for a type As tympanogram is less than 0.25 mmho/cc/ml for children and 0.3 mmho/cc/ml for adults. The value of the ECV in a type As tympanogram is also typically normal (from 0.3 ml to 1.0 ml in children and from 0.65 to 1.75 ml in adults [Alencar et al., 2005]). If you look at the pattern shown in Figure 9.20B, you will see that the peak value of pressure is again within the normal limits defined, but the height of that peak is significantly reduced.

The significance of this finding is that there is a stiff middle ear system, with reduced or restricted mobility of the eardrum (as illustrated by the shallow peak). Some of the conditions that can cause a tympanogram to be shallow include otosclerosis (abnormal bone growth around the ossicles, typically the stapes), middle ear effusion, severely scarred eardrum, or plaque on the eardrum (the latter two sometimes are caused by a history of excessive ear infections). A type As tympanogram is often accompanied by a hearing loss. Regardless of whether your patient has passed a pure tone screening, if you perform a tympanometry screening and get this result, a referral needs to be made to an audiologist and/or otologist.

Type Ad Tympanogram

The subscript *d* in the classification of a type Ad tympanogram refers to the fact that the compliance represented in this pattern is very *"deep"*. The pressure peak continues to occur in the normal range (between $+50$ daPa/mm H_2O and -100 daPa/mm H_2O [Margolis & Hunter, 2000]), but the peak compliance is excessive. The value of the ECV in a type Ad tympanogram is typically normal (from 0.3 ml to 1.0 ml in children and from 0.65 to 1.75 ml in adults [Alencar et al., 2005]). Refer to Figure 9.20C and you will notice that the height of the peak is much higher and exceeds the normal value.

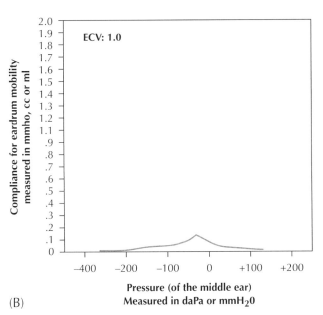

(B)

Figure 9.20B A shallow type As tympanogram, which is consistent with a stiff middle ear system.

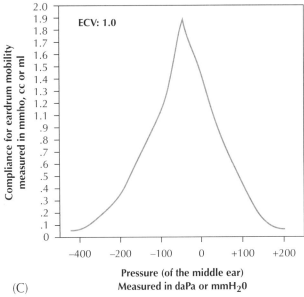

(C)

Figure 9.20C A very deep type Ad tympanogram, which is consistent with a hypermobile middle ear system.

The significance of the type Ad tympanogram is that there is a hypermobile (excessively flaccid) middle ear system. Some of the conditions that can cause a type Ad tympanogram include a disarticulation of the middle ear ossicles (disconnected), minor scar tissue, and a very thin or monomeric (single layer) eardrum. As with any abnormal tympanogram, regardless of whether the pure tone screening has been passed, this requires a referral to an audiologist and/or an otologist.

Type B Tympanogram

The type B tympanogram is a flat pattern; that is, there is no peak at all, only a flat line. The ECV is a key finding with the type B tympanogram, and can be either normal (from 0.3 ml to 1.0 ml in children and from 0.65 to 1.75 ml in adults [Alencar et al., 2005]), exceedingly small, or excessively large. Refer to Figure 9.20D and you will notice that there is no clearly defined pressure peak to this pattern, and there is essentially no compliance either; it is basically a completely flat or near flat line.

Regardless of the ear canal size (the ECV measure), a flat type B tympanogram generally suggests that no eardrum movement can be detected (as illustrated by the flat line). This can occur for a variety of reasons. In order to properly interpret a type B tympanogram, one must look to the ECV measure along with a visual inspection of the ear canal. Visual inspection (otoscopy) often helps us decipher the

meaning of the tympanometric findings: that there is an occluding plug of wax, a large hole in the eardrum, a patent (open and properly functioning) PE tube, or a bulging fluid-filled space beyond the eardrum, as in the case of otitis media. Combining these pieces of information can not only assist us in establishing the significance of the type B pattern, but also enable us to make the appropriate recommendations.

A type B tympanogram is often associated with a conductive and sometimes mixed hearing loss. As with the previously discussed abnormal tympanogram findings, regardless of whether the pure tone screening has been passed, a referral to an audiologist and/or an otologist is required.

Type C Tympanogram

As you will notice, the pattern of the type C tympanogram is one in which the pressure peak is in the abnormally negative range. Peak pressure values that fall beyond -200 daPa/mm H_2O are considered outside the normal range (Margolis & Hunter, 2000). The compliance of a type C tympanogram typically falls within normal limits (between 0.25 mmho/cc ml and 1.05 mmho/cc/ml for children and between 0.3 and 1.7 for adults), although slightly reduced compliance with the Type C is not terribly uncommon. The value of the ECV in a type C tympanogram is typically normal (from 0.3 ml to 1.0 ml in children and from 0.65 to 1.75 ml in

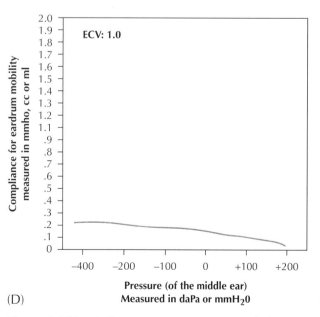

(D)

Figure 9.20D   A flat type B tympanogram, which is consistent with abnormal middle ear function.

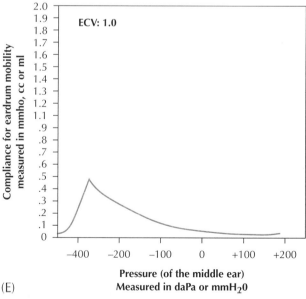

(E)

Figure 9.20E   A type C tympanogram, which shows significant negative middle ear pressure.

adults [Alencar et al., 2005]). A type C tympanogram is illustrated in Figure 9.20E.

A type C tympanogram reflects a retraction of the eardrum and a system of negative pressure in the middle ear space. This condition can be caused by a partially blocked Eustachian tube, and is often seen with allergies, or the developing or resolving of an ear infection. These individuals need to be monitored, and referral to an audiologist and/or otologist is recommended.

Otoacoustic Emission (OAE) Interpretation

In addition to its utility in estimating the presence or absence of auditory dysfunction, there are many other clinical applications for OAEs. However, much of this information is beyond the intended scope of this text. We are, therefore, limiting our discussion to what is most appropriate and necessary for you within your scope of practice as an SLP.

To reiterate, OAE testing is not actually a hearing test; rather, it assesses the functional health of the structures in the cochlea. When the cochlea is functioning properly, the OAE response is observed. In the majority of the population, this presence of a normal OAE response also means that the person has normal or near normal hearing. However, because a person can have a normally functioning cochlea and then have a physical anomaly further along the auditory pathway that may produce a hearing loss, OAE results, viewed *alone,* should never be the determining factor in the diagnosis of hearing loss. Auditory neuropathy syndrome disorder (ANSD) is an example of such retrocochlear pathology.

With that caveat in mind, the OAE is an immensely useful tool; it allows us to glean the presence of normal hearing and alerts us to potential impairments. The first thing we can establish based on the presence of an OAE response is that there is no conductive pathology, regardless of whether it is the transient evoked otoacoustic emission (TEOAE) or the distortion product otoacoustic emission (DPOAE) that has been tested. This means that the conductive mechanism (outer ear and middle ear) is free and clear of blockage and dysfunction. The reason we know this is quite simple—a pathology or blockage would physically prevent the forward and reverse transmission of sound on which the test is based.

Now, let us consider the additional significance of a response from each of the two separate types of OAE; that

is, the TEOAE and the DPOAE. The presence of a TEOAE response means that the outer hair cells in the sensory organ of the cochlea are working; in most cases, this means normal/near normal hearing sensitivity as well, or at least not poorer than approximately 30 dB HL (the mild range of hearing loss) (Hoth, Polzer, Neumann, & Plinkert, 2007). The significance of the DPOAE response is also that of a functioning cochlea, specifically the outer hair cells; however, in the case of the distortion product the response can be seen with hearing levels up to approximately 40 dB HL to 50 dB HL (in the mild to moderate range) (Schmuziger, Patscheke, & Probst, 2006). Therefore, the DPOAE response generally suggests hearing levels no poorer than the mild to moderate range, with no evidence of conductive (outer/middle ear) pathology. **Figure 9.21** illustrates a normal DPOAE result.

Finally, there are common findings of both types of emissions that must be remembered. Specifically, conditions beyond the level of the cochlea can leave the OAE response intact, such as in the case of a child with auditory neuropathy syndrome disorder (ANSD). This can give a family a false sense of security about their child or loved one's hearing status. This is one reason why newborn hearing screening programs utilize a combination of both OAE and the ABR. When reviewing the history and test results, if your patient passed the OAE screening, yet concerns remain, a referral to an audiologist for a complete diagnostic workup is essential.

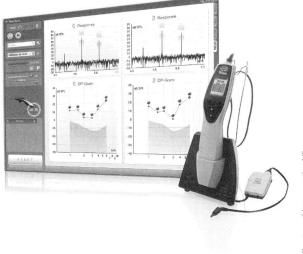

Courtesy of Interacoustics A/S

Figure 9.21 An illustration of distortion product otoacoustic emission results with the Interacoustics Titan DPOAE system.

Auditory Brainstem Response (ABR)

The auditory brainstem response (ABR) has multiple clinical applications, most of which fall outside the scope of this text. For our purposes we will again be limiting our discussion to what is most appropriate and necessary for you within your scope of practice as an SLP. It bears repeating that the ABR response is not a direct measure of hearing sensitivity; rather, it is a measure of the functional integrity of the auditory nerve up to and including the brainstem. Based on the information the test yields, we can glean estimates of hearing sensitivity that can later be confirmed with additional test procedures.

The types of ABR response modes we see employed when the test is done to estimate audiometric function are either the screening "pass" or "refer" type responses, or diagnostic decibel threshold search results. When the results of an ABR screening indicate the individual has passed the test, it is assumed that the screened ear is functioning normally and that further testing is not warranted. When a refer response is obtained, further diagnostic assessment is necessary, and referral to an audiologist for a complete evaluation is recommended. When the refer result is obtained, no conclusions should be drawn beyond the need for referral; there can be many reasons for someone not passing the ABR screening, ranging from the existence of a hearing loss to simple testing inaccuracies. **Figure 9.22** illustrates normal ABR threshold search results.

When a diagnostic ABR has been done for the purpose of a threshold search, the results may be reported in a decibel reference known as dB n HL, with *n* signifying above normal hearing level. A response in dB n HL is within approximately 10 dB to 20 dB of the person's behavioral response to sound (dB HL). Therefore, if results show, for example, an ABR response is at 65 dB n HL we can assume that the behavioral hearing threshold will be at perhaps 45 dB HL to 55 dB HL, which is at the level of a moderate hearing loss (refer to the earlier section on moderate hearing loss).

Questions to Guide Your Interpretation

You should now have enough information to understand the meaning of the results in front of you. By asking yourself a few simple questions you should be able to have a confident understanding of the implications of these results. Ask

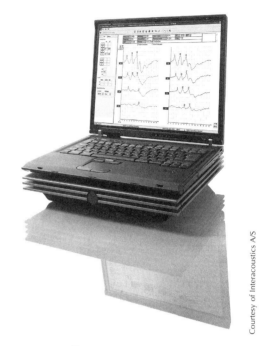

Courtesy of Interacoustics A/S

Figure 9.22 An illustration of the results of auditory brainstem response (ABR) testing with the Interacoustics Eclipse ABR system.

yourself each of the following questions and then refer back to the individual sections as necessary.

Can You Identify Behavioral Versus Nonbehavioral Results?

At first glance, the obvious implication of this question is: Can you distinguish between those tests that require a behavioral response and those that do not? The tests that require a behavioral response include, for example, pure tones and speech audiometry; the nonbehavioral tests include tympanometry, electroacoustic and electrophysiologic procedures. The implication that may be less obvious is: Do the specific procedures employed make sense based on the patient's chronological age?

Let us consider the situation in which a child has been referred to you for a speech-language evaluation and in preparation you are reviewing the audiologic report. You notice that the procedures completed include tympanometry, acoustic reflex testing, and OAE. Now you take note of the date of birth and calculate that the patient is 9 years of age. The knowledge of the child's age and that the tests employed are all nonbehavioral objective types of procedures should immediately raise the question of whether pure tone testing was attempted, what this youngster's developmental age might be, and so on. The mere knowledge of the difference between what is behavioral and what is not can quickly guide you and assist in establishing your differential diagnosis.

Is There a Hearing Loss?

Whether there is the presence or absence of hearing loss, of any degree or type, must be ascertained. Speech-language services should not commence until you know the answer to this question, and the questions that follow should a hearing loss exist. If there is no hearing loss, yet there is still concern about speech-language development, a referral for a complete audiologic evaluation should be made because there are many etiologies for progressive and late onset hearing loss. Do not let the fact that a child may have passed a newborn infant hearing screening create a false sense of security regarding hearing status.

What Are the Type and Degree of Hearing Loss?

Assuming you have established that your patient has a hearing impairment, what is the nature of the hearing loss? Is it conductive, sensorineural, or mixed? What is the degree? Remember, especially in the case of children, a slight or mild degree of hearing loss does not equate with a slight or mild communication impairment. Refer back to the appropriate sections to review information about each of these categories and characteristics.

What Are the Speech Audiometry Findings?

You have determined the nature and the severity of the hearing loss for this patient. Look now at the results of speech audiometry, and consider the following questions:

- What is the SRT? Is it in agreement with the PTA?
- If an SRT could not be obtained and an SDT was obtained instead, why?
- What is the WDT score in each ear, and at what dB presentation level was the test performed?
- Does the presentation level of WDT and the score obtained make sense based on the pure tone findings?
- Look at the WDT score one ear at a time and together. Knowing that these scores represent the best possible speech discrimination skills, what does it say about this patient's potential communication ability?
- Was the WDT test done with the addition of background noise? If so, what are the findings (i.e., will this patient have additional difficulties in noisy settings)? If so, what additional accommodations might need to be made?
- Is there a normal or restricted dynamic range for speech? For a normal hearing person, the value is typically no less than 100 dB. In the presence of a hearing loss, this range can be significantly reduced. View the UCL level and subtract the SRT value. Does the patient have a very narrow difference between the softest level for speech (SRT) and the threshold of discomfort (UCL)? The reader should note that there is a considerable variability in the definition of the term "narrow," as it is based on subjective measures. A key factor may be the complaint that hearing aid use is difficult and/or a report of a low tolerance for loud sounds.

Now look at the MCL for speech. In the presence of normal hearing sensitivity, the MCL should fall between 45 dB HL and 55 dB HL (with only minimal variability). The MCL value will increase in dB HL with the presence of hearing loss. However, if the MCL and UCL are in close dB level of each other, the patient may again experience difficulty in using amplification successfully.

What Are the Diagnostic Findings for the Outer Ear?

The initial consideration might involve the results of visual inspection of the pinna: Are there any malformations or abnormalities; such as, atresia, microtia, ear tags or keloids? What are the results of otoscopy? Is there any indication of excessive wax or other foreign body in the ear canals? Is there a pressure equalization tube visible in the ear canal or tympanic membrane? Has the tympanic membrane been visualized? Were any abnormalities noted in its appearance? If the diagnostic findings show evidence of the possibility of any outer ear pathology, has a medical/otologic referral been recommended?

What Are the Diagnostic Findings for the Middle Ear?

When considering diagnostically significant findings related to the middle ear, how do they relate to the results of the otoscopy? Is there any indication that there is perhaps occluding or partially occluding cerumen, a perforation of the eardrum, a meniscus (fluid line) visible on the eardrum, bulging and/or pus-filled outer/middle ear, or the like? These otoscopy findings will manifest themselves in the tympanometry results as well.

What do the results of tympanometry reveal? What type or configuration of tympanogram is reflected in the report? Is it a type A, As, Ad, C, or B? Do the tympanometry findings corroborate the presence of either a conductive or mixed hearing loss? Any abnormal tympanometric findings, individually or in combination with abnormal otoscopy results, can indicate the possibility of middle ear pathology and a recommendation for a medical/otologic examination should have been made in the report.

Do tympanometry results match the audiogram? Normal (type A tympanograms) tympanometric findings are associated with normal hearing and sensorineural hearing loss; whereas abnormal tympanometric results are associated with conductive and mixed types of hearing loss.

Are There Other Nonbehavioral Diagnostic Findings, and If So, Do They Match the Audiogram?

Are there other audiometric findings, such as OAEs, acoustic reflexes, ABR? Each of these procedures may potentially add significant diagnostic information. Carefully review the audiogram, the evaluation report (if supplied), and any other information provided and then refer to the appropriate section of this chapter for additional guidance.

What Is the Reported Reliability?

Each time the patient is tested, the audiologist should make a statement regarding the reliability of behavioral results. This information is very important and—in and of itself—may provide valuable insight into the patient. When reliability is judged to be very good, this tells us that the examiner trusts the information obtained. Conversely, if reliability is poor, one must then look further. For example, if a patient is a young child or a child with multiple disabilities, has further testing been recommended (e.g., additional test sessions, sedated diagnostic ABR study, and the like)? If a patient is an adult with poor reliability, one must also investigate why this is possibly the case. Such reasons might include pseudohypacusis (see the following section), multiple impairments, developmental delays, and so on.

Pseudohypacusis

Pseudohypacusis is one of many terms used to refer to a false or exaggerated hearing loss; that is, one that is not organic in nature. The numerous terms used that can be found in the literature may reflect the many reasons why a person might present with a hearing loss, either wittingly

or not, when a loss does not exist. Some of the other terms found include *nonorganic hearing loss*, *psychogenic hearing loss*, *malingering*, and *functional hearing loss*. Regardless of the reasons why this type of hearing loss might exist—a topic that is interesting but beyond the scope of this chapter—it is critical that the audiologist and SLP be alert to the signs that a true organic hearing loss might not exist or at least not to the degree shown. There are many indicators of pseudohypacusis; we will discuss some of them in this section.

An alert clinician will be able to glean much diagnostically useful information before the actual testing procedures begin. Some mannerisms frequently observed in such cases are exaggerated difficulty hearing during the case history interview, such as leaning one's ear in toward the audiologist speaking, squinting of the eyes, or frequently asking "huh" or "what." Alternatively, the patient may not appear to experience difficulty communicating during the interview process, but may present with a significant handicapping hearing loss during behavioral testing. Either way, there is an unexplained discrepancy. Another red flag is whether the individual is anxious to have insurance or disability paperwork completed by the examiner.

Results of behavioral audiometry can also provide strong indications of pseudohypacusis. For example, if the pure tone responses are inexplicably poorer than the results of speech audiometry (SRT and/or WDT scores), pseudohypacusis should be strongly suspected (refer to **Figure 9.23**). Similarly, if a person claims not to be able to respond to pure tones until a very intense 100 dB HL, but then is able to repeat back words (for WDT) with excellent accuracy when the words are presented at the much lower average conversational level of 50 dB HL, a case of pseudohypacusis must be suspected. Another indication that this type of condition may be present is when a person shows normal hearing in one ear and a total loss of hearing in the other ear, *before* the masking process has been performed (**Figure 9.24**). This would not be possible, because cross-hearing/crossover would occur. In a *real* case of normal hearing in one ear with a profound hearing loss in the other ear, hearing test results before masking (refer back to Figure 9.12) would show a shadow curve. Additionally, these individuals will also frequently show very poor test–retest reliability; that is, the results obtained from one session may be significantly different from those obtained even 1 hour later.

Other indications of pseudohypacusis include differences between the behavioral and nonbehavioral test results. For

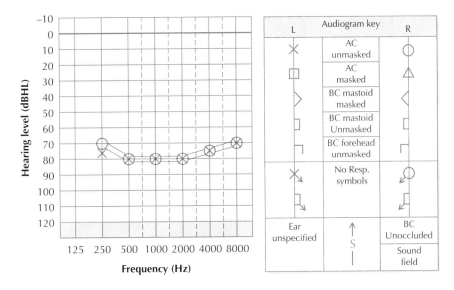

Figure 9.23 An audiogram illustrating an example of pseudohypacusis. Notice the inconsistency between the pure tone averages and the results of SRT and WRT testing.

example, if a patient is volitionally showing a severe to profound hearing loss in both ears when tested using pure tones, and then the OAEs are all completely within normal limits and the ABR is also normal, pseudohypacusis must immediately be suspected.

A number of tests can be done proving the presence of pseudohypacusis. Frequently, when a false or exaggerated hearing loss is suspected a clinician will turn to the nonbehavioral measures such as the OAE and ABR; however, there are several behavioral test techniques specifically

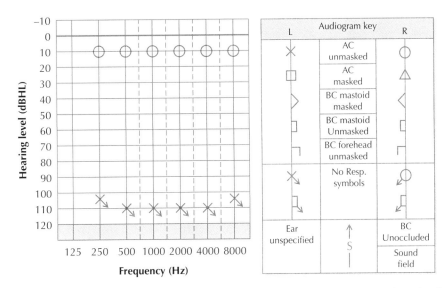

Figure 9.24 An audiogram illustrating another example of pseudohypacusis. Notice the lack of a shadow curve before masking has been performed.

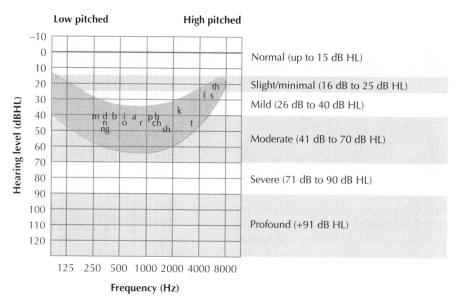

Figure 9.25   The speech banana audiogram, charting the typical frequency and intensity locations of the phonemes of speech.

designed for this purpose, relegated to the practice of audiology, that can provide the information necessary to establish that the hearing loss has a nonorganic cause.

Whenever there is the suspicion of pseudohypacusis, or the results do not appear to make sense for whatever reason, a referral is essential.

Counseling with Your Audiogram

A comprehensive presentation of the role of the communication disorders specialist in counseling is far beyond the scope of this chapter; some of the components of the counseling process include psychosocial support, individual and family counseling, and assertiveness training in addition to the need for informational counseling and guidance. We strongly encourage all SLPs and audiologists to further explore this area on their own. Nevertheless, this is a very appropriate time to point out that the audiogram itself may be very instrumental in the informational portion of the counseling process. The following sections present two tools that the SLP may find useful when working with patients and their families and loved ones.

Speech Banana Audiogram

One of the methods used to convey the significance and impact of a person's hearing loss is to use the **speech banana**

audiogram (see Figure 9.25), which is a typical audiogram with a shaded banana-shaped area on it that is positioned in such a way as to represent the *approximate* frequency and intensity of most common speech sounds. Some professionals find it useful to superimpose a patient's hearing test results onto this type of audiogram to visually explain the impact the hearing loss will have on his or her ability to hear normal conversational speech. When the Xs and Os of the audiogram fall well above the banana-shaped area, the person should be hearing speech sounds comfortably. However, if the Xs and Os fall below, this suggests that the sounds of average-level conversational speech are inaudible to him or her.

Familiar Sounds Audiogram

Like the speech banana audiogram, the **familiar sounds audiogram** (see Figure 9.26) is another tool that may be used to help explain to patients and their families what kind of impact the hearing loss may have on their ability to function and respond to sounds that are routinely encountered in everyday life. Although the placement of the objects on the familiar sounds audiogram is *approximate*, the form is a very useful tool, particularly when dealing with a patient who has been newly diagnosed with hearing impairment. It may be desirable to use a form that contains both familiar sounds and the speech banana. An example of this type of audiogram is shown is Figure 9.27.

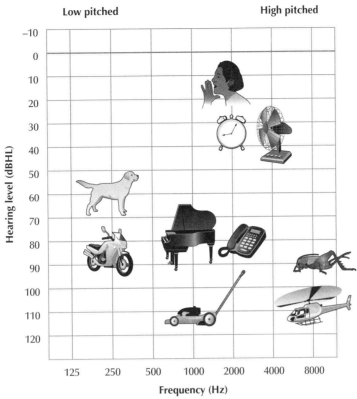

Figure 9.26 An example of a familiar sounds audiogram, displaying the approximate frequency and intensity of several everyday sounds.

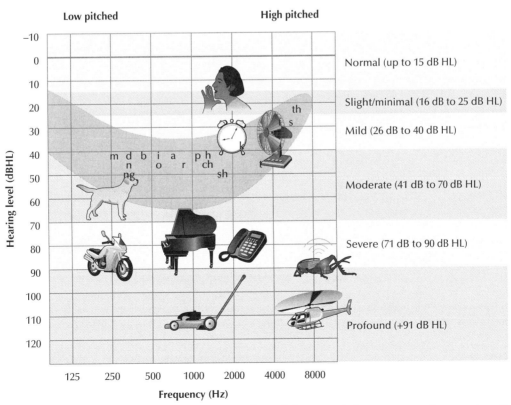

Figure 9.27 An audiogram with both familiar sounds and the speech banana superimposed on it.

Summary

In this chapter we have described the results of the evaluation process: typical results and their interpretation. It bears repeating that the most comprehensive picture of an individual's functional ability can be obtained only by reviewing the results in their entirety. The SLP must have a secure understanding of how to go about the process of interpreting the information in order to best understand the implications and appropriately utilize the information in the implementation of intervention strategies.

It is important to reiterate that the goal of this particular chapter is to help the SLP gain a secure and comfortable understanding of the test results and their implications. If the test results don't make sense to you, find an audiologist with whom you can network. If your interpretation of the results has left you with more questions than answers, *do not* proceed with inaccurate information or results that you either don't understand or with which you do not feel confident. Inaccurate results and/or misdiagnoses happen; although we hope they are infrequent, they do occur.

Discussion Questions

1. A child is referred to you by his kindergarten teacher. She indicates that an audiological evaluation was recently completed (within 1 month), revealing a mild sensorineural hearing loss. Describe some behaviors that the teacher should expect from such a student. What are some questions you would ask the parents of this child?

2. What are the reliability measures between pure tone audiometry and speech audiometry that you should always double check?

3. If a child has a moderate conductive hearing loss based on pure tone and speech audiometry, what findings would you expect to see for tympanometry? For otoacoustic emissions?

4. Why would the familiar sounds audiogram and the speech banana be useful counseling tools for the speech-language pathologist?

5. You have received an audiological report and attached audiogram from an unknown clinical facility. Your personal clinical judgment tells you that two of the test results just don't corroborate each other. Hypothetically, choose those two measures. Why don't they make sense? What is your next step?

References

Alencar, A. P. T., Iorio, M. C. M., & Morales, D. S. (2005). Equivalent volume: Study in subjects with chronic otitis media. *Brazilian Journal of Otorhinolaryngology,* 71(5): 644–648.

American Academy of Audiology (AAA). (2008). *Effort aims to curb number of kids who suffer from noise-induced hearing loss.* Available from http://www.audiology.org/news/pr/pages/pr20080116.aspx.

American Speech-Language-Hearing Association. (1988). *Determining threshold level for speech.* Available from http://www.asha.org/policy.

American Speech-Language-Hearing Association. (1990). Guidelines for audiometric symbols. *ASHA, 32*(Suppl. 2): 25–30.

American Speech-Language-Hearing Association. (1999). *Joint audiology committee clinical practice statements and algorithms.* Available from http://www.asha.org/policy.

Anderson, K., & Matkin, N. (1991). *Relationship of long term hearing loss to psychosocial impact and educational needs, revised 2007.* Available from http://successforkidswithhearingloss.com/uploads/SIFTER.pdf

Brackenbury, T., Ryan, T., & Messenheimer, T. (2006). Incidental word learning in a hearing impaired child of deaf adults. *Journal of Deaf Studies and Deaf Education,* 11(1): 76–93.

Brandy, W. T. (2002). Speech audiometry. In Katz, J. (ed.), *Handbook of clinical audiology* (5th ed., pp. 96–110). Baltimore: Lippincott, Williams and Wilkins.

Brannstrom, K. J., & Lantz, J. (2010). Interaural attenuation for Sennheiser HDA 200 circumaural earphones. *International Journal of Audiology,* 49: 467–471.

Center for Disease Control and Prevention (2013). *Noise induced hearing loss.* Available from: http://www.cdc.gov/healthyyouth/noise/

Clark, J. G. (1981). Uses and abuses of hearing loss classification. *ASHA,* 23: 493–500.

Felix-Trujillo, M. M., Valdez-Martinez, E., Ramirez, J. E., & Lozano-Morales, R. (2009). Surgical and medical treatment of hearing loss in mixed otosclerosis. *Annals of Otology, Rhinology & Laryngology,* 118(12): 859–865.

Finitzo-Hieber, T., & Tillman, T. W. (1978). Room acoustics effects on monosyllabic word discrimination ability for normal and hearing-impaired children. *Journal of Speech and Hearing Research,* 21(3): 440–458.

George, P, Farrell, T. W., & Griswold, M. F. (2012). Hearing loss: Help for the young and old. *Journal of Family Practice,* 61(5): 268–277.

Goldberg, L. R., & Richburg, C. M. (2004). Minimal hearing impairment: Major myths with more than minimal implications. *Communication Disorders Quarterly,* 25(3): 152–160.

Hornsby, B. W. Y., & Ricketts, T. A. (2005). The effects of hearing loss on the contribution of high and low frequency speech information to speech understanding. II. Sloping hearing loss. *Journal of the Acoustical Society of America,* 119(3): 1752–1763.

Hoth, S., Polzer, M., Neumann, K., & Plinkert, P. (2007). TEOAE amplitude growth, detectability, and response threshold in linear and nonlinear mode and in different time windows. *International Journal of Audiology,* 46: 407–418.

Jerger, J. F. (1970). Clinical experience with impedance audiometry. *Archives of Otolaryngology,* 92: 311–324.

Joint Committee on Infant Hearing. (2007). *Year 2007 position statement: Principles and guidelines for early detection and intervention.* Available from http://www.asha.org/policy.

Jubas, K. (2011). Everyday scholars: Framing informal learning in terms of academic disciplines and skills. *Adult Education Quarterly,* 61(3): 225–243.

Levey, S., Fligor, B. J. H., Ginocchi, C., & Kagimbi, L. (2012). The effects of noise-induced hearing loss on children and young adults. *Contemporary Issues in Communication Science and Disorders,* 39: 76–83.

Liden, G. (1969). The scope and application of current audiometric tests. *Journal of Laryngology and Otology,* 83: 507–520.

Margolis, R. H., & Hunter, L. L. (2000). Acoustic immittance measurements. In R. J. Roeser, M. Valente, and H. Hosford-Dunn (eds.), *Audiology diagnosis* (pp. 381–423). New York: Thieme.

Martin, F. N., & Clark, J. G. (2012). *Introduction to audiology* (11th ed.). Boston: Pearson Education.

National Institute on Deafness and Other Communication Disorders (NIDCD). (1997). *Presbycusis.* NIH Pub. No. 97-4235. Available from http://www.nidcd.nih.gov/health/hearing/Pages/presbycusis.aspx.

National Institute on Deafness and Other Communication Disorders (NIDCD). (2002). *Noise-induced hearing loss.* NIH Pub. No. 97-4233. Available from http://www.nidcd.nih.gov/health/hearing/pages/noise.aspx.

Neuman, A. C., Wroblewski, M., & Rubinstein, A. (2010). Combined effects of noise and reverberation on speech recognition performance of normal-hearing children and adults. *Ear and Hearing,* 31(3): 336–344.

Pennings, R. J. E., Gulliver, M., & Morris, D. P. (2011). The importance of an extended preoperative trial of BAHA in unilateral sensorineural hearing loss: A prospective cohort study. *Clinical Otolaryngology,* 36: 442–449.

Penrod, J. P. (1994). Speech threshold and word recognition/discrimination testing. In Katz, J. (ed.), *Handbook of clinical audiology* (4th ed., pp. 147–164). Baltimore: Williams and Wilkins.

Robinson, J. D., Baer, T., & Moore, C. J. (2007). Using transposition to improve consonant discrimination and detection for listeners with severe high-frequency hearing loss. *International Journal of Audiology,* 46: 293–308.

Rothpletz, A. M., Wightman, R. L., & Kistler, D. J. (2012). Self-monitoring of listening abilities in normal-hearing children, normal-hearing adults, and children with cochlear implants. *Journal of the American Academy of Audiology,* 23(3): 206–221.

Roup, C. M., & Noe, C. M. (2009). Hearing aid outcomes for listeners with high-frequency hearing loss. *American Journal of Audiology,* 18: 45–52.

Ruscetta, M. N., Arjmand, E. M., & Pratt, S. R. (2005). Speech recognition abilities in noise for children with severe-to-profound unilateral hearing impairment. *International Journal of Pediatric Otorhinolaryngology,* 69(6): 771–779.

Schmuziger, N., Patscheke, J., & Probst, R. (2006). Automated pure-tone threshold estimations from extrapolated distortion product otoacoustic emissions (DPOAE) input/output functions. *Journal of the Acoustical Society of America,* 119(4): 1937–1939.

Schow, R. L., & Nerbonne, M. A. (2007). *Introduction to audiologic rehabilitation* (5th ed.). Boston: Pearson Education.

Yoshinaga-Itano, C. (2008). Outcomes of children with mild bilateral hearing loss and unilateral hearing loss. *Seminars in Hearing,* 29(2): 196–211.

Chapter 10

Hearing Aids and Hearing Assistance Technology for Children and Adults

Donna M. Goione Merchant, AuD
Private Practice Audiologist
Assistant Professor, Montclair State University, Montclair, NJ

Key Terms

Assistive listening devices (ALDs)

Behind-the-ear (BTE) hearing aid

Bone-anchored hearing aid (BAHA)

Captioned telephone (CapTel)

Cochlear implant

Completely-in-canal (CIC) hearing aid

Direct audio input (DAI)

Hearing assistance technology (HAT)

In-the-ear (ITE) hearing aid

Invisible-in-canal (IIC) hearing aid

Middle ear implant (MEI)

Telecoil

Text telephone (TTY)/ telecommunication device for the deaf (TDD)

Objectives

- Gain a historical perspective of hearing aids from pre-electric to digital devices.
- Identify the different styles of hearing aids available to address hearing loss including devices worn on the ear, in the ear, and those that are surgically implanted
- Illustrate the tools needed to troubleshoot and maintain hearing aids
- Identify appropriate use of additional assistive and alerting devices
- Identify the specialized listening devices available for classroom instruction

Introduction

Hearing loss presents communication challenges across many listening conditions and to varying degrees. The impact of a hearing loss on an individual's ability to function day to day will vary from person to person and situation to situation. Because each person is unique in how he or she will cope with hearing loss, many factors should be considered in order to determine the appropriate interventions needed to improve a person's function and quality of life. These factors include skills related to communication, social interaction, independent functional capacity, vocational needs, and academic needs. Further consideration should include general safety and alerts to one's auditory environment.

First and foremost in this process is the purchase of hearing aids. These devices provide personal amplification to address the specific configuration and severity of hearing loss. The style of the hearing aid—behind the ear or in the ear; large or small; analog or digital signal processing; large device controls, regular controls, or no controls at all; large batteries or small; and whether the battery compartment is easily accessible or locked—are just a few considerations that need to be taken into account by the hearing aid dispenser or audiologist during the hearing aid fitting process. The more thorough this process is, the higher the likelihood that the patient will be happy with the device(s). The first step to being a *happy* hearing aid user is *to be* a hearing aid user. Unfortunately, when this process is not done with fortitude, hearing aids remain in their boxes, on dressers, or in drawers, providing none of the intended benefit.

Hearing aid technology is just one option for managing a hearing loss. In many instances, and in specific situations, additional assistance is needed to help a person manage his or her auditory environment. A myriad of hearing assistance and altering technologies are available to help in special and often very specific situations. These devices can be used directly attached to hearing aids or as accompanying devices.

Historical Background

Perhaps the first hearing aid in use was the hand cupped behind the ear. This "aid" to hearing is still in use today, and sometimes is the preferred method of amplification for some. Early pre-electric devices to aid in the enhancement of sound can be traced back to the seventeenth century. Ear trumpets and cones of the day were designed to rest above the ear and collect and transmit sound to the ear canal.

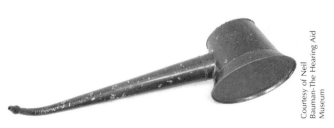

Courtesy of Neil Bauman-The Hearing Aid Museum

Figure 10.1 The Dipper Ear Trumpet, circa 1880, was 16 1/2 inches long and looked like a water barrel dipper, hence its name. It was known as the power aid of its time.

Through the following centuries, this method of collecting sound and channeling it to the ear via a tube was a common design. Devices ranging from larger tabletop units to ear trumpets and cones (**Figures 10.1** through **10.3**) can be traced through the Victorian era. At the time, society placed a great importance on hiding hearing loss, because it was seen as a disability (Healthy Hearing, 2011).

The second industrial revolution greatly changed the face of technology around the world. Hearing aids were no exception to technological advancements during this time period. Famous for his invention of the telephone,

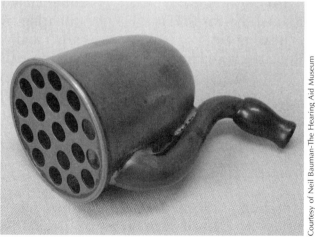

Courtesy of Neil Bauman-The Hearing Aid Museum

Figure 10.2 The Tiny London Dome, circa 1900, was 2 1/2 inches in size and named for St. Paul's Cathedral in London, because it was thought to have the same shape as the cathedral's dome. It was designed to fit in the palm of the hand while holding it up to the ear, so it would be "invisible."

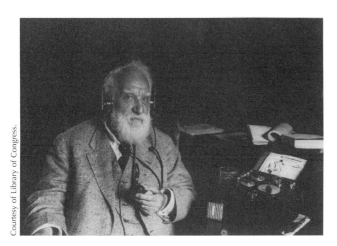

Courtesy of Neil Bauman-The Hearing Aid Museum

Figure 10.3 The traditional ear trumpet, circa 1900, measured 15 inches long.

Alexander Graham Bell (**Figure 10.4**) played a pivotal role in the invention of the hearing aid. Bell's grandfather, father, and brother worked in the study of elocution and clarity of speech, which culminated in some of the earliest publications regarding the correction of speech disorders. The invention of the phonetic alphabet is attributed to Melville Bell, Alexander's father. Alexander Graham Bell's wife and mother were both deaf. Bell's preoccupation with his mother's deafness led him to the study of acoustics. It was Bell's early work in the amplification of sound and manipulation of intensity and frequency that eventually led to the invention of the telephone. Many regard Bell's invention of the telephone to be the result of seeking to amplify the hearing ability of his beloved wife and his mother (Winefield, 1987). The Alexander Graham Bell Association for the Deaf and Hard of Hearing, located in Washington, D.C., continues to support individuals with hearing loss and their families today.

Advancements by another famous inventor of the time, Thomas Edison (**Figure 10.5**), brought the world closer to the invention of the electric hearing aid. Although not deaf himself, he was quoted as stating, "I have not heard a bird sing since I was 12 years old." In contrast to Bell, Edison saw

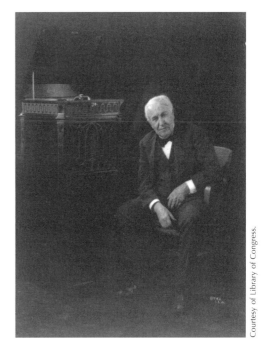

Courtesy of Library of Congress.

Figure 10.5 Thomas Alva Edison.

his hearing loss as an advantage, allowing him to concentrate on his inventions by blocking out what he referred to as "the babble of ordinary conversation" (National Park Service, 2013). It was Edison's invention of the carbon transmitter, which, used in combination with an electric current, transformed a weaker signal into a stronger signal, thus paving the way for an electronic device to amplify sound.

Several companies, including George P. Pilling and Sons of Philadelphia and Kirchner and Wilhelm of Stuttgart, Germany, combined the technologies from Bell and Edison to produce devices that amplified sound for individuals with hearing loss. In 1898, the Dictograph Company, also the inventors of the classic-style rotary phone, introduced the first commercial carbon-type hearing aid. In 1899, Miller Reese Hutchison, working for Akouphone in Alabama, patented the first practical electrical hearing aid, which used a carbon transmitter and battery. This aid for the hearing impaired was so cumbersome that it had to sit on a table. It sold for $400 (Watson, 2013) (Miller, 2011).

In an effort to reduce the weight of hearing aid devices, the vacuum tube hearing aid was introduced during the 1920s. These units were smaller and lighter, making them easier to carry. As manufacturers were able to create smaller vacuum tubes, hearing aids also could be reduced in size. By the end of World War II and the late 1940s, more advances in hearing

Courtesy of Library of Congress.

Figure 10.4 Dr. Alexander Graham Bell.

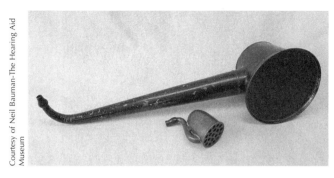

Figure 10.6 Tiny London dome and dipper size comparison.

technology were emerging, and hearing aids continued to be reduced in size for wearability. Transistors replaced vacuum tubes in hearing aids, and improvements to hearing aid function and structure continued (Mills, 2011).

Vanity Thy Name Is Hearing Aid

The inherent desire by many to hide hearing loss has had a significant influence on hearing aid manufacturing. Even with pre-electric devices, trumpets and domes were designed with size and "invisibility" in mind (see Figure 10.6).

This desire for invisibility drove advances in electronic hearing aids through the twentieth century as well. During the middle part of the century, once technological advances reduced the size of electric devices from the top of the table to the top of the ear, the push to create a smaller, less visible hearing aid sparked the creation of some fascinating devices (Figures 10.7 through 10.9). Multiple options were offered, including hiding the devices in clothing and accessories. Attempts were even made to hide hearing aids in pieces of furniture.

For individuals with a significant degree of hearing loss, the microphone and receiver had to be placed sufficiently apart

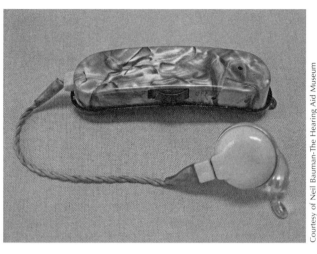

Figure 10.8 Faux pearl barrette-style hearing aid.

to decrease feedback (a high-pitched whistling sound) caused when the two are placed in close proximity during high levels of amplification. Although not as cosmetically appealing, the body aid became the common style of hearing aid for severe and profound hearing losses (Figures 10.10 and 10.11). Attempts were made to create camouflaged cases for these devices, in the form of a woman's pressed powder make-up compact and flesh-toned case appropriately sized to fit inside a man's shirt pocket (Figure 10.12).

Analog Technology

The development of the microprocessor during the 1970s made it possible to consider miniaturizing the circuitry for wearable hearing aids (Mills, 2011). From this point to the

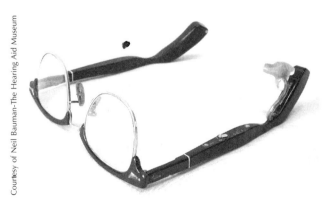

Figure 10.7 Eyeglass-style hearing aid.

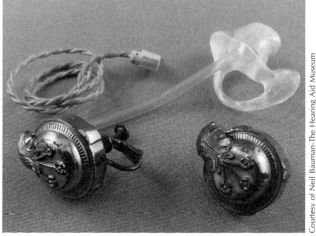

Figure 10.9 Hearing aids made into earrings.

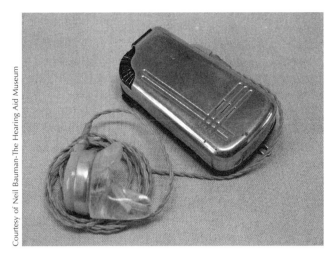

Courtesy of Neil Bauman-The Hearing Aid Museum

Figure 10.10   Metal cased body-style hearing aid.

present, the technological advances came at a rapid pace. Conventional analog hearing aids were the primary device of choice through the late twentieth century. These devices were manufactured with circuitry that provided amplification based on the person's degree of hearing loss. Hearing aid manufacturers/distributors would provide large notebooks with the specifications of each hearing aid produced by their company. Hearing aids were selected based on manufacturer, then on specifications of gain (volume), output (maximum power of the aid, also known as SSPL90), and frequency response (adding and subtracting base and treble sounds). Potentiometers (small dials inside of the devices) allowed for adjustment and minor changes in the amount of volume, SSPL90, and frequency response by the professional fitting the device for the comfort of the user.

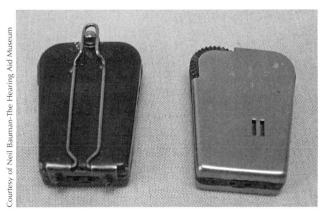

Courtesy of Neil Bauman-The Hearing Aid Museum

Figure 10.11   Body-style hearing aid with clip for placement in hair or pocket.

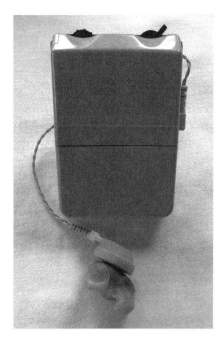

Figure 10.12   Plastic flesh tone body-style hearing aid.

Digital Technology

Bell Telephone Laboratories introduced digital hearing aid technology, the current technology used today, during the early 1960s. The ability to digitize a sound wave and analyze it via a computer chip for clarity and specificity made the technology very desirable for hearing aid manufacturers. However, due to the physical space needed to house the technology, the overall size of a digital system was not practical at the time to fit into wearable hearing aids. A second drawback to the technology was a slight but noticeable time delay while the digital signal was being processed through the computer chip.

By the 1980s, a fully digital hearing aid encompassing real-time processing technology was invented. It was not until 1987, however, that the first commercially available digital hearing aid was introduced. This was a body-worn hearing aid that required an earpiece connection. Customers viewed this style as a flashback to the technology of the 1950s. Although not well received by consumers, it allowed other hearing aid manufacturers to develop systems that would be more aesthetically appealing to the public. By 1989, the first behind-the-ear digital hearing aid was introduced. Since that time, numerous advancements and improvements have been incorporated into the hearing aids, with the first fully digital behind-the-ear (BTE) style hearing aid being introduced for research in 1995. Demand for this product was so strong that the first fully digital BTE hearing aid was commercially available one year later in 1996 (Healthy Hearing, 2011).

Conventional Hearing Aids

Personal hearing amplification defines both hearing aids and implantable devices. Conventional hearing aids are considered personal listening devices that provide frequency-based amplification to manage hearing loss. These devices are customized to address the specifics of an individual's hearing loss once it has been determined by an audiologic evaluation and are commercially available for purchase through dispensing audiologists, hearing aid dispensers, and (although not encouraged by this text) even mail order. Implantable devices (discussed later in this chapter) are obtained through medical facilities via consultation with otolaryngology/otology practices and in consultation with an audiologist (National Institute on Deafness and Other Communication Disorders [NIDCD], 2007).

Hearing aids are made up of three primary parts: a microphone, an amplifier, and a receiver or speaker. Sound from an individual's environment enters the microphone. The microphone then changes the sound's energy into a form that the amplifier can recognize. The amplifier, which connects to a speaker, takes the information from the microphone, processes and amplifies the sound, and sends it to the receiver, which in turn channels the amplified sound into the ear (NIDCD, 2007). Hearing aids use batteries as their energy source.

Conventional Hearing Aid Styles

The styles of devices in common use today vary greatly from the hearing aids used in the mid-twentieth century. Devices of the twenty-first century include a variety of options in terms of size and capability to more efficiently address the personal needs of the individual with hearing loss.

Behind-the-Ear (BTE) Hearing Aids

Behind-the-ear (BTE) hearing aids are devices that are worn over the top of the ear. All components of the BTE hearing aid are housed in the casing that sits on the ear. An ear hook on the top of the hearing aid is connected to an earpiece called an earmold that is placed into the ear canal (**Figure 10.13**). An earmold is custom molded to the specific shape of the individual's ear dimensions. Plastic tubing runs through the earmold and is then attached to the earhook of the hearing aid.

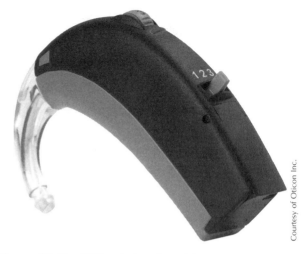

Courtesy of Oticon Inc.

Figure 10.13 BTE style hearing aid.

Sound travels from the hearing aid through the earhook, tubing, and earmold and into the ear. Earmold shapes are chosen with specific consideration given to the severity and configuration of a hearing loss. For example, an individual with a severe to profound hearing loss may need an earmold that fills the entire concha of the ear, whereas a less severe hearing loss may have a more open concha area (**Figure 10.14**).

In some cases, the BTE hearing aid is connected to a thin tube, which may have a small plastic dome on the end that sits in the ear canal. This alternative type of BTE is called a receiver-in-the-ear (RITE)/receiver in canal (RIC) (**Figure 10.15**).This unit removes the receiver component of the hearing aid from the enclosed casing and places it at the end of thin tubing. A dome is placed over the receiver, which sits just inside the entrance to the ear canal.

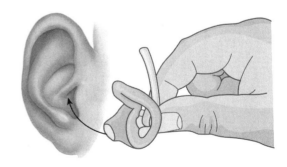

Figure 10.14 Proper earmold insertion.

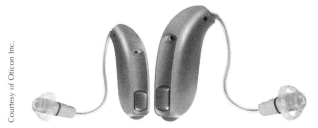

Courtesy of Oticon Inc.

Figure 10.15   RITE (RIC) style BTE hearing aid.

In-the-Ear(ITE) Hearing Aids

In-the-ear (ITE) hearing aids are custom molded to fit the shape of the individual's ear. These are one-piece amplification devices with all components housed in a hard shell shaped to the contours of the individual's ear. Three styles of ITE hearing aids are available based on the hearing aid user's degree of hearing loss and cosmetic preference. The first device fills the entire concha portion of the outer ear completely and is generally referred to as a full-shell ITE (Figure 10.16). The second ITE, referred to as a half-shell, fills only half of the concha portion of the outer ear (Figure 10.17). The third device, referred to as an in-the-canal (ITC) aid, is smaller than the half-shell device and can only be seen in the opening of the concha (Figure 10.18).

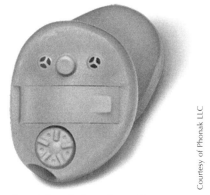

Courtesy of Phonak LLC

Figure 10.18   ITC-style hearing aid.

Completely-in-Canal (CIC) and Invisible-in-Canal (IIC) Hearing Aids

Completely-in-canal (CIC) and **invisible-in-canal (IIC) hearing aids** are also custom molded to fit the shape of the individual's ear; however, these are designed to be inserted deeper into the ear canal to be less noticeable. These devices are characterized by a small line of filament with an attached ball so that the user can grasp the ball between two fingernails to remove the device from its placement deep in the ear canal (Figures 10.19 and 10.20).

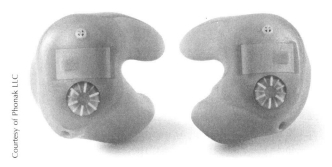

Courtesy of Phonak LLC

Figure 10.16   Full-shell ITE style hearing aid.

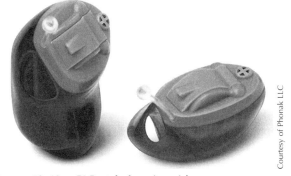

Courtesy of Phonak LLC

Figure 10.19   CIC-style hearing aid.

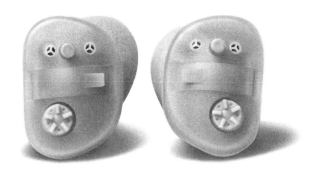

Courtesy of Phonak LLC

Figure 10.17   Half-shell ITE style hearing aid.

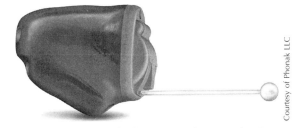

Courtesy of Phonak LLC

Figure 10.20   IIC-style hearing aid (note the longer filament than the CIC device).

Anatomy of a Conventional Hearing Aid

Conventional hearing aids have a variety of standard and special functions to allow flexibility in their sound enhancement capabilities as well as for maintenance and ease of use. These features give the hearing aid user options to manage the sound in a variety of situations, and can include power source options, on–off switches, volume controls, push-button controls, direct audio input circuitry, and telecoil circuitry.

Power Source Options

All hearing aids draw from a power source. This power source is in the form of button-style batteries that come in a variety of sizes. The larger the battery is, the greater potential power storage capacity and the longer it will last. Conversely, the smaller the battery, the less power and life it will have. Hearing aids that provide high levels of amplification, such as in the case of severe to profound hearing loss, will use larger #675 or #13 button batteries; devices designed for lesser degrees of hearing loss may use a smaller #312 or #10A battery. Larger BTE-style hearing aids can accommodate a larger battery size, whereas CIC or IIC devices will use only the smallest of batteries. Hearing aid button batteries are color coded based on their size—#675 are blue, #13 are orange, #312 are brown, and #10A are yellow. This color coding makes for ease of purchase and distinction between sizes. Conversely, button batteries for other devices such as watches and timers do not carry the same color coding.

A hearing aid user's ability to manipulate smaller size batteries should be taken into consideration during the hearing aid selection process. An older adult may want a cosmetically appealing hearing aid but may not have the dexterity to change very small batteries. For ease of management, some hearing aids come with a magnetic accessory tool to aid in manipulating small batteries (**Figure 10.21**).

Button battery safety should also be taken into consideration. All hearing aid batteries are small and round. So are many medications and types of favorite candy. If a hearing aid user (a small child, an individual with cognitive impairment, or those with low vision) is at possible risk for swallowing hearing aid batteries, a tamper-resistant battery door can be installed on the device on request. Button battery warning literature can also be provided to the guardian of a patient to heighten awareness to this risk.

On–Off Control Switch

An on–off control switch is an option that allows the user to manually turn the hearing aid on or off. These can be in the form of a small sliding switch or incorporated into a volume

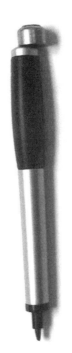

Figure 10.21   Battery magnet.

control wheel. In the case of many digital hearing aids, the on–off function is controlled by opening the battery door. When a hearing aid does not have an on–off switch, once a battery has been inserted the unit is turned on by closing the battery door. To turn off the hearing aid, the wearer opens the battery door to deactivate the battery.

Volume Control

A volume control allows the individual to raise or lower the overall volume of sound around them. This means both speech and background sounds are raised or lowered equally. These controls are sometimes found as a wheel on the hearing aid or in some cases they are a toggle switch. However, not all hearing aids have the option of a volume control. This typically depends on the size of the hearing aid and whether there is room internally for the circuitry.

Telecoil Circuitry

A **telecoil**, also referred to as a T-coil, is circuitry found inside many but not all hearing aids. This magnetic coil is designed to pick up and connect wirelessly to an external magnetic signal. Telecoils are most often found in the ITE- and BTE-style hearing aids; the smaller CIC styles typically do not have enough room to accommodate the circuitry. Activation of the T-coil can be through a switch on the hearing aid specifically designated for the T-coil feature (**Figure 10.22**) or by using a program button that has been

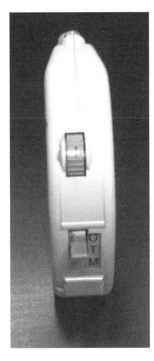

Figure 10.22   M-T-O switch on conventional BTE device.

activated when the aid is programmed through a computer at the time of dispensing (**Figure 10.23**) (Morris, 2011).

The telecoil was originally designed to make sounds clearer to the listener over the telephone, but it can now be used with multiple assistive listening devices when activating the magnetic hearing loop (or induction loop) of the device. The telecoil will pick up an electromagnetic signal only, in contrast to the hearing aid microphone, which picks up all sounds (Morris, 2001).

Direct Audio Input

Direct audio input (DAI) can be found in the form of cords that connect directly into the hearing aid, providing a direct

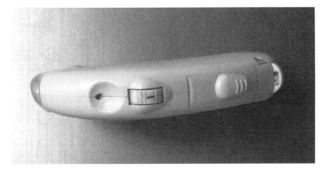

Figure 10.23   MTO press button on conventional BTE device (button has been programmed at the time of dispensing for T-coil functionality).

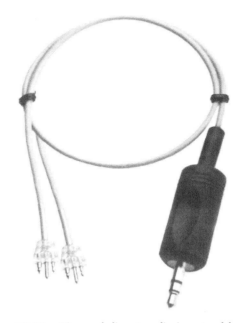

Figure 10.24   Binaural direct audio input cables.

audio cable connection between the hearing aid and an external auditory device (**Figure 10.24**). Such circuitry may also be included in many BTE hearing aids. It allows an external source or device to be connected directly to the hearing aid as an input that bypasses the microphone; for example, a hearing aid with DAI can allow direct access to a television, telephone, computer, CD player, microphone, or assistive listening device to allow a signal to be sent directly into the hearing aid. DAI is not available on smaller ITE, ITC, or CIC hearing aids, because these hearing aids are typically not large enough to accommodate the necessary circuitry.

The DAI connects with the aid through a special connection. The circuit connection can be found on the bottom of the hearing aid or on the back portion of the BTE case. Some hearing aids have a dedicated connection; others use a "boot" that is snapped onto the end of the aid and electronically connects the source to the aid through three tiny brass dots on the underside of the BTE.

The DAI boot (or other connector) may use a wire and a miniplug to plug into the audio source (Tye-Murray, 2009), or it may even have a tiny FM radio receiver attached to the boot with no wires required (**Figure 10.25**). The signal is typically improved because it goes directly into the hearing aid. Some hearing aids allow the microphone to be active along with the DAI. In some instances the hearing aid's microphone is disabled, thus eliminating the amplification and input of background noise. Continued activation of the microphone while the DAI circuitry is engaged allows the listener to access environmental information as a secondary input.

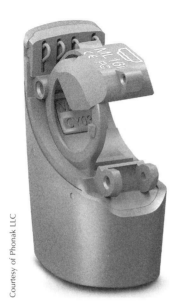

Courtesy of Phonak LLC

Figure 10.25 Direct audio input boot.

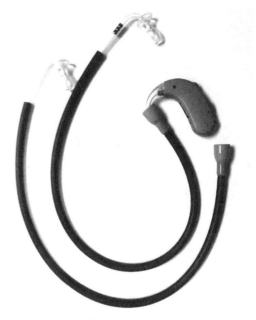

Figure 10.27 Listening tube.

Bluetooth Compatibility

Bluetooth technology is now being incorporated into many new hearing aids to allow wireless connectivity to a variety of Bluetooth-enabled devices. Hearing aid manufacturers provide different wireless options including remote control-type devices that allow audio output to stream from the device directly into an individual's hearing aid (Figure 10.26). With the appropriate devices, hearing aids without Bluetooth capability have the ability to connect to landline telephones, televisions, cell phones, computers, personal digital assistants (PDAs), and MP3 players and iPods.

Hearing Aid Care, Maintenance, and Troubleshooting

As with any other form of electronic assistive technology, a hearing aid must be in good working condition to be of benefit

to the user. Although an individual with hearing loss will hopefully already have amplification when he or she enters into a therapeutic relationship with a speech-language pathologist, in order for the hearing aids to benefit that individual they must be functioning appropriately. The assumption should never be made that a device or devices are working simply based on the fact that they are in the individual's ear(s).

Having the hearing aids present at a therapy session is only the first step in guaranteeing that they are in good working condition. Basic daily hearing aid maintenance can ensure that hearing aids are working properly and efficiently. There are several different cleaning and maintenance tools that can assist in monitoring the hearing aid's function and keeping hearing aids clean, free of debris and wax, and clear of moisture. These tools include the following:

- A hearing aid listening tube to listen to the hearing aid (Figure 10.27) A parent, guardian, or spouse with normal hearing should become accustomed to listening to the device's output. Signal distortion and static can be confounding factors to clear amplification.
- A hearing aid air blower to remove any moisture buildup in the earmold tubing or in the earmold itself, and to assure patency of the tubing (Figure 10.28)
- A battery tester to determine if the battery is good or has completely discharged (Figure 10.29)
- Wax removal tools to remove any cerumen or debris from the earmold of a BTE device or from the vent and/or receiver tube of an ITE device (Figure 10.30)

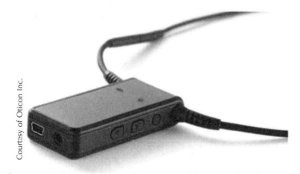

Courtesy of Oticon Inc.

Figure 10.26 Bluetooth connectivity: Amigo Arc.

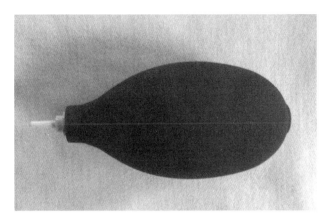

Figure 10.28   Hearing aid air blower.

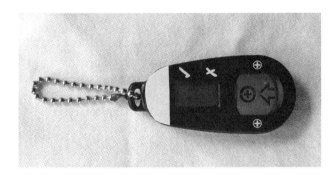

Figure 10.29   Hearing aid battery tester.

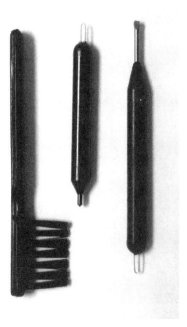

Figure 10.30   Hearing aid cleaning tools.

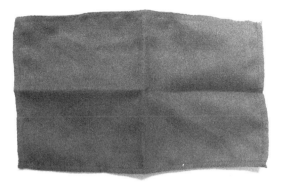

Figure 10.31   Microfiber cloth.

Only the tools provided by the hearing aid manufacturer should be used to clean ITE devices. Features of these tools, such as the loop of wire at the end of the wax removal tool, are specifically measured and designed so as not to do damage to any internal components of the device. The hearing aid user should always refer to the reading materials that accompany a device or are available from the manufacturer online for further instruction.

- A microfiber cloth can be used to remove any debris from the device itself. Hearing aids should never be washed with soap and water (Figure 10.31)
- A hearing aid dehumidifying kit removes moisture buildup from the circuitry of the hearing aid itself. This is especially important in humid climates or during the summer when the weather is warm. Because a hearing aid touches the body, it is subject to absorbing moisture from the body itself. Placing a hearing aid in a dehumidifier overnight draws the moisture from the device, significantly prolonging

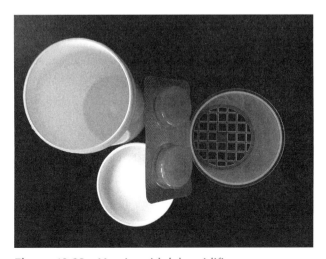

Figure 10.32   Hearing aid dehumidifier.

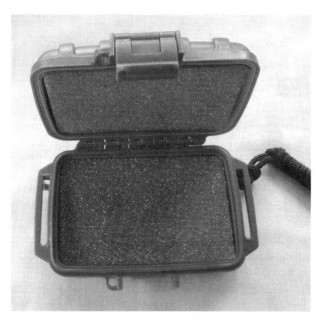

Figure 10.33 Waterproof hearing aid case.

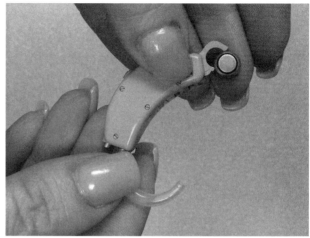

Figure 10.34 Changing the battery of a conventional BTE.

the life of the circuit board (**Figure 10.32**) Most hearing aid manufacturers recommend that the battery of the hearing aid be removed and the earmold of a BTE device be detached prior to placing the hearing aid into the dehumidifying unit.

- A waterproof storage box is another option for individuals who spend time involved in sports activities or around water (**Figure 10.33**). In many instances, hearing aids are removed when the user participates in sports (e.g., swim team) or other recreational activities. Cases can be attached to gym bags or backpacks as a visual reminder that hearing aids should be put away properly when not in the ear. Waterproof boxes are also sand-proof, which makes them a nice addition to the beach bag as well. Hard plastic construction makes it easy to put an individual's name and telephone number on the box in case it should become lost or misplaced.

Routine care and maintenance of hearing aids should be reinforced by the speech-language pathologist and in some cases may need to be retaught during the therapeutic sessions. However, it should ultimately become a responsibility of the patient or primary caretaker of the individual with hearing loss.

Troubleshooting

The speech-language pathologist working with a deaf or hard of hearing individual should be comfortable performing basic troubleshooting when a hearing aid is not functioning

properly. Although not every malfunction of a hearing aid can be anticipated, the following are common problems that may be encountered and can be resolved with some easy troubleshooting tips (see **Figures 10.34** through 10.42).

Common Problem: Hearing Aid Is Dead.

- Check for a dead battery. Replace if necessary.
- Earmold (BTE) or receiver tube (ITE) is completely blocked with cerumen or other matter. Remove wax with a wax-cleaning tool. Hairspray can also easily clog a microphone. Individuals should be advised to finish using all hair care products before putting their hearing aid on.

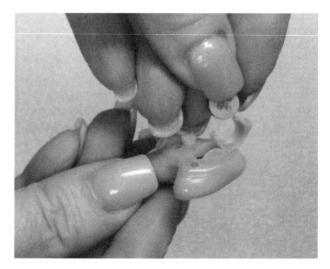

Figure 10.35 Changing the battery of a conventional ITE.

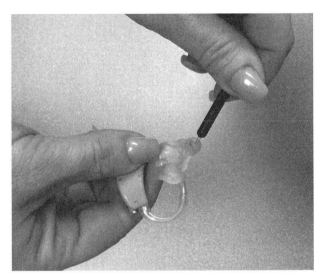

Figure 10.36 Cleaning an earmold with a wax loop.

Common Problem: Hearing Aid Is Emitting Feedback.

- Volume of the hearing aid is turned up too high. Review the recommended volume settings with the individual or guardian. Turn the volume down appropriately. If the hearing aid is programmable with no volume control, this conversation should take place with the audiologist or hearing aid dispenser.
- Earmold is not seated properly in the concha portion of the outer ear. Remove and reseat earmold.
- Earmold is too small for the ear. Children can grow out of their earmolds as quickly as every 3 months

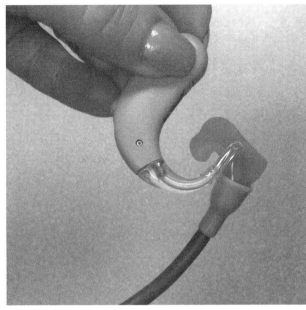

Figure 10.38 Listening to a BTE device.

during periods of extreme growth spurts. Older adults can lose the rigidity of the pinna, causing loosening of the fit. The individual must return to the audiologist or hearing aid dispenser to have new earmolds made or, in the case of an ITE, the device recased.

- Inspect earmold tubing/ear hook for cracks or holes. Tubing becomes stiff over time as it absorbs natural

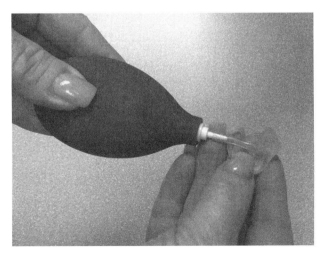

Figure 10.37 Hearing aid air blower cleaning moisture from earmold tubing.

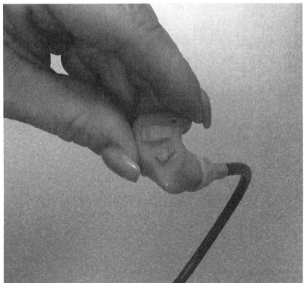

Figure 10.39 Listening to an ITE device.

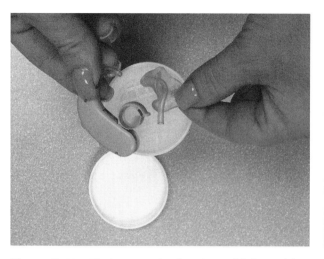

Figure 10.40 Placing a BTE in a hearing aid dehumidifier.

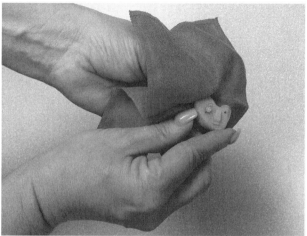

Figure 10.42 Cleaning the case of an ITE with a microfiber cloth.

oils from contact with skin. To determine if there is a crack or hole, place one finger over the receiver of the hearing aid or the hole at the end of the earmold. If the feedback continues, it suggests a hole somewhere in the earmold tubing or earhook. The individual must return to the audiologist or hearing aid dispenser to have the tubing replaced.

- Inspect the ITE casing for cracks. Over time the plastic housing of an ITE can become brittle and is subject to cracking. Again, place one finger over the receiver hole of the device. If the feedback continues, it suggests a crack in the casing. The individual must return to the audiologist or hearing aid dispenser to have the device recased.

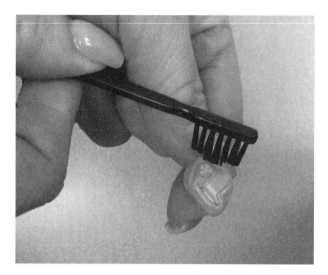

Figure 10.41 Cleaning an ITE with a cleaning brush.

Common Problem: Signal Is Distorted or Intermittent

- Inspect earmold for moisture buildup or partially occluding cerumen. Use an earmold hearing aid air blower to dry moisture buildup and/or a wax loop to remove cerumen. Hearing aid air blowers cannot be used on ITE devices, but the hearing aid should still be checked for cerumen, which should be removed if necessary.
- Use a listening tube to inspect signal clarity. On occasion, the individual may have complaints regarding the signal clarity, which may not be a problem with the hearing aid at all, but rather a change in hearing loss. If a problem with the signal cannot be identified by an unimpaired listener, the individual should immediately be referred back to his or her audiologist.
- If the complaint is persistent during hot and humid times of the year, recommend use of a hearing aid dehumidifier to draw moisture from the circuit board.

When counseling the individual with hearing loss and/or the family members, encourage daily cleaning and maintenance of the device(s) when they are removed from the ear(s).

External Bone Conduction Hearing Aids and Implantable Hearing Devices

A bone conduction hearing aid is a device that is considered preferable amplification when a conductive or mixed type of hearing loss (occurring due to disorders of the

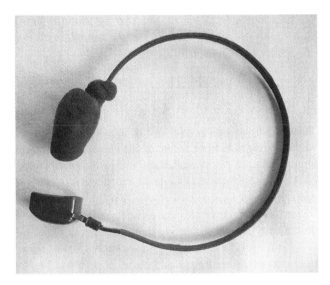

Figure 10.43 Bone conduction hearing aid.

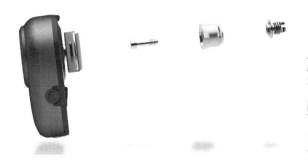

Figure 10.44 Bone-anchored hearing aid (BAHA).

inserted into the middle ear (Ross, 2000). For sensorineural hearing loss it delivers vibratory mechanical energy to the small bones (ossicular chain) located in the middle ear system and then sends mechanical energy to the cochlea at the round window via motion of the stapes. Devices for conductive or mixed hearing losses that involve damaged or a poorly functioning middle ear system send mechanical energy directly to the cochlea through direct bone conduction, circumventing the three tiny bones (ossicular chain) in the middle ear.

Cochlear Implants

Cochlear implants are surgically implanted devices that can enhance hearing and speech abilities for individuals with severe to profound hearing loss. More recently, these devices

middle ear) is identified and neural hearing (cochlear and beyond) is intact. This type of hearing aid bypasses the outer and middle ears, eliminating the need for an earmold. It can also address individuals with single-sided deafness/ unilateral hearing loss.

Headband-style bone conduction hearing aids (**Figure 10.43**) were frequently used in the mid-twentieth century, when middle ear infections were more common and very difficult to treat (Ross, 2000). Years ago, when a person had a problematic conductive (outer and/or middle ear) pathology that precluded the use of an earmold (perhaps due to drainage or atresia/microtia), a bone conduction (externally fit) hearing aid was used.

Bone-Anchored Hearing Aids (BAHAs)

A newer option for such hearing losses is the **bone-anchored hearing aid (BAHA)**, which can be worn externally or surgically implanted. BAHAs are basically a logical progression of the older-style bone conduction device. The BAHA involves surgically anchoring a screw into the skull behind the ear, to which an external device is connected, and directly stimulating the cochlea by bone conduction (**Figure 10.44**) (Ross, 2000). These devices can also be used externally on children, using a band to secure the device without surgery and implantation (**Figure 10.45**).

Middle Ear Implant (MEI)

The **middle ear implant (MEI)** is basically a hearing aid, but one in which the receiver or the entire hearing aid is

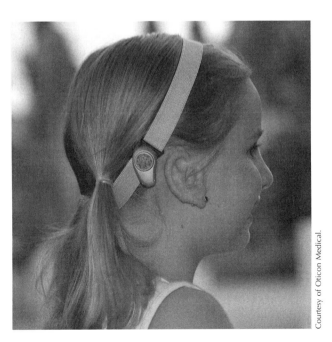

Figure 10.45 BAHA worn externally with a headband.

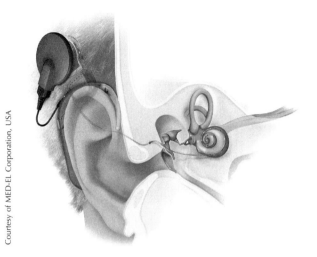

Courtesy of MED-EL Corporation, USA

Figure 10.46 Internal and external view of a cochlear implant.

have been used to address some individuals diagnosed with auditory neuropathy or auditory dys-synchrony.

A cochlear implant system is made up of an external speech processor, a transmitting coil and wire, and an internal receiver/stimulator. The receiver (which is magnetic) is surgically implanted into the temporal bone above the mastoid process, and the stimulator (or electrode array) is surgically inserted into the cochlea.

The external speech processor, which looks similar to a conventional BTE-style hearing aid, lies behind the helix of the pinna, and attaches via a transmitter cord to the transmitter coil, which magnetically attaches itself to the internal receiver. The external cochlear implant device (speech processor) picks up sound from the environment via a microphone. It then selects and arranges the sounds based on the preset programs (called maps) individual to the cochlear implant user. That signal is then sent to the internal transmitter via the transmitter coil, which receives signals from the speech processor and converts them into electric impulses. The transmitter then sends them to the electrode array, which collects the impulses from the stimulator and sends the message along to the central auditory pathway (**Figure 10.46**).

Hearing Assistance Technology (HAT)

Hearing assistance technology includes a variety of devices that help an individual with or without hearing loss communicate more effectively in adverse listening situations.

For individuals with hearing loss that significantly limits their ability to access auditory events, amplified and/or visual alerting systems are also available.

Assistive Listening Devices (ALDs) and Auditory Trainers

These devices help to modify the acoustic environment when hearing aids alone are inadequate to augment the listening situation. Personal devices work with hearing aids, cochlear implants, and bone-anchored devices to provide more direct access to a speaker. Whether the individual has a hearing loss or other disorders of auditory attention, these devices play an important role in increasing the signal-to-noise difference, thus making the speaker's voice louder than the background noise and more accessible to the listener. Group devices are designed to work in larger areas including classrooms, theaters, meeting and conference rooms, courtrooms, museums, and other group-gathering facilities. These devices fall into several categories including frequency-modulated (FM) amplification systems, induction loop systems, and infrared systems. Whether personal or group, assistive device or auditory trainer, there are three main components that make up a system—a transmitter that includes a microphone, a signal transmitting modality, and a receiver.

A Word on Terminology

The term *assistive listening device* encompasses all technology used to enhance the auditory environment of a listener, regardless of whether that person has a hearing loss. Frequently, the term *auditory trainer* is used to make the distinction between a device used by an individual with hearing loss to "train" their auditory system to listen and attend and one that merely enhances the auditory environment. However, these terms often, perhaps incorrectly, are used interchangeably. Similarly, the term *FM system* refers to a device that transmits its signal via an FM radio signal (described in detail later in this chapter). However, the term *FM system* is frequently used in the educational realm to refer to any device placed in a classroom that enhances classroom acoustics, regardless of how that signal is transmitted through the air. For the purpose of this chapter, we will be specific with the terminology as follows:

- *Assistive listening device* will be used to refer only to a unit with a limited amount of gain (volume) that is used for individuals with auditory attention difficulties within the classroom or for those with minimal hearing loss.

- *Auditory trainer* will be used to refer only to a unit designed to train an impaired auditory system. These devices have high levels of gain that must be adjusted to meet the needs of a specific hearing loss or are coupled directly to the hearing aid, taking on the amplification and acoustical characteristics of that device. It is in the best interest of the user to have an auditory training device selected and fit by an audiologist.

The way in which each device sends the signal from the transmitter to the receiver will also be specified, as well as how the receiver is coupled to the individual user. The speech-language pathologist working with assistive technology is encouraged to use the proper terminology when referring to a specific device. This assists in more accurate knowledge transfer between professionals and assures that the proper device is selected based on the needs of the individual. Again, the reader is encouraged to meet and consult with their friendly neighborhood audiologist whenever possible regarding assistive devices, their selection, and proper use.

Personal and Sound Field Systems

Background noises can include a myriad of sound sources. Internal and external noises have the potential to complicate the listening environment and the speech message, especially for a child in a learning environment. Environmental noises may include heating, ventilation, and air conditioning systems (HVAC); student and teacher movement; desks and chairs scraping on the floor; fans blowing; fish tank filters; hamster wheels; and computers, to name just a few. Additional sources of noises are generated outside the classroom in the hallways and include office announcements through the loudspeakers, schedule bells ringing, conversations, class movement, and noise generated from classrooms on the floors above or below. External noises might include students on the playground, parking lot noises, and traffic noise if the school is located near busy roads, lawn mowers and maintenance machines, nearby railroad crossings, and airports. It is safe to say that classrooms are very noisy places in which to learn.

Acoustic barriers to communication in the classroom can make listening and learning more complicated for an individual with hearing loss, (central) auditory processing disorder and with students struggling with auditory attention. Personal FM amplification systems allow the individual to hear, listen, and attend to the teacher more directly, as if they are standing close by. These systems are designed to manage the impact of background noise, reverberation, and distance factors that can degrade or alter the speech message being

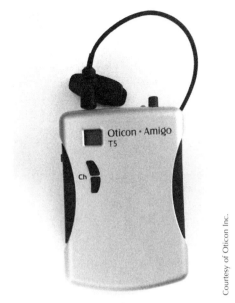

Figure 10.47 FM transmitter.

presented. This allows the teacher to move around the classroom while the individual continues to hear the teacher's voice at the same level and without interference from noises that may be between the teacher and the individual.

Personal FM Systems

Frequency-modulated (FM) systems are used to transmit a speaker's voice or a specific sound source directly to an individual. The receiver device can couple directly to the ear via earphones, induction loop, or earbuds, or couple through a hearing aid, cochlear implant, or BAHA (Figures 10.47 and 10.48). These devices are often found in academic settings to allow a student direct access to a teacher's voice while

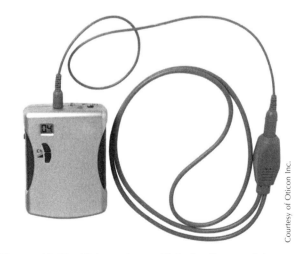

Figure 10.48 FM receiver with induction neck loop.

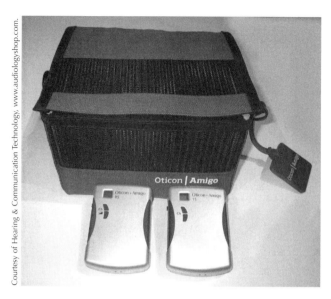

Courtesy of Hearing & Communication Technology, www.audiologyshop.com.

Figure 10.49   FM system with tabletop speaker.

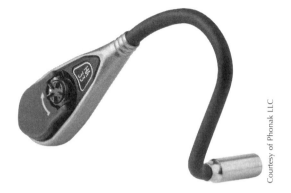

Courtesy of Phonak LLC

Figure 10.50   Ear-level assistive listening device.

diminishing the effects of background noise, reverberation impact (the echo effect when sound bounces off hard surfaces), and the impact of distance between a listener and speaker or sound source. The frequency transmission for these devices is regulated by the Federal Communications Commission (FCC), which has designated the bandwidths near 72 MHz and 216 MHz to be used only for FM systems (Tye-Murray, 2009). Personal FM devices are available from several manufacturers and in numerous forms of connectivity. Some devices are used as an assistive listening devices for individuals with minimal hearing loss (where hearing aids may or may not be required) or when auditory attention issues are being addressed in the classroom.

An additional option available for an individual when a receiver is not worn is a tabletop speaker unit used to provide amplification in close proximity to the listener (**Figure 10.49**). These tabletop devices can easily move with a student from classroom to classroom (e.g., students who are in inclusive settings, pulled out to resource rooms or departmentalized). These devices are the unit of choice when a student is unwilling or unable to tolerate earphones, or when the device needs to be out of reach (e.g., multiply impaired children or children with autism spectrum disorder). Personal FM assistive listening devices are also available in the form of ear-level units, which may be more cosmetically appealing to adolescents and teenagers because they draw less attention to the use of such a system (**Figures 10.50** and **10.51**).

Personal FM auditory training devices are available for individuals with hearing loss (**Figure 10.52**). These devices

come with many different coupling options. Connectivity decisions are based on a number of variables including type of hearing aid and preferred methodology adopted by the school or facility. Connecting hearing aids directly to FM systems, referred to as direct audio input (DAI), can be accomplished in one of three ways: using an audio shoe or audio boot, an integrated FM system, or a dedicated FM system. Certain hearing aids have been designed to work directly with specific FM systems, typically manufactured within the same company. An integrated FM system includes the receiver circuitry within the actual hearing aid. A dedicated FM system allows the FM receiver to attach directly to the hearing aid, cochlear implant, or bone-anchored hearing device without the use of an audio shoe/boot. When a hearing aid is not manufactured by the same FM manufacturer, an audio shoe or audio boot is used as an interface connector for the hearing aid to receive the signal from the receiver (**Figure 10.53**).

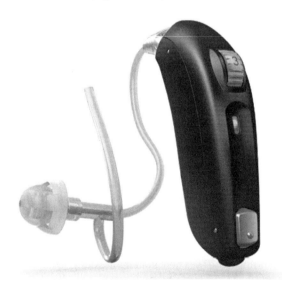

Courtesy of Oticon Inc.

Figure 10.51   Ear-level assistive listening device.

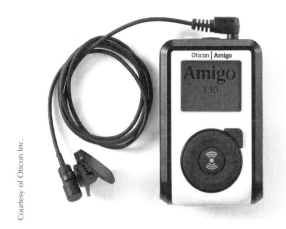

Courtesy of Oticon Inc.

Figure 10.52 FM auditory trainer transmitter and microphone.

FM systems can transmit signals up to 300 feet and can be used in many public places. However, because radio signals are able to penetrate walls, each transmitter is assigned an FM channel on which to operate and send the signal to the receiver. The devices are paired or linked according to the frequency on which the transmitter operates (Figure 10.54). Frequencies can either be preset by the manufacturer or be set by the facility using the devices.

To ensure there is no cross-contamination of signals in a facility, each classroom or meeting hall must use a different frequency band on which to communicate. An assigned staff member typically tracks these frequencies to assure that each channel is used only once in a single building.

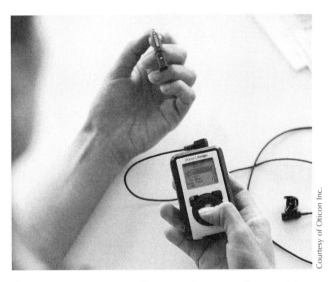

Courtesy of Oticon Inc.

Figure 10.54 FM auditory trainer receiver pairing with transmitter.

Induction Loop Coupling for Personal FM

People with hearing aids and cochlear implants with telecoil circuitry also have the option of using an induction loop FM system that can be worn around the neck (a neckloop; see Figure 10.55) or behind their aid or implant (called a silhouette inductor). The telecoil circuit picks up a magnetic signal from the induction loop and transmits the signal to the hearing aid. Individuals whose hearing aids or

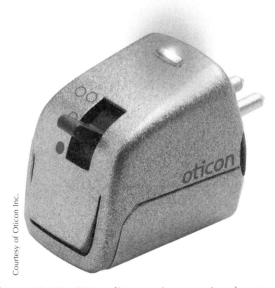

Courtesy of Oticon Inc.

Figure 10.53 FM auditory trainer receiver boot.

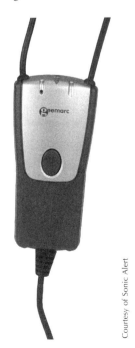

Courtesy of Sonic Alert

Figure 10.55 Bluetooth-compatible neck loop.

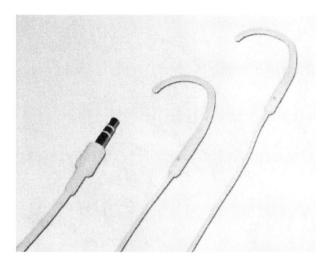

Figure 10.56   T-coil sillouettes.

cochlear implants have a telecoil may also wear a silhouette inductor to change an infrared signal into a signal recognized by a telecoil circuit (**Figure 10.56**).

Sound Field Systems

Sound field systems (**Figure 10.57**) are designed to provide an increased signal-to-noise ratio throughout a single

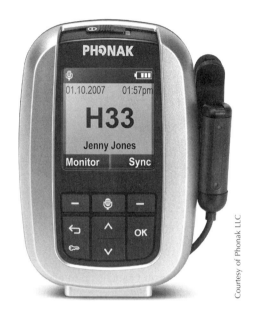

Courtesy of Phonak LLC

Figure 10.58   Dynamic SoundField assistive listening device (transmitter).

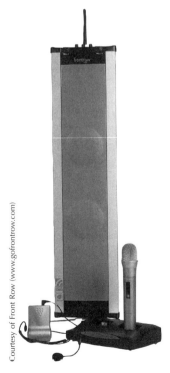

Courtesy of Front Row (www.gofrontrow.com)

Figure 10.57   FM portable sound field assistive listening device.

room, whether a classroom or meeting hall. These systems distribute sound evenly around the room, providing all listeners in the room an improved signal-to-noise ratio by making the speaker's voice equally loud in all areas of the room. These systems are often used in classrooms to combat the effects of background noise, reverberation, and speaker distance, all of which may have a negative impact on a person's ability to understand speech clearly.

Some sound field systems are FM systems transmitting on assigned frequencies between the transmitter device and the receiver base. Digital technology is used in newer types of signal transmission such as Dynamic SoundField (**Figures 10.58** and **10.59**). In this type of FM sound field device, the audio signals are digitized and packaged in very short digital bursts of code and broadcast several times at different channels between 2.4000 and 2.4835 GHz. This frequency-hopping technology avoids interference issues, and repetition of the broadcast ensures correct reception. Unlike older FM technology, with digital modulation (DM), no frequency planning to specific classrooms is required.

Sound field devices can also be infrared-based, which means they do not require a dedicated frequency to transmit a signal. A speaker-worn transmitter changes sound into a light signal that is then sent to a receiver. The receiver changes the light signal back to a sound signal. These

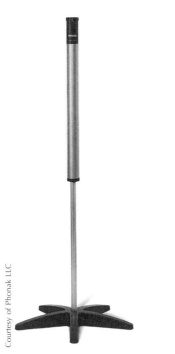

Figure 10.59 Dynamic SoundField assistive listening device (receiver speaker).

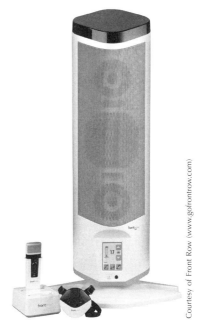

Figure 10.61 Infrared portable sound field system with lesson capture.

signals can be distributed through wall-mounted speakers that are spaced to disperse the sound evenly throughout the room, through a ceiling-mounted speaker, or through a free-standing speaker placed strategically in the classroom to disperse the sound evenly. The infrared signal cannot pass through walls or be used in direct sunlight (**Figures 10.60** and **10.61**).

Induction Loop Systems for Sound Fields

Induction loop systems are another type of sound field system that is used in large meeting halls and commercial theaters. Although less frequently used in educational facilities, induction loop systems allow large groups of hard of hearing individuals to connect via the telecoil circuitry of their personal hearing aids or cochlear implants. Induction loop

systems create an electromagnetic field that is picked up by the telecoil. In a large room such as a theater, a thin loop of wire is placed around the room. The hearing aid user activates their telecoil and the signal is picked up and directed into their hearing aid. This can directly connect the listener through their hearing aid telecoil to a variety of audio sources including public address systems (NIDCD, 2011).

Assistive Technologies for Sound Enhancement and Alerting Devices

Although the advanced digital technology found in hearing aids provides greatly improved communication ability, there are still times when the hearing aid or cochlear implant alone is not enough. Hearing and distinguishing speech in noisy situations, when watching television, or hearing and communicating over the telephone may still be challenging. In addition, we depend on a variety of devices to help us function in our environments and alert us to dangers or auditory events. In our auditory environment, a doorbell alerts us to a visitor and a fire or smoke alarm lets us know there is danger; however, these devices may not be sufficiently loud to provide an alert to a person with a significant degree of hearing loss. As technology advances, a wide range of devices are now available to enhance signals from audio devices as well as to alert individuals who are deaf or hard of hearing to sounds in their environment (NIDCD, 2011).

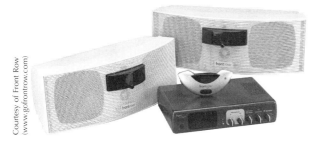

Figure 10.60 Infrared sound field system with speakers.

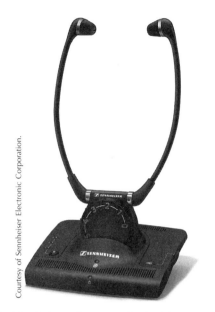

Courtesy of Sennheiser Electronic Corporation.

Figure 10.62 Infrared personal television amplifier.

Television Amplification

There are currently several options for television amplification systems. Such amplifiers plug directly into the television and use FM or infrared signals that are transmitted to the listener (Figure 10.62). Some devices use an induction loop worn around the listener's neck with the signal transmitted via the telecoil in the hearing aid. An additional and more recent technological option is a Bluetooth connection with a television device (Figure 10.63). Hearing aids that are Bluetooth compatible have the option to patch into the television using auxiliary devices. The Bluetooth remote system allows a signal to be transmitted directly to the individual's hearing aid(s).

Closed Captioning

Closed captioning for television programs allows the viewer to read the text and sounds related to the audio portion of a program. This feature is typically controlled by the user's television remote control. All televisions now sold with screens of at least 13 inches must have built-in closed captioning

reception technology; however, it should be noted that the individual using closed captioning must have a certain level of reading ability to use this functionality appropriately. An individual with hearing loss must not only have a reading ability commensurate with the content of the program they are watching, but also have the ability to read the captioning at the speed of conversational speech. Therefore, when recommending closed captioning to a hard of hearing or deaf individual, the speech-language pathologist is advised to take into consideration the individual's receptive language abilities, as well as their ability to read and comprehend written text at a rapid rate. A common misconception regarding closed captioning is, if the program is age appropriate for the individual, they will be able to comprehend its content using the closed captioning feature of their television.

Telephone Amplifiers

Telephone amplifiers and amplified telephones are available in the form of landline units (Figure 10.64) or can attach to an existing landline-based unit. These devices allow the listener to increase the speaker's voice using a volume control (Figure 10.65) and also have a built-in visual alerting system, typically a flashing light, to indicate that there is an incoming call.

Hearing aids that have telephone coils but not Bluetooth technology can be paired with a neck loop apparatus that converts a Bluetooth signal to a telecoil signal, which transmits into the hearing aids. These devices are especially useful with mobile phones, which typically come enabled with Bluetooth technology but have advanced away from magnet T-coil technology (Figure 10.66).

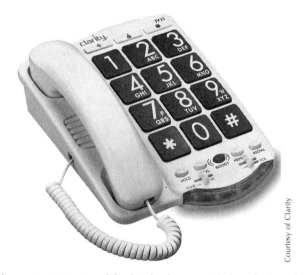

Courtesy of Clarity

Figure 10.64 Amplified Telephone with handset and ring alert.

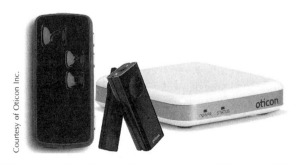

Courtesy of Oticon Inc.

Figure 10.63 Bluetooth personal television amplifier.

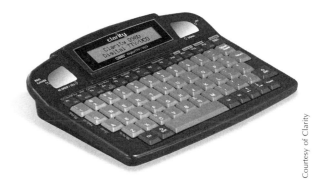

Courtesy of Clarity

Figure 10.67 Telecommunication device for the deaf (TDD).

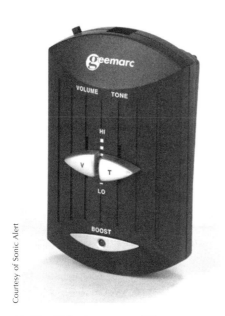

Courtesy of Sonic Alert

Figure 10.65 Telephone amplifier.

Text Telephones (TTYs)/Telecommunication Devices for the Deaf (TDDs)

Text telephones (TTYs), also known as **telecommunication devices for the deaf (TDDs)**, are a system of communication via the telephone by using typed messages instead of speaking and listening. In order to use this system, typically

both parties must have a device. The TTY has a keyboard for typing out messages and a display to read the incoming messages (Figure 10.67). This allows a phone conversation to be typed and read rather than spoken and heard. Some units also have printer capabilities to print messages for a hard copy. The TTY/TDD system can also be used if one party does not have a device by calling the Telecommunications Relay Service (TRS). The speaker's message is typed by a third-party operator so that the individual with the TTY/TDD can read the message. This national service is available free of charge, 24 hours a day, 365 days a year, by dialing 711.

Although texting is now the choice of many individuals over using a TTY/TDD, these devices are still used throughout the country. In fact, many of our common texting abbreviations came out of the TTY/TDD messaging era of deaf telecommunication.

Video Relay Service Devices (VRS)

As an alternative to the TTY/TDD or TRS, video relay service (VRS) was developed to allow individuals with hearing loss who utilize sign language to communicate directly over the telephone (Figure 10.68). This system provides the individual with hearing loss the ability to communicate using video devices. Such devices can also be linked with a TRS operator called a communications assistant (CA). This CA uses sign language to translate oral conversation into sign and vice versa. The system is facilitated by an Internet connection and requires that the CA be a qualified sign language interpreter. There is no typing or written text. The service can be accessed by either the user with hearing loss or a hearing individual, and is typically provided through a toll-free phone number via an Internet connection.

CapTel: Captioned Telephone

The **captioned telephone (CapTel)** system is a type of telephone that provides a display of written text or captions

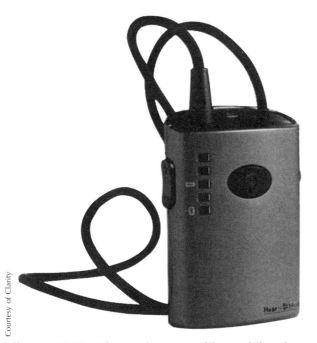

Courtesy of Clarity

Figure 10.66 Bluetooth-compatible mobile phone amplifier.

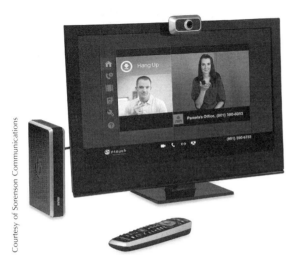

Courtesy of Sorenson Communications

Figure 10.68   Videophone.

along with the audible telephone conversation—in essence, a dictation of everything the caller says (**Figure 10.69**). Similar to a TTY/TDD device, a captioned telephone uses an intermediary operator to key an auditory message into the visual display (**Figure 10.70**). This allows the user to hear and see what the speaker is saying simultaneously (**Figure 10.71**).

Skype and FaceTime

The capability to communicate face to face over the Internet is becoming more popular in the deaf community as a way of interacting visually in real time. Computers connected to the Internet can access services such as Skype and FaceTime. A Universal Serial Bus (USB) device (**Figure 10.72**) is available

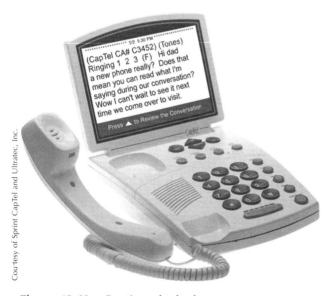

Courtesy of Sprint CapTel and Ultratec, Inc.

Figure 10.69   Captioned telephone.

to visually alert a deaf or hard of hearing individual so they can see the simulated ring that indicates a call is coming through.

Visual Listening Systems and Note Taking Service

For a student with hearing loss, listening in general can be fatiguing. Different lecture formats may require an individual to listen and respond, and/or listen and write information down. This is seen daily in secondary schools as well as colleges and universities as students are required to take notes from a verbal lecture format of instruction. The dual function of listening to a speaker and responding and/or taking notes or writing information down can be overwhelming as well as fatiguing. Information presented orally can be missed and/or misinterpreted. For these situations, special note-taking systems are available to assist the hearing-impaired student, allowing him or her to focus on the auditory while also getting the information in a written format.

The first system is communication access real-time translation (CART), also known as real-time captioning. A CART system requires special training because it uses a stenocode similar to the language coding used by a court stenographer. The caption writer or stenographer types what the speaker is saying into a stenotype device. This information is typically an abbreviated or condensed version of what is spoken, and is typed in an outline format. This is then translated into captions sent to an LCD projector or laptop computer. A software program with a dictionary of terms, as well as the accuracy of the typist, determines the accuracy of the translated stenographic codes.

The second method is a computer-assisted note-taking system (CAN). This system requires the typist to have good note-taking skills as well as the ability to type accurately and quickly. Additional special training is not required. This method is most often helpful for situations in which the listener needs basic information and some visual information to keep track of what is being presented, but is not completely dependent on verbatim transcription.

For both CART and CAN, the Americans with Disabilities Act (ADA) requires the educational system, business, or other public entity to employ an individual to provide the service, which can be costly.

Lesson Capture Devices

As technology advances, so does the ability to add additional functionality to existing equipment. Lesson capture devices allow for the recording of lecture format instruction for review at a later time. One such device (**Figure 10.61**)

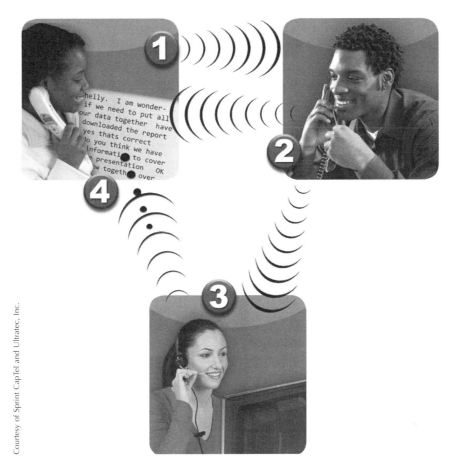

Courtesy of Sprint CapTel and Ultratec, Inc.

Figure 10.70   The captioned telephone triangle.

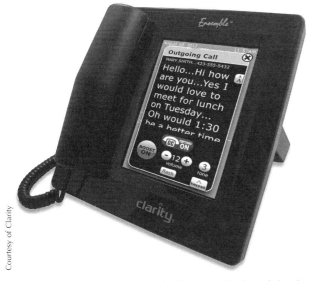

Courtesy of Clarity

Figure 10.71   Captioned telephone with digital display.

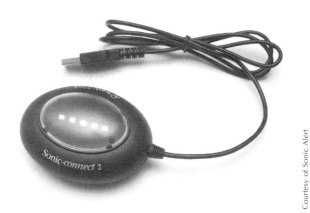

Courtesy of Sonic Alert

Figure 10.72 USB visual signaling for computer-generated alerts.

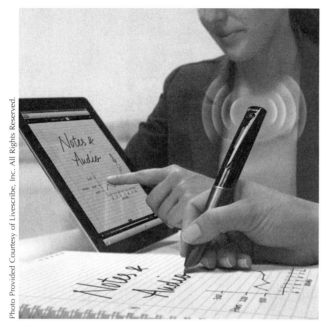

Figure 10.73   Smart pen (personal lecture-capturing device).

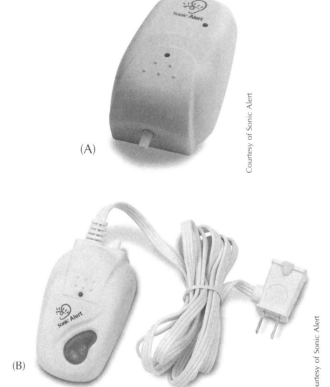

(A)

(B)

Figure 10.74   (A) Baby cry alert transmitter.   (B) Baby cry alert receiver.

combines the ability to record the auditory lecture and pair it with visual material from an interactive white board. This information is stored via computer software and can then be uploaded to the Internet for future review on a password secure site. This type of device also becomes very useful when students are absent. Missed classes can be viewed in their entirety when a student cannot attend the class.

A second, more affordable option is a smart pen (**Figure 10.73**). This device allows an individual to take notes on digitized paper using a specialized pen. The device records the lecture while simultaneously visually recording the location of the pen on the specialized paper. During the lecture, the pen records what is said based on the specific digital location on the paper. Regardless of the person's note-taking ability, following completion of the lecture the individual can return to their notes and review the auditory lecture using the device's headphone jack. This jack can also be adapted to be used with DAI auxiliary cables and an individual's personal hearing aids. Notes can also be uploaded to a computer or a tablet for review with the audio recording, revision, and printing.

Alerting Systems

Alerting or alarm devices use amplified sound, light, vibrations, or a combination of these to make the hearing-impaired individual aware of an event occurring in their

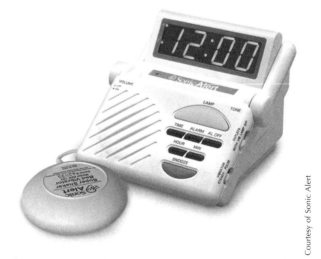

Figure 10.75   Vibrating alarm clock.

auditory environment. These visual alerting systems are used for various household devices, including doorbells, fire alarms, timers, and alarm clocks (**Figures 10.74** through **10.80**). When an auditory event occurs, a light flashes or a vibration is generated in the device, alerting the individual with hearing loss. In some instances, both a visual and a vibratory alert can be activated. Devices are also available to alert a parent or caregiver to a baby's cry. In many instances, portable pagers can be worn or a lighted system can be connected in multiple rooms to respond in conjunction with a single alerting system (NIDCD, 2011).

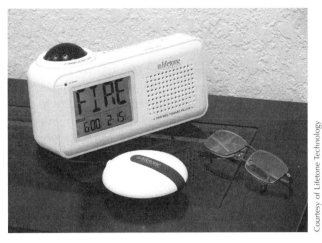

Figure 10.78 A visual alert system with visual, amplified auditory and vibratory alerts.

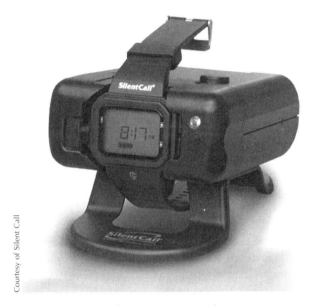

Figure 10.76 Vibrating wristwatch.

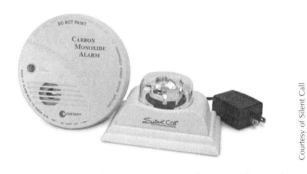

Figure 10.79 Carbon monoxide alarm with strobe alert.

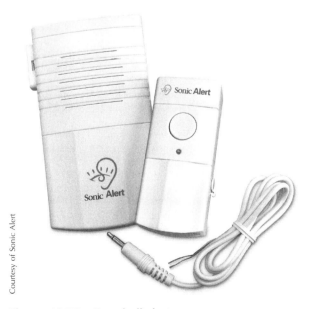

Figure 10.77 Doorbell alert.

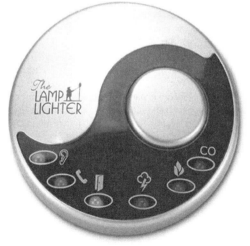

Figure 10.80 Multiple signal alert system.

Summary

A component of any auditory intervention program for hearing loss includes a wide variety of amplification choices. There are several different styles and technology options for hearing aids, including those worn in the ear and on the ear. When hearing aids are not appropriate, alternatives may include surgical placement of instrumentation to stimulate the auditory system. In some instances, hearing aids, cochlear implants, BAHA's, or middle ear implants may not be enough to address specific communication, academic, and safety needs. For these situations, hearing assistance technology (HAT); assistive listening devices (ALDs) and alerting devices are available. The combination of hearing aids with hearing assistance technology can greatly enhance the quality of life for an individual with hearing loss through a wide variety of technologically advanced devices and services.

Discussion Questions

1. Why are age, cognitive ability and dexterity important considerations when choosing a hearing aid?
2. A client on your caseload has a hearing aid. She complains that it is not always working and sounds "weird." Describe the steps you would take to troubleshoot this device.
3. What HAT devices would be useful for a child with a cochlear implant in the 4th grade?
4. What assistive listening device might you recommend for a 17-year-old student who has significant difficulty with auditory attention? What elements are important to consider when selecting a device for an individual of this age?
5. Research one type of alerting device. In what situation would this device be most beneficial? What difficult listen situation does this device overcome for a deaf or hard of hearing individual?

References

Healthy Hearing. (2011, Feb. 21). *Hearing aid history: From ear trumpets to digital technology*. Available from http://www.healthyhearing.com/content/articles/Hearing-aids/Types/47717-Digital-hearing-aid-history.

Miller, F., Vandome, A., & McBrewster, J. (2011). *Miller Reese Hutchison*. Saarbrücken, Germany: Alphascript.

Mills, M. (2011). Hearing aids and the history of electronics miniaturization. *IEEE Annals of the History of Computing, 33*(2): 24–44.

Morris, R. (2001). *Telecoils in plain language*. Available from http://www.beyondhearingaids.com/resource/aldarticles/telecoils.htm.

National Institute on Deafness and Other Communication Disorders. (2011). *NIDCD fact sheet: Assistive devices for people with hearing, voice, speech, or language disorders*. Available from http://www.nidcd.nih.gov.

National Park Service. (2013). *Thomas Edison National Historic Park, New Jersey*. Available from http://www.nps.gov/edis.

Ross, M. (2000, Nov./Dec.). Implantable hearing aids. *Volta Review*. Available from http://www.hearingresearch.org/ross/hearing_aids/implantable_hearing_aids.php.

Tye-Murray, N. (2009). *Foundations of aural rehabilitation: Children, adults and their family members*. Clifton Park, NJ: Delmar-Cengage Learning.

Watson, S. (2013). *Hearing Aid Basics : Hearing Aid History*. Available from http://health.howstuffworks.com/medicine/modern-technology/hearing-aid6.htm

Winefield, R. (1987). Alexander Graham Bell. (1847–1922). In J. V. Cleve (Ed.), *Gallaudet encyclopedia of deaf people and deafness* (Vol. 1, pp. 135–141). New York: McGraw-Hill.

Chapter 11

Laws, Standards and Guidelines

Arsen Zartarian, Esq.
President, New Jersey Association of School Attorneys (2013–2015)
Deputy General Counsel Newark Public Schools

Key Terms

Accreditation norm
Best practice

Certification norm
Guidelines

Standards or norms

Objectives

- Gain a fundamental understanding and working knowledge of the laws governing individuals with disabilities, including those that govern deaf and hard of hearing individuals
- Provide an overview of agencies and regulations that govern standards of practice in the field of audiology

Introduction

A myriad of laws, regulations and guidelines—on both the federal and state levels—impact the lives of adults and children with disabilities, including those who are deaf or hard of hearing. As we will examine in this chapter, these laws, regulations and guidelines run the gamut:

- they mandate that institutions take preventive measures to guard against individuals incurring possible hearing loss;
- they affirmatively afford rights to individuals with disabilities to ensure that those individuals are on an even playing field with their non-disabled peers, whether at work, school or another institution open to the public; or
- they might simply require the regular maintenance and calibration of appropriate or necessary audiological equipment and supports.

This chapter will review some of the more prevalent laws, regulations and guidelines of which the speech-language pathologist should be aware. Although this chapter will focus primarily on federal standards, the reader is also encouraged to review all applicable state or local legislation, regulations and guidelines, given that the states may afford individuals even greater rights or protections than those set forth in federal law.

Individuals with Disabilities Education Act (IDEA)

In 1975, Congress enacted the Education for All Handicapped Children Act ("EHA") which guaranteed a "free appropriate public education" to every child with a disability (as defined in that law) in every state across the country. The law was a federal legislative response to an increasing number of children with disabilities who were either excluded entirely from the education system or were only provided restricted access to the education system. As articulated in the EHA itself, the four purposes of the law were: (1) "to assure that all children with disabilities have available to them . . . a free appropriate public education ("FAPE") through an individualized education program ("IEP") which emphasizes special education and related services designed to meet their unique needs"; (2) "to assure that the rights of children with disabilities and their parents . . . are protected"; (3) "to assist States and localities to provide for the education of all children with disabilities"; and (4) "to assess and assure the effectiveness of efforts to educate all

children with disabilities." The EHA established mandatory programs for children with disabilities from age 3 to 21, and its subsequent amendments supported extended protections to additional populations of children such as early intervention, refined procedures for discipline of special education children, and, most recently, emphasized preparation of students for vocational and transition programs. The 1990 amendments to the EHA revised the name of the law to the Individuals with Disabilities Education Act (IDEA), which imposes even greater obligations on state and local education agencies, and confers substantive and procedural protections to qualified persons.

Referral, Evaluation, Eligibility, and IEP Services

As a threshold matter, school districts have "child find" obligations under the IDEA that obligate them to locate, identify and evaluate children suspected of having disabilities, including homeless children, highly mobile or migrant children, and wards of the state. This obligation even extends to parentally placed children in private schools located in the school district served by the local education agency (LEA).

Once a referral is made to the local education agency, a meeting is held at which a determination is made by appropriate persons on whether to evaluate the student. If evaluation is deemed warranted, any agreed upon assessments must be "administered in the language and form most likely to yield accurate information on what the child knows and can do academically, developmentally, and functionally, unless it is not feasible to so provide and administer." (IDEA regulations, 2006).

Consent by the parent/guardian/adult student/other qualified individual is required prior to the school district's initial evaluation, as well as before the initial provision of special education services (if the parent refuses to provide consent, the school district will not be deemed to be in violation of the IDEA). The initial evaluation must be conducted within 60 days of receiving parental consent, unless a state establishes a different timeline for completion or certain exceptions allow the school to claim an excusable delay (e.g., the parent of a child refuses to produce the child for evaluation) (IDEA regulations, 2006).

Parents/guardians of special education students are afforded numerous rights and procedural protections under the IDEA regulations and corresponding state regulations. These rights include:

- A very detailed notice to be provided before the school proposes or refuses to initiate or change the identification,
- Notice of evaluation,
- Provision of FAPE,
- Notice regarding specifying actions proposed or refused, and an explanation therefore;
- A description of each evaluation procedure,
- Provision of Assessment reports,
- Record or report used for the proposed or refused action, along with options considered and the reasons they were rejected;
- A statement of all procedural safeguards;
- Sources for parents to contact to obtain assistance.

The notices must be written in language "understandable to the general public" or "in the native language of the parent or other mode of communication by the parent, unless it is clearly not feasibly to do so." If the native language or other mode of communication of the parent is not a written language, the IDEA regulations provide that the school must maintain "written evidence that it had taken steps to ensure that the notice was translated orally or by other means to the parent in his or her native language or other mode of communication, and that the parent understood the content of the notice" (IDEA regulations, 2006).

Also, with regard to the evaluation process, the IDEA regulations provide that a parent/guardian has a right to an "independent educational evaluation" at public expense by an evaluator not employed by the school district if the parent disagrees with an evaluation by the school district, unless the school district files a court application to show that its evaluation is appropriate. The school district may not impose "conditions or timelines" related to obtaining an independent evaluation and the criteria under which the independent evaluation is obtained, including the location of the evaluation and the qualifications of the examiner, must be the same as the school district uses when it initiates an evaluation. Once the independent evaluation is completed, it must be considered by the school district in any decision regarding the provision of FAPE to the student (IDEA regulations, 2006).

Under the IDEA, after the school district completes the initial evaluation process, the "IEP team" must convene to determine if the student is eligible for special education and related services. While the definition of "IEP team" varies from state to state, according to the IDEA federal regulations, the IEP team must include: (1) the parent(s); (2) not less than one regular education teacher of the child (if the child is, or may be, participating in the regular education environment); (3) not less than one special education teacher of the child; (4) a school representative who is qualified to provide or supervise the provision of specially designed construction to meet the unique needs of the child with a disability, is knowledgeable about the general education curriculum, as well as the availability of the school's resources; (5) an individual who can interpret the instructional implications of evaluation results; (6) at the discretion of the parent or school, other individuals who have knowledge or special expertise regarding the child, including related services personnel as appropriate; and (7) whenever appropriate, the child (IDEA regulations, 2006).

Under the IDEA regulatory framework, a student may be deemed eligible for special education and related services upon finding that the student has one of thirteen (13) conditions that designate that student as a "child with a disability." For example, "specific learning disability" is defined as "a disorder in one or more of the basic psychological processes involved in understanding or in using language, spoken or written, that may manifest itself in the imperfect ability to listen, think, speak, read, write, spell, or to do mathematical calculations, including conditions such as perceptual disabilities, brain injury, minimal brain dysfunction, dyslexia, and developmental aphasia." Expressly excluded from the federal regulatory definition of "specific learning disability" are "learning problems that are primarily the result of visual, hearing, or motor disabilities, of mental retardation, of emotional disturbance, or of environmental, cultural, or economic disadvantage" (IDEA regulations, 2006).

Other definitions of disabling conditions establishing eligibility for special education and related services which may be of interest to the reader include:

1. **Autism**: "A developmental disability significantly affecting verbal and nonverbal communication and social interaction, generally evident before age three, that adversely affects a child's educational performance . . . Other characteristics often associated with autism are engagement in repetitive activities and stereotyped movements, resistance to environmental change or change in daily routines, and unusual responses to sensory experiences;"
2. **Deaf-blindness**: "Concomitant hearing and visual impairments, the combination of which causes such severe communication and other developmental and educational needs that they cannot be accommodated in special education programs solely for children with deafness or children with blindness;"

3. **Deafness**: "A hearing impairment that is so severe that the child is impaired in processing linguistic information through hearing, with or without amplification, that adversely affects a child's educational performance;"

4. **Hearing impairment**: "An impairment in hearing, whether permanent or fluctuating, that adversely affects a child's educational performance but that is not included under the definition of deafness in this section;"

5. **Multiple disabilities**: "Concomitant impairments (such as mental retardation-blindness or mental retardation-orthopedic impairment), the combination of which causes such severe educational needs that they cannot be accommodated in special education programs solely for one of the impairments, but not including deaf-blindness;"

6. **Speech or language impairment**: "A communication disorder, such as stuttering, impaired articulation, a language impairment, or a voice impairment, that adversely affects a child's educational performance."

If the student is found eligible for special education services, he or she is provided with an IEP that must include, among other things, a statement of the student's present levels of academic achievement and functional performance (PLAAFP); measurable academic and functional goals; a statement of special education and related services and supplementary aids and services to be provided to the student, as well as program modifications or supports; an explanation of the extent, if any, to which the child will not participate with nondisabled children in regular classes and activities; and a statement of individualized appropriate accommodations necessary to measure the academic achievement and functional performance of the student on state and district assessments (IDEA regulations, 2006).

In order to receive funding under the IDEA, the IEP must be designed to confer FAPE in accordance with the standards of the state education agency and controlling law. In *Board of Ed. v. Rowley* (1982), the United States Supreme Court interpreted "free and appropriate public education," finding that an IEP need not *maximize* the potential of a disabled student, but nevertheless must consider the potential of the student and provide "meaningful" access to education and confer "some educational benefit" necessary to satisfy IDEA. Certain federal courts have demanded a higher level of scrutiny. For example, United States Court of Appeals for the Third Circuit, governing Pennsylvania, New Jersey, Delaware and the Virgin Islands, has found that

IDEA requires that an IEP confer more than "trivial educational benefit," but rather must confer "significant learning" and confer "meaningful benefit," and also noted that "when students display considerable intellectual potential, IDEA requires a great deal more than a negligible benefit" (*Ridgewood Bd. of Ed. v. N.E.*, 1999). Nevertheless, this means that the school district is required, by law, to provide services that are "appropriate" for the child to gain meaningful educational benefit. However, many times, there may be a significant discussion at the IEP meeting between what the school district deems as appropriate and what the parents/guardians/advocate or others may desire as optimal.

Certain students may require additional home services (such as applied behavior analysis or related services) after school (extended day), or even on weekends or holidays if those services are required for the student to receive FAPE. As such, students may also be eligible for extended school year services (e.g., summer) if that additional instruction is required for the student to receive FAPE; and it must be tailored to the individual needs of the student, as opposed to a one size fits all approach or a "that's what we have available" program.

Along with the academic program, an IEP also may include related services that have been determined necessary to confer FAPE to the student. *Related services* are defined in the IDEA regulations as "transportation and such developmental, corrective, and other supportive services as are required to assist a child with a disability to benefit from special education." These services include speech-language pathology and audiology services, interpreting services, psychological services, physical and occupational therapy, recreation, counseling, orientation and mobility services, school health services, and parent counseling and training.

Under the IDEA regulations, each school must ensure that hearing aids worn in school by children with hearing impairments are functioning properly and that external components of surgically implanted medical devices (including cochlear implants) are functioning properly. However, related services do *not* include the optimization of a surgically implanted device's functioning (e.g., mapping), maintenance of that device, or the replacement of that device.

Other definitions of individual related services that may be of interest to the reader include:

1. **Audiology**: "Identification of children with hearing loss; determination of range, nature, and degree of

hearing loss, including referral for medical or other professional attention for the habilitation of hearing; provision of habilitative activities, such as language habilitation, auditory training, speech reading (lip-reading), hearing evaluation, and speech conservation; creation and administration of programs for prevention of hearing loss; counseling and guidance of children, parents, and teachers regarding hearing loss; and determination of children's needs for group and individual amplification, selecting and fitting an appropriate aid; and evaluating the effectiveness of amplification;"

2. **Interpreting services**: "Oral transliteration services, cued language transliteration services, sign language transliteration and interpreting services, and transcription services, such as communication access real-time translation (CART), C–Print, and TypeWell when used with respect to children who are deaf or hard of hearing; special interpreting services for children who are deaf-blind; and assisting in developing positive behavioral intervention strategies;"

3. **Speech-language pathology services**: "Identification of children with speech or language impairments; diagnosis and appraisal of specific speech or language impairments; referral for medical or other professional attention necessary for the habilitation of speech or language impairments; provision of speech and language services for the habilitation or prevention of communicative impairments; and counseling and guidance of parents, children, and teachers regarding speech and language impairments;"

4. **Parent counseling and training**: "Assisting parents in understanding the special needs of their child; providing parents with information about child development; and helping parents acquire the necessary skills that will allow them to support the implementation of their child's IEP or IFSP."

5. **Rehabilitation counseling services**: "Services that focus specifically on career development, employment preparation, achieving independence, integration in the workplace, and vocational rehabilitation" (IDEA regulations, 2006).

As IDEA has evolved, so have its standards on transition services, which have become more detailed and comprehensive. The 2004 IDEA amendments instituted a requirement that, beginning at age 16, an IEP include "appropriate measurable postsecondary goals based upon age appropriate transition assessments related to training, education, employment, and where appropriate, independent living skills." Some states, such as New Jersey, require transition services to commence at age 14 (New Jersey Department of Education Special Education Code, 2006).

The IDEA regulations define transition services as "a coordinated set of activities for a child with a disability that . . . is designed to be within a results-oriented process . . . focused on improving the academic and functional achievement of the child to facilitate the child's movement to post-school activities," which must be based on the child's individual strengths, preferences, and interests, including instruction, related services, community experiences, development of employment and other post-school adult living objectives, and, if appropriate, acquisition of daily living skills through functional vocational evaluation" (IDEA regulations, 2006).

Least Restrictive Environment

Additionally, IDEA requires that FAPE be provided in the least restrictive environment ("LRE"), meaning that: (1) to the maximum extent appropriate, children with disabilities, including children in public or private institutions or other care facilities, are educated with children who are nondisabled; and (2) special classes, separate schooling, or other removal of children with disabilities from the regular educational environment occurs only if the nature or severity of the disability is such that education in regular classes with the use of supplementary aids and services cannot be achieved satisfactorily. This general rule applies with equal force to arrangements concerning the provision of nonacademic and extracurricular services and activities. Unless the IEP requires some other arrangement, the child should be educated in the school he or she would attend if not disabled. Further, the child should not be removed from education in age-appropriate regular classrooms solely because of needed modifications to the general education curriculum (IDEA regulations, 2006).

Although IDEA imposes least restrictive environment requirements and a preference for mainstream placements, the laws and regulations acknowledge that some students with disabilities may require additional instruction at home or at hospitals or institutions. Similarly, a private day school or even a residential placement may be appropriate if a student cannot "reasonably be anticipated to benefit from instruction without such a placement." In that analysis, it must be determined whether the full-time residential placement is considered necessary for educational purposes, or whether the residential placement is a response to medical, social or emotional problems segregable from the learning process (IDEA regulations, 2006).

Discipline of Special Education Students

One common challenge for school administrators, parents/guardians, and educators/service providers is navigating the rules pertaining to the discipline of children eligible for special education services, as this cohort of students is afforded significant procedural and substantive protections under the law. As a result, IDEA disciplinary requirements may lead to friction between: (1) school officials seeking to take swift action and utilize any flexibility in the disciplinary authority they possess, with (2) those parents or guardians who are aware of their child's IDEA discipline rights and seek to interpret those rights broadly or expansively. It should be noted that these disciplinary protections apply to not only those students who are already classified, but those "potentially classifiable" students not yet deemed eligible for services, but for whom the parent or teacher has requested an evaluation or expressed concern in writing that the child is in need of services (IDEA regulations, 2006).

In general, school personnel may remove a child with a disability who violates a code of student conduct from his or her current placement to an appropriate interim alternative setting or suspension for not more than 10 consecutive or cumulative school days in a school year, to the extent those alternatives are applied to children without disabilities. More significant and substantial removals require additional actions, such as a "functional behavioral assessment" (an examination of when and under what circumstances the misbehavior occurs) and "behavior intervention services" or a "behavior intervention plan"—an outlined strategy based on rewards or consequences that attempts to reduce the instances of misbehavior (IDEA regulations, 2006).

Further, if the school has proposed significant discipline beyond the 10 days, a meeting must be held to conduct a manifestation determination, (i.e., "to determine whether the conduct in question was caused by, or had a direct and substantial relationship to, the child's disability," or if the conduct was the result of a failure to implement the IEP). If the conduct *was* a manifestation of the disability, the student must be returned to the previous placement (IDEA regulations, 2006).

Under three "special circumstances," a school district may change a student's program unilaterally: (1) if the student possesses a "weapon" (as that term is defined in the IDEA) in school or at a school function; (2) if the student knowingly possesses, uses or sells a "controlled substance" (as that term is defined in the IDEA) in school or at a school function; or (3) if the student has inflicted "serious bodily injury" (as that term is defined, and a difficult standard to

meet) in school or at a school function. All other significant changes of placement require either parental consent or a court application, including a 45-day interim alternative educational setting if the school contends that continuing the child's placement is "substantially likely to result in injury to the child or to others" (IDEA regulations, 2006).

Disagreements Under IDEA and Due Process Proceedings

It should be no surprise that, on occasion, there may be disagreements between the parent/guardian and the school district regarding the identification, evaluation, or educational placement of a student, imposition of discipline or conclusions regarding the manifestation determination, or the content of an IEP necessary to confer provision of FAPE. If that occurs, in accordance with the IDEA regulations, a parent or school district may file a due process complaint with the state within 2 years from the date the parent or school "should have known about the alleged action that forms the basis of the complaint." The parties may voluntarily participate in mediation before a state mediator, a "resolution" session without a state mediator, or proceed directly to an impartial hearing officer.

In *Schaffer v. Weast* (2004), the United States Supreme Court placed the burden of proof at due process hearings on the parent. Nevertheless, some states (e.g., New Jersey) have enacted laws placing the burden of proof on school districts to demonstrate that they have offered FAPE, thereby allowing a parent/guardian to proceed against the school district essentially on what may be a general allegation that FAPE has not been provided, without the need for an expert to explain the manner of the alleged deprivation or failure (New Jersey L. 2007, ch. 331, sec. 1).

During the pendency of the due process proceedings, the child is afforded "stay put protection," meaning that he or she remains in the current educational placement until the matter is resolved. Also, the court may award reasonable counsel fees to the parent or guardian who is a prevailing party in the litigation, or to the school district if it can demonstrate that the application was "frivolous, unreasonable or without foundation" or if it was brought to "harass, cause unnecessary delay, or needlessly increase the cost of litigation." (IDEA regulations, 2006).

Numerous issues may form the basis of a disagreement under IDEA and resultant due process filing. One area of disagreement that might form the basis of the complaint could be that the school has declined to evaluate the student, or, alternatively, has evaluated the student and found the student ineligible for special education services. Another area might be a parent/guardian's disagreement with the proposed disabling condition (e.g., "other health impaired" vs. "emotionally disturbed") or proposed program ("self-contained," segregated special classes vs. a mainstream class). Additionally, the parent may challenge the type, frequency or duration of a related service—for example, the parent may request more goals and objectives regarding emphasis on speech articulation or auditory processing services in the IEP; individualized speech rather than group speech; speech in a segregated area rather than in the classroom; speech three times a week instead of once a week; or speech for 40-minute sessions rather than 20-minute sessions.

In addition to seeking evaluations or a change in the proposed program, another mode of relief requested by a parent may be compensatory services or compensatory education if services were not provided as set forth in the IEP, if a parent contends the IEP was not designed to confer FAPE, or if an unlawful exclusion from school (through inappropriate discipline or for another reason) deprived the student of FAPE. If a student did not receive occupational/physical therapy or speech sessions for some reason through no fault of the student or parent, the school district might be compelled to make up the undelivered service sessions unless an alternate means of service is more appropriate or the student no longer requires the service. An award of compensatory education—such as additional instruction after school, during the summer, placement in a private school, or services continuing after the age of 21—is a court-recognized remedy that allows the student to make up for an earlier deprivation of FAPE. (*Carlisle Area School District*, 1995).

Services Plan

A school district can also develop a services plan that sets forth the special education and related services that the district provides to a parentally placed private school children with disabilities. Those services, however, are conditioned upon availability of funding pursuant to federal budgetary formulas and allotments, and are different than the services provided to the students in public schools, because the requirement of a free and appropriate public education does not apply to those students (IDEA regulations, 2006).

Early Intervention

Although school districts have the obligation to provide a free and appropriate education and provide an IEP that commences at age 3 and lasts until graduation or through the age of 21, Part C of the IDEA also mandates that states implement a "statewide, comprehensive, coordinated, multidisciplinary, interagency system that provides early intervention services for infants and toddlers with disabilities and their families." An infant and toddler with disability is defined as an individual under 3 years of age who needs early intervention services because the individual is experiencing a developmental delay, as measured by appropriate diagnostic instruments and procedures, in one or more of the following areas: (1) cognitive development; (2) physical development, including vision and hearing; (3) communication development; (4) social or emotional development; (5) adaptive development; or (6) has a diagnosed physical or mental condition that has a high probability of resulting in developmental delay, including conditions such as chromosomal abnormalities, genetic or congenital disorders, sensory impairments, inborn errors of metabolism, disorders reflecting disturbance of the development of the nervous system, congenital infections, severe attachment disorders, and disorders secondary to exposure to toxic substances, including fetal alcohol syndrome (IDEA regulations, 2006).

Under this framework, states must implement a public awareness program and a comprehensive child find system, coordinated with multiple agencies and programs established under, among other enactments, the Head Start Act, Social Security Act, Child Abuse Prevention and Treatment Act, Developmental Disabilities Assistance and Bill of Rights Act, Family Violence Prevention Act, and various other state laws. After a multi-disciplinary assessment of the child and family is conducted, a meeting is scheduled to determine if the child is eligible for early intervention services. Similar to other IDEA disputes, a parent has the option to appeal eligibility determinations by filing for due process or mediation (IDEA regulations, 2006).

If the child is deemed eligible, an Individual Family Service Plan (IFSP) is prepared that includes: (a) a statement of the child's present levels of physical development (including vision, hearing, and health status), cognitive development, communication development, social or emotional development, and adaptive development; (b) a statement of the family's resources, priorities, and concerns related to enhancing the development of the child as identified through the assessment of the family; (c) a statement of the measurable results or measurable outcomes expected to be achieved for the child and family, and the criteria, procedures, and timelines used to determine the degree to which progress toward achieving the results or outcomes identified in the IFSP is being made and whether modifications or revisions of the expected results or outcomes, or early intervention services identified in the IFSP are necessary; (d) a statement of the specific early intervention services necessary to meet the unique needs of the child and the family to achieve the results or outcomes identified, including the length, duration, frequency, intensity, and method of delivering the early intervention services and a statement that each early intervention service is provided in the natural environment for that child or service to the maximum extent appropriate; (e) identification of medical and other services that the child or family needs or is receiving through other sources, but that are neither required nor funded under this early intervention, and if those services are not currently being provided, a description of the steps the service coordinator or family may take to assist the child and family in securing those other services; (f) dates and duration of services; (g) identification of the service coordinator; and (h) transition from early intervention services. The regulations also require periodic review and evaluation of the IFSP, as well as transition to preschool and other programs prior to the child's third birthday (IDEA regulations, 2006).

Audiology services are specifically included as a type of early intervention service within the federal regulatory definition, and include: (1) identification of children with auditory impairments, using at-risk criteria and appropriate audiologic screening techniques; (2) determination of the range, nature, and degree of hearing loss and communication functions, by use of audiological evaluation procedures; (3) referral for medical and other services necessary for the habilitation or rehabilitation of an infant or toddler with a disability who has an auditory impairment; (4) auditory training, aural rehabilitation, speech reading and listening devices, orientation and training, and other services; (5) services for prevention of hearing loss; and (6) determination of the child's individual amplification, including selecting, fitting, and dispensing appropriate listening and vibrotactile devices, and evaluating the effectiveness of those devices. Speech-language pathology services are also listed as early intervention services, and include: (1) identification of children with communication or language disorders and delays in development of communication skills, including the diagnosis and appraisal of specific disorders and delays in those skills; (2) referral for medical or other professional services necessary for the habilitation or rehabilitation of children with communication or language disorders and

delays in development of communication skills; and (3) provision of services for the habilitation, rehabilitation, or prevention of communication or language disorders and delays in development of communication skills (IDEA regulations, 2006).

Standards for Acoustics in the Classroom

Services under IDEA may be affected by the physical layout or construction of a classroom, often leading to such requests as follow-up observations by educational audiologists when, for example, a student with a central auditory processing disorder is moved to another location or program. It is fairly common for acoustics to vary from classroom to classroom, depending on, among other factors, the location of the building; the size, shape, and design of the classroom; and the construction composition of the walls, floor or ceiling. Further, each classroom is affected by background noise, whether the result of external sounds such as planes, trains, and automobiles; noises from the hallways or other classrooms, whether next door or on higher or lower floors; and building utilities and services, such as heating, ventilation and air conditioning (HVAC) units. All of these factors have an influence on the direct sound made by a teacher's instruction and create reflected sound", and affect the classroom's reverberation level and signal-to-noise ratio (e.g., the teacher's voice as the [signal] to the background sound level [noise] at the target location, such as the student's ear), which, in addition to speaker-to-listener distance, contribute to the listening environment. It is fairly self-evident that any of these factors can lead to missed instruction for all students, in particular non-native speakers or children with learning disabilities and hearing impairments (Guckelberger, 2002).

Family Educational Rights and Privacy Act (FERPA)

The IDEA incorporates the student privacy protections set forth in the Family Educational Rights and Privacy Act of 1974 (FERPA), which, among other things, protects the confidentiality of all students' educational records and prohibits release without the written authorization of a parent or adult student, subpoena or at times under state law, a court order. Under FERPA, an *educational record* is defined as "those records, files, documents, and other materials which: (1) contain information directly related to a student; and (2) are maintained by an educational agency or institution or by a person acting for such agency or institution."

Thus, special education records, such as IEPs and evaluations, or service delivery logs, summary of contents, and anecdotal notes, fall within that definition.

Certain organizations, however, are listed as exemptions and allowed access to the records in any event, including: (1) other school officials, including teachers within the educational institution or local educational agency; (2) officials of other schools or school systems in which the student seeks or intends to enroll, upon the condition that the student's parents be notified of the transfer; (3) certain designated government agencies or state and local officials or authorities to whom such information is specifically allowed to be reported or disclosed pursuant to state statute; (4) organizations conducting studies for, or on behalf of, educational agencies or institutions for the purpose of developing, validating, or administering predictive tests, administering student aid programs, and improving instruction; (5) accrediting organizations in order to carry out their accrediting functions; or (6) parents of a dependent student (FERPA, 1974).

Section 504 of the Rehabilitation Act

The IDEA is often referenced as a funding statute (i.e., a statute that provides federal funding to public agencies such as school districts so that they can provide services to students with disabilities who fall within the designated disabling conditions). The next statute we will review is considered an "anti-discrimination" statute, which obligates certain affirmative actions to individuals with disabilities so that the end result will be equality of opportunity. Although considered by many in the school district environment as an alternative to the IDEA, the statute applies to both students and adults.

By way of brief history, shortly after the Civil Rights Act of 1964, Congress enacted the Rehabilitation Act of 1973 as a vehicle to extend protection to persons with disabilities. In particular, Title V of that act was fashioned to ensure that all programs receiving federal money would be accessible to persons with disabilities. Section 501 of the act applies to federal employment hiring practices, and mandates an affirmative action plan for persons with disabilities; Section 502 applies to all federally funded buildings and public transportation to ensure full accessibility to persons with disabilities; Section 503 applies to employers who have a contract or subcontract with the federal government to require an affirmative action plan for employment of persons with disabilities; and finally, Section 504 prohibits discrimination against federally qualified persons with disabilities by federally assisted programs.

Application of Section 504

In pertinent part, Section 504 of the Act provides:

> No otherwise qualified individual with a disability . . . shall, solely by reason of her or his disability, be excluded from the participation in, be denied the benefits of, or be subjected to discrimination under any program or activity receiving Federal financial assistance or under any program or activity conducted by any Executive agency.

As far as "any program or activity" covered by the law, federal regulations implementing Section 504 were passed in 1977, applying the law to all entities receiving federal funds. Additional regulations cover public preschool, elementary, and secondary schools. In general, the program or services must be a "recipient of federal financial assistance," including public school districts and other public or private agencies that receive federal financial assistance directly or through another recipient (Section 504 regulations, 1977).

Court decisions have extended application of Section 504 to, among other entities: private school placements approved by the state (*P.N. v. Greco*, 2003); parochial schools, through participation in national lunch and e-rate programs (*Rosso v. Diocese of Greensburg*, 2010); after school childcare programs (*Conejo Valley*, 1995), including a program providing afterschool care to children based in a public school but paid for through tuition (*K.G. v. Morris*, 2007); and recreation programs where the school provided only facilities and distributed applications for the programs (*Arlington County*, 1990).

For purposes of Section 504, an "individual with a disability" is defined as an individual who has: (1) a physical or mental impairment that substantially limits one or more major life activities, (2) a record of such an impairment, or (3) is regarded as having such an impairment. A "physical or mental impairment" includes neurological; musculoskeletal; special sense organs; respiratory, including speech organs, cardiovascular, reproductive, digestive, genitourinary, hemic, and lymphatic disorders; skin, and endocrine disorders; any mental or psychological disorder or cognitive impairment; organic brain syndrome; emotional or mental illness; and specific learning disabilities (Section 504 definitions, 1977).

An individual who "has a record of such an impairment" is defined in Section 504 as an individual who "has a history of, or has been misclassified as having, a mental or physical impairment that substantially limited one or more major life activities." If an individual establishes that he or she has been subject to a prohibited action because of an actual or *perceived* physical or mental impairment, whether or mot that impairment limits or is perceived to limit a major life activity, an individual meets the requirements of "being regarded as having an impairment." (Section 504 regulatory definitions, 1977).

"Major life activities" within the meaning of Section 504 include, but are not limited to, caring for oneself, performing manual tasks, seeing, hearing, eating, sleeping, walking, standing, lifting, bending, speaking, breathing, learning, reading, concentrating, thinking, communicating, and working. The term also includes "the operation of a major bodily function, including but not limited to functions of the immune system, normal cell growth, digestive, bowel, bladder, neurological, brain, respiratory, circulatory, endocrine and reproductive functions." (Section 504 regulatory definitions, 1977).

Expanded Coverage and Broad Interpretations

The Americans with Disabilities Amendments Act of 2008 (ADAA) amended the Rehabilitation Act to include the ADAA's definitions of "disability." As a result of that amendment, it was easier for an individual seeking the benefits of the law to claim that he or she had a disability, provided that the definition of disability was to be construed in favor of broad coverage, and adding "the question of whether an individual's impairment is a disability under the ADA should not demand extensive analysis" (ADA amendments, 2008).

Although Section 504 does not define the term "substantially limited," the amendments rejected the Equal Employment Opportunity Commission (EEOC) regulatory definition of "substantially limited" as "significantly restricted," as well as the United States Supreme Court's restrictive definition of "substantially limited" as "prevented or severely restricted" from performing the major life activity (*Toyota v. Williams*, 2002). The ADAA amendments also rejected a Supreme Court decision which found that the determination as to whether an impairment substantially limits a major life activity is to be determined with respect to the ameliorative effects of mitigating or corrective measures (*Sutton v. United Air Lines*, 1999).

Accordingly, under the law, the ameliorative effects of medication, medical supplies or equipment, prosthetic limbs and devices, hearing aids and cochlear implants or other implantable hearing devices, mobility devices, oxygen therapy equipment and supplies, assistive technology, auxiliary aides or services, learned behavioral or adaptive neurological modifications, psychotherapy, behavioral therapy and physical therapy are all *not* to be considered if determining whether an impairment or disability "substantially limits a major life activity." Additionally, any side effects of a mitigating measure can be taken into consideration in determining whether an individual meets the definition of a "disability." Further, an individual cannot be required to use a mitigating measure (ADA amendments, 2008).

The ADAA regulations provide that in making the "substantial limitation" determination, the individual's ability to perform the major life activity should be compared to that of "most people in the general population." Considerations may include the difficulty, effort, or time required to perform a major life activity, pain experienced when performing a major life activity, the length of time in which a major life activity can be performed, and/or the way an impairment affects the operation of a major bodily function. The analysis should focus on the manner that the activity is substantially limited, as opposed to the outcomes the individual may achieve. The regulations illustrate, by example, that deafness substantially limits hearing; blindness substantially limits seeing; intellectual disability, cerebral palsy, cognitive impairment, obsessive compulsive disorder, major depressive disorder, bipolar disorder, schizophrenia and autism substantially limit brain function; partially or completely missing limbs or mobility impairments substantially limit musculoskeletal function; epilepsy, multiple sclerosis, and muscular dystrophy substantially limit neurological function; and cancer substantially limits normal cell growth (ADA amendments, 2008).

Discrimination Under Section 504 and Required Services

An entity covered by Section 504 discriminates against a covered individual if, in "providing any aid, benefit, or service . . . directly or through contractual, licensing, or other arrangements, on the basis of handicap," proceeds to, among other things: (1) deny a qualified handicapped person the opportunity "to participate in or benefit from the aid, benefit, or service"; (2) afford a qualified handicapped person "an opportunity to participate in or benefit from the aid, benefit, or service that is not equal to that afforded others;" or (3) "provide different or separate aid, benefits or services to handicapped persons . . . unless such action is necessary to provide [those] persons with aid, benefits, or services that are as effective as those provided to others." Section 504 specifically provides that "a recipient to which this subpart applies that employs fifteen or more persons shall provide appropriate auxiliary aides persons with impaired hearing or vision, [which] may include brailled and taped material, interpreters, and other aids." (Section 504 regulations, 1977).

For example, an institution of higher learning covered under Section 504 is required to provide interpreter services to a deaf graduate student (*Camenisch v. University of Texas*, 1980). A hospital must provide an effective means of communication to a deaf patient and her deaf husband, otherwise it will be deemed to have denied the benefits of services to those individuals (*Borngesser v. Jersey Shore Medical Center*, 2001). A school district has been found to violate Section 504 by failing to name an eligible student the sole valedictorian (*Hornstine v. Township of Moorestown*, 2003) or by failing to provide support in honors or world language classes (*Washington Twp. School District-Sewell*, 2006) if those services are required to have the students participate in those programs on an "even playing field" with nondisabled peers. Similarly, school districts cannot condition an eligible student's participation in class, afterschool activities, or field trips on parent's attendance. Hearing-impaired parents are deemed otherwise qualified individuals with disabilities for school-sponsored events, and thus are entitled to sign language interpreters for school activities concerning their child's education (*Rothschild v. Grottenhaler*, 1990). Students attending private schools would be deemed otherwise qualified individuals if they meet the "essential eligibility requirements" for those services from the private school (*St. Johnsbury Academy v. D.H.*, 2001).

In other areas, such as health care, for example, the Office of Civil Rights (OCR) has determined that hospitals must provide qualified interpreters and telecommunication devices for the deaf (TDD) to hearing-impaired clients, finding that "it would be extremely difficult for the health care provider to demonstrate in certain service settings that effective communication is being provided in the absence of . . . interpreters" (OCR, 1982). OCR has determined that critical points of inpatient or outpatient medical treatment and hospitalization include admission, explanation of medical procedures, when informed consent is required for treatment, and discharge (OCR, 1991). OCR has also determined that written notes given to the patient, or even interpreters not versed in American Sign Language (ASL), will not suffice as effective communication for those deaf persons who use ASL, because its "idioms and concepts are not directly translatable into English" (OCR, 1991).

Americans with Disabilities Act (ADA)

Nearly 20 years after the Rehabilitation Act, the Americans with Disabilities Act (ADA) of 1990 expanded the rights of persons with disabilities to the private sector. Title II of the ADA, governing state and local government activities, requires that state and local governments provide people with disabilities an equal opportunity to benefit from all of their programs, services, and activities, including education, employment, recreation, and social services. In that regard, state and local governments are required to follow certain architectural barrier-free standards in new construction or alterations. (Department of Justice, 2009). State and local governments must also relocate programs or otherwise provide access in accessible older buildings, and communicate effectively with people who have hearing, vision, or speech disabilities. (Department of Justice, 2009). For example, persons who are deaf or hard of hearing may need to be provided with computer-assisted transcription services, assistive learning systems, auxiliary aides, or qualified interpreters who are able "to interpret effectively, accurately, and impartially, using any specialized vocabulary" (ADA regulations, 2008).

Similarly, Title III of the ADA, governing public accommodations, applies to businesses and nonprofit service providers; privately operated entities offering certain types of courses and examinations, privately operated transportation, and commercial facilities such as restaurants, retail stores, hotels, movie theaters, private schools, convention centers, doctors' offices, homeless shelters, transportation depots, zoos, funeral homes, day care centers, fitness clubs, and sports stadiums (ADA regulations, 2008). Not only must these public accommodations comply with basic nondiscrimination requirements that prohibit exclusion, segregation, and unequal treatment, they must also comply with ADA's architectural standards and provide other access requirements, such as effective communication with people who have hearing, vision, or speech disabilities (ADA regulations, 2008).

Title IV of the ADA concerns telephone and television access for people with hearing and speech disabilities, and requires common carriers/telephone companies to establish telecommunications relay services (TRSs) 24 hours a day, 7 days a week. The TRS enables callers with hearing and speech disabilities who use a teletypewriter or text telephone (TTY)—a type of a telecommunication device for the deaf (TDD)—and callers who use voice telephones to communicate through a third-party assistant. The law is overseen by the Federal Communication Commission (FCC), which sets minimum standards for the TRS services (ADA regulations, 2008).

Health Insurance Portability and Accountability Act (HIPAA)

The Health Insurance Portability and Accountability Act (HIPAA) was enacted on August 21, 1996. Title II of HIPPA establishes policies, procedures and guidelines for maintaining the privacy and security of individually identifiable health information and requires the Department of Health and Human Services (DHHS) to draft rules aimed at increasing the efficiency of the healthcare system by creating standards for the use and dissemination of protected health information (PHI), any information held by a covered entity within the meaning of the law that covers health plans, provision of health care, or payment for health care that can be linked to an individual (HIPAA regulations, 2002).

Covered entities may include healthcare clearinghouses, employer-sponsored health plans, health insurers, and medical service providers that engage in certain transactions. The confidentiality obligations are extended to independent contractors of covered entities that fit the definition of *business associates* (HIPAA regulations, 2002).

HIPAA imposes very strict conditions on disclosure. Protected health information may be disclosed to facilitate treatment, payment, or healthcare operations without a patient's express written authorization. All other circumstances require written authorization for disclosure, and even in that circumstance, the covered entity must make a reasonable effort to disclose only the minimum necessary information required to achieve its purpose. Covered entities do have an obligation to disclose protected health information when required to do so by law, such as reporting suspected child abuse to state child welfare agencies (HIPAA regulations, 2002).

Covered entities must take reasonable steps to ensure the confidentiality of communications with individuals. All disclosures of PHI, as well as privacy policies and procedures, must be documented. Further, a privacy official must be appointed, as well as a designee responsible for receiving complaints and training all members of the workforce regarding implementing procedures governing disclosure and confidentiality of protected health information (HIPAA regulations, 2002).

HIPAA also mandates that covered entities disclose protected health information to the individual within 30 days of request, and individuals are given the right to request that a covered entity correct any inaccurate information. Further, an individual who believes that his or her privacy rights have been violated by a covered entity can file a complaint with the Office of Civil Rights within the United States Department of Health and Human Services (HIPAA regulations, 2002).

Civil Rights of Institutionalized Persons Act (CRIPA)

The Civil Rights of Institutionalized Persons Act (CRIPA) was enacted in 1997 for the purpose of protecting person's rights of health and safety while residing in an institution. CRIPA authorizes the filing of civil rights complaints with the Office of the United States Attorney General, which investigates questionable conditions of confinement and or imprisonment at state and local government institutions, such as county and state prisons, local municipality jails, holding cells in public courthouses, juvenile correctional facilities, publicly operated nursing homes, inpatient psychiatric institutions, and facilities servicing residents with developmental disabilities.

Although the Attorney General's office does not have authority under CRIPA to investigate isolated incidents or to represent individual institutionalized persons, it does have the authority to investigate and correct widespread infringement of rights in such facilities. Infringement of civil rights must cause "grievous harm", or be proven by reasonable cause in such cases proved to be "egregious or flagrant," or a "pattern or practice" (CRIPA, 42 USC, 1997).

Social Security Act: Medicare and Medicaid

In 1965, the Social Security Amendment Act to the Social Security Act of 1935, also known as Title XVIII of the Social Security Act, established the Medicare and Medicaid programs. These programs were originally administered through two agencies organized under the Department of Health, Education and Welfare, later renamed the Centers for Medicare and Medicaid Services, which is now located within the United States Department of Health and Human Services. Although both programs provide medical and health-related services to a designated cohort of individuals and have similar names, often leading to confusion, the programs are very different.

Medicare

Medicare is a social health insurance program that covers individuals 65 years of age or older, as well as individuals under age 65 with certain disabilities such as amyotrophic lateral sclerosis (ALS or Lou Gehrig's disease) and end-stage renal disease (i.e., permanent kidney failure requiring dialysis or a kidney transplant). Medicare has four different "parts" covering different services: (1) Part A, hospital insurance, covering hospital inpatient care, nursing home care, home healthcare, or hospice; (2) Part B, medical insurance, covering health care provider or doctor services, outpatient care, durable medical equipment, and home health care, as well as certain preventive services to help maintain health or prevent acceleration of certain diseases; (3) Part C Medicare Advantage, which offers health plan options run by Medicare-approved private insurance companies; and (4) Part D, Medicare prescription drug coverage, also run by Medicare-approved private insurance companies.

Medicaid

Medicaid is a health and medical services program available to qualified individuals with low incomes and limited resources. Although primary oversight of the program is administered at the federal level, each state administers its own program, and establishes its own eligibility standards; determines the type, amount, duration and scope of services, and fixes the rate of payment for services. To qualify for federal funding, however, all states must provide certain mandatory services, including, but not limited to, inpatient/outpatient hospital services; prenatal care; children's vaccines; physician, nurse/midwife, family nurse, and pediatrician care; and family planning services and supplies. States may also provide certain Medicaid-approved optional services, such as diagnostic and clinic services; prescribed drugs and prosthetic devices; optometrist services and eyeglasses; rehabilitation and physical therapy services; speech pathology and audiology services;

community-based care; and transportation services. Of particular relevance, "services for individuals with speech, hearing, and language disorders" is defined in the Medicaid regulations as "diagnostic, screening, preventive, or corrective services provided by or under the direction of a speech pathologist or audiologist, for which a patient is referred by a physician or other licensed practitioner of the healing arts within the scope of his or her practice under state law" (ASHA, 1997–2013).

Special Education Medicaid Initiative (SEMI)

Some state education agencies, such as the New Jersey Department of Education (DOE), have mandated that the local districts initiate appropriate steps to increase revenue generated from the Special Education Medicaid Initiative (SEMI) by maximizing participation in that program. New Jersey DOE regulations governing "fiscal accountability, efficiency and budgeting procedures", for example, require that each school district or county vocational school district "strive to achieve" a 90% return rate of parental consent forms for all SEMI-eligible students in addition to mandated submission of documentation of services to students by Medicaid-qualified practitioners such as nurses, occupational and physical therapists, psychologists, social workers, and speech therapists. In that regard, speech therapists are required to submit a copy of their state DOE certification and either their past or present license, American Speech-Language-Hearing Association (ASHA) certification, or documentation that the equivalent educational requirements and work experience necessary for ASHA certification have been met. Speech correctionists, similar to occupational or physical therapist assistants, even though not Medicaid-qualified, can render services under the direction of Medicaid-qualified practitioners (New Jersey DOE regulations, 2008), (ASHA, 2004).

American National Standards Institute (ANSI)

The American National Standards Institute (ANSI), a not-for-profit 501(c)(3) organization founded in 1918, is the official organization representing the United States to the International Organization of Standardization (ISO), an international standard-setting entity located in Geneva, Switzerland. Located in both Washington, D.C. and New York City, ANSI's official mission statement reads: "To enhance both the global competitiveness of U.S. business and the U.S. quality of life by promoting and facilitating voluntary consensus standards and conformity assessment systems, and safeguarding their integrity."

ANSI is a voluntary organization which oversees the creation and dissemination of a wide variety of norms and guidelines that regulate and certify many of the products and services around us. ANSI also provides monitoring and auditing programs to ensure that services are maintained (ANSI, 2013).

ANSI is an active part of our everyday lives. From audiological equipment to car design, from computer standards to wiring specifications, the establishment of a product standard allows goods and services to be uniform across all 50 states. In 2011, ANSI also began accreditation of Health Information Technology (HIT). This accreditation process will allow standardization of the United States Department of Health and Human Services, national medical data recording system, Electronic Health Record Technology (EHR) as a nationwide medical database for all American residents (ANSI, 2013).

In the field of audiology, ANSI provides the following standard specifications: ANSI S3.6-2010 Audiometer Specification; ANSI S3.7-1995 (R 2008) Method for Coupler Calibration of Earphones; ANSI S3.39-1987 (R 2007) Immittance Specifications; ANSI S.322-2009 Hearing Aid Specification; ANSI S3.46-1997 (R 2007) Real Ear Specifications; ANSI S3.45-2009 Vestibular Testing Specifications; ANSI S3.1-1991 Maximum permissible ambient noise levels for audiometric test rooms; ANSI S3.21-2004 Method for manual pure-tone threshold audiometry. As with all standards and guidelines, ANSI updates its standardization methods and principles as technology develops.

For example, with regard to schools and education, in 2002 ANSI and the Acoustical Society of America (ASA) jointly developed a standard for acoustical design, ANSI/ASA S12.60-2002, "Acoustical Performance Criteria, Design Requirements, and Guidelines for Schools." ANSI/ASA S12.60-2002 sets forth acoustical performance criteria for different categories of learning spaces, and establishes maximum limits for each. Under the standard, the maximum permissible reverberation time in an unoccupied, furnished classroom with a volume under 10,000 cubic feet is 0.6 to 0.7 seconds, and the maximum level of background noise allowed in the same classroom is 35 decibels. However, these standards are voluntary recommendations, unless adopted by state code or otherwise mandated on a local level (Acoustical Society of America, 2002).

Occupational Safety and Health Act (OSHA)

The Occupational Safety and Health Act of 1970 created the Occupational Safety and Health Administration (OSHA), an agency within the United States Department of Labor that was authorized to "assure safe and healthful working conditions for working men and women by providing training, outreach, education and assistance." Among other things, OSHA regulations require that employers impose a "hearing conservation program" consisting of noise exposure assessment, audiometric testing, hearing protection and staff development/training for employees exposed to noise at 85 decibels or above as an 8-hour time-weighted average sound level. OSHA also imposes an "employee alarm systems" standard that mandates emergency actions and alarm systems should be perceived by all employees—including those employees who are deaf or hearing impaired—thus requiring visual or flashing lights, instant messaging, vibrations, or similar alerting device options in the case of hearing-impaired employees (US Department of Labor, OSHA).

The Joint Commission

A speech pathologist's job is not only the provision of services, but also the tracking of services delivered and efficient, complete record-keeping. These obligations are not only essential for maintaining confidentiality and preparation for possible legal issues, they also are crucial for federal and state monitoring of the entities for which the speech pathologist is providing services. This may be the federal or state Departments of Education, or another agency may be conducting accreditation checks for the facility of employment.

For example, the Joint Commission, created in 1951 and formerly known as The Joint Commission on the Accreditation of Healthcare Organizations (JCAHO), is a federal non-profit organization that accredits and certifies more than 20,000 healthcare organizations and programs across the United States. Many hospitals and healthcare organizations that receive Joint Commission accreditation must pass rigorous inspections of facility practices and adhere to certain performance standards.

In order to achieve the Joint Commission accreditation, hospitals and medical facilities must prove they have strong, evidence-based practices, a strong commitment to patient outcomes, clinical care, and promotion of patient safety. An appointed group of Joint Commission members assigned to accredit the facility undertakes an extensive evaluation process. Joint Commission inspections can take several weeks to complete, at which time standards of practice are evaluated and scrutinized. A speech pathologist working in a healthcare facility at some time in his or her career will participate in a Joint Commission accreditation inspection (The Joint Commission, 2013).

Summary

In order for the field of speech-language pathology to maintain homogony, speech-language pathologists must be held to a high standard of practice. First and foremost is the professional's ethical commitment to the profession. Following that, laws, guidelines and standards direct our daily activities of quality service provision. We find these regulations and directives in a variety of places, depending on the professional setting. Whether it is in a school system or a medical center, laws, standards, and guidelines enable us to serve the public in a uniform fashion across the country. Our clients, students, and patients are afforded their rights as well, to assure that they are receiving the best of care possible. The symbiotic relationship between civil rights and standards of practice drive best practices within the field of speech-language pathology.

Discussion Questions

1. A parent/guardian disagrees with the school district's determination of eligibility or proposed frequency of speech therapy. What law applies, and what are the parent's rights? How can the parent/guardian demonstrate that more service or a different service is warranted?

2. A school district proposes suspending a deaf student for 20 days for failing to follow verbal directions. What are the student's rights? What would the school have to demonstrate?

3. A hearing-impaired employee attends a professional development day and is unable to understand the presentation. What law applies? What are the employee's rights? What would be the employer's obligations?

4. What is the difference between Medicare and Medicaid?

5. True or False: Federal laws and regulations are the only mandates that apply to the hearing-impaired population; once familiarity with them is mastered, there is no need to review state or local standards. Explain your answer.

References

Acoustical Society of America, 2002. ANSI S12.60-2002: Acoustical Performance Criteria, Design Requirements, and Guidelines for Schools (Melville, NY: ASA)

A Guide to Disability Rights Laws, U.S. Department of Justice. Civil Rights Division, Disability Rights Section, July 2009)

American National Standards Institute (ANSI), 2013. New York, NY, www.ANSI.org/overview

American Speech-Language-Hearing Association (1997-2013) Introduction to Medicaid. Available from www.ASHA.org/practice/reimbursement/medicaid/medicaid_intro.htm

American Speech-Language-Hearing Association. (2004). *Medicaid guidance for speech-language pathology services: addressing the "under the direction of" rule* [Position Statement]. Available from www.asha.org/policy. D. Guckelberger, A New Standard for Acoustics in the Classroom, Engineers Newsletter, Vol. 32, No. 1 (2003)

National Archives and Records Administration Federal Register (2006) "Assistance to States for the Education of Children with Disabilities and Preschool Grants for Children with Disabilities."

National Archives and Records Administration Federal Register (2010) "Nondiscrimination on the Basis of Disability in State and Local Government Services."

Notice of Exercise of Authority Under 45 CFR 84.52(d)(2) Regarding Recipients With Fewer Than Fifteen Employees

Section 594, Effective Communications, and Health Care Providers, U.S. Department of Health and Human Services, Region III, Regional Technical Assistance Staff (January 1982)

U.S. Department of Health and Human Services, Office for Civil Rights, Region III, Letter of Findings, Ref. No. 03913037 (Dec. 12, 1991). US Department of Labor, Occupational Safety and Health Administration. www.osha.gov/pls/oshaweb/owadisp.show_document?p_table=stardards&p_id=9735

The Joint Comission 2013. www.jointcommission.org/accreditation

Cases

Arlington County (VA) Pub. Sch., 16 EHLR 1190

Borngesser v. Jersey Shore Med. Ctr., 340 N.J. Super. 369 (App. Div. 2001)

Camenisch v. University of Texas, 616 F.2d 127 (5th Cir. 1980)

Carlisle Area Sch. Dist. V. Scott P., 62 F.3d 520 (3d Cir. 1995)

Conejo Valley Unified Sch. Dist., 23 IDELR 448 (1995)

Hornstine v. Township of Moorestown, 263 F.Supp. 2d 887 (D.N.J. 2003)

K.G. v. Morris Board of Education, OAL Dkt. EDS-11872-06 (Aug. 10, 2007)

M.C. v. Central Reg. Sch. Dist., 81 F.3d 389 (3d Cir. 1996)

Oberti v. Board of Ed. of the Bor. of Clementon School District, 995 F.2d 1204 (3d Cir. 1993)

P.N. v. Greco, 282 F. Supp. 221 (D.N.J. 2003)

Rosso v. Diocese of Greensburg, 55 IDELR 98 (W.D. Penn. 2010)

Rothschild v. Grottenhaler, 907 F.2d 286 (2d Cir. 1990)

Schaffer v. Weast, 546 U.S. 49 (2004)

St. Johnsbury Academy v. D.H., 240 F.3d 163(2d Cir. 2001)

Sutton v. United Air Lines, Inc., 527 U.S. 471 (1999)

Toyota Motor Manufacturing v. Williams, 534 U.S. 184 (2002)

Washington Township (NJ) School District-Sewell, 48 IDELR 80 (OCR Oct. 19, 2006)

Wilson County (TN) Sch. Dist. 50 IDELR 230 (OCR 2007)

Regulations

28 CFR 35.104
29 CFR 1630.2
29 CFR 1630.2
29 CFR 1910.95
29 CFR 1910.165
34 CFR 104.3
34 CFR 104.31
34 CFR 300.34
34 CFR 300.132
34 CFR 300.138
34 CFR 300.502
34 CFR 300.506
34 CFR 300.507
34 CFR 300.510
34 CFR 300.511
34 CFR 300.517
34 CFR 300.518
34 CFR 300.530
34 CFR 300.532
34 CFR 303.1
34 CFR 303.13
34 CFR 303.21

34 CFR 303.209
34 CFR 303.302
34 CFR 303.321
34 CFR 303.322
34 CFR 303.342
34 CFR 303.343
34 CFR 303.344
42 CFR 440.70
42 CFR 440.110
45 CFR 84.52
45 CFR 164.501
45 CFR 160.102
45 CFR 160.103
45 CFR 160.306
45 CFR 164.502
45 CFR 164.512
45 CFR 164.522
45 CFR 164.524
45 CFR 164.526
45 CFR 164.528
45 CFR 164.530
NJAC 6A:23A-5.3

Statutes

29 USC 651
29 USC 794
20 USC 1232
42 U.S.C. § 1997 et seq.
42 USC 42642

42 USC 12101
42 USC 12102
42 USC 1395
NJSA 18A:46-1.1

Chapter 12

Understanding Auditory Development and the Child with Hearing Loss

Christina Barris Perigoe, PhD, CED, CCC-SLP, LSLS-Cert. AVT
Coordinator, Graduate Program in Early Oral Intervention
Associate Professor, Department of Speech and Hearing Sciences
The University of Southern Mississippi

Marietta M. Paterson, EdD, CED
Director, Education of the Deaf
Associate Professor, Department of Speech and Hearing Sciences
The University of Southern Mississippi

Key Terms

Auditory access
Auditory environment
Closed-set assessment
Comprehension

Detection
Discrimination
Functional auditory
  assessment

Hearing age
Identification
Open-set assessment
Telescope vocal development

Objectives

- Understand how auditory skills develop in typically developing children with normal hearing
- Understand and describe the relationship between listening and spoken language
- Understand the elements that need to be in place for a child with hearing loss to learn language through audition, and the rationale for doing so
- Describe functional auditory assessment, and the tools and methods available to complete it

Introduction

Spoken language acquisition happens for the typically developing hearing child in such an integrated, progressive manner that how the child receives, perceives, and processes the auditory sensory input from his or her environment may be taken for granted. In the case of children with hearing loss, a strong understanding of the impact of hearing loss on auditory spoken language acquisition is essential, as well as how to optimize the listening capacity and auditory skills development for the individual child who is deaf or hard of hearing. Just as for the hearing child, the mother language can be learned through the primacy of the auditory channel; the brain can learn to use an auditory signal that arrives through hearing instruments and auditory development can be followed. The concept that spoken language is primarily an auditory event underlies the practices of professionals who provide early auditory-based intervention and auditory–verbal education to children with hearing loss who are learning to listen and speak. How do we use our understanding of typical auditory learning to assist children with hearing loss to access the auditory code-cracking potential of their brains?

This chapter will present an overview of the following topics: auditory development in typically developing children with normal hearing, auditory development in children with hearing loss, a model for auditory work with children with hearing loss, the use of developmental hierarchies and checklists in tracking auditory skills, and functional auditory skills assessment tools. We will also provide several resources at the end of the chapter.

Auditory Development in Typically Developing Children

In the past 20 years, there has been a great deal of research concerning the prenatal auditory environment and the earliest weeks and months of auditory development. These findings confirm the importance of paying attention to the earliest stages of auditory development (Boothroyd, 1997). There are several general assumptions that inform us about early auditory pathway development and ongoing auditory learning. First, we now assume the innate capacity of the human brain to perform categorical speech perception (Owens, 2012). Second, the timetable of auditory development needs to be considered from the formation of the auditory system in utero and the auditory experiences with sounds that are possible through the uterine wall. We can assume that, even before birth, a child is listening to it's mother's heartbeat and attending to mother's voice, music, and other speech and nonspeech sounds and even stories that are loud enough to be heard (Saffran, Werker, & Werner, 2006). Third, research into auditory pathway development in utero and the first few years of life emphasizes the critical period for auditory neural pathway development (Sharma, Dorman, & Kral, 2005). Fourth, cross-linguistic research on auditory perceptual abilities of infants in the first days and weeks of life informs us that the neonate is indeed an amazing sound processor and can perform a larger variety of perception tasks than previously thought. Auditory abilities that are more complex than auditory awareness are already present at birth (Welling, 2010). The presence of a hearing loss at birth, therefore, means that the auditory brains of these children have not benefited from diverse auditory input and listening practice; hence the crucial need for early detection and early intervention.

What do we know about auditory development and the typical child with normal hearing, and how does that inform us about the child with hearing loss? For the child whose hearing loss is detected early and who is able to access sufficient auditory input, we would want to follow a developmental model. It is useful to think about how the auditory–verbal link develops and how auditory input is linked to speech and spoken language output. The following is a useful way to conceptualize this:

Input

1. Auditory perception (ability of the ear to hear the speech signal)
2. Auditory processing (ability of the brain to understand speech and spoken language)

Output

1. Speech and spoken language organization (ability of the brain to organize speech and spoken language)
2. Speech and spoken language production (ability to produce nonmeaningful speech sounds and meaningful speech in spoken language)

As we observe children at various ages and stages of development, our observations of their speech and spoken language output can be an indicator of the auditory input they are receiving and how they are processing that input. If the auditory input is compromised, then spoken language output will be negatively impacted.

Table 12.1 contains a list of aspects of auditory development related to concurrent attainments in speech production and spoken language. This developmental information is a reference for later discussion of how listening and speaking can be developed in hearing loss. For further details the reader is referred to Owens (2012), Cole and Flexer (2011), Oller (1986), and Hall and Moats (1998).

Auditory Development of Children with Hearing Loss

Understanding the course of auditory development in the typically hearing child should inform best practices of speech pathologists, audiologists, teachers of the deaf, auditory-verbal therapists, early interventionists, and listening and spoken language specialists. Our challenge in working with children who are deaf or hard of hearing is to ensure early identification of hearing loss, early and consistent use of advanced hearing instruments, early access to auditory-based language learning in the home environment, and access to knowledgeable and skilled professionals.

Children born with hearing loss, even a minimal hearing loss, are at risk for not achieving all the essential auditory abilities outlined in Table 12.1. Early identification of hearing loss through newborn hearing screening, and the provision of early intervention programs and advanced hearing technologies, have played a part in changing our expectations of children with all levels of hearing loss and of the age of attainments. The mission of the state Early Hearing Detection and Intervention (EHDI) programs is: detection of hearing loss by 1 month of age, diagnostic audiology and hearing aid wearing by 3 months of age, and

enrollment of the child and family in an early intervention program by 6 months of age (Joint Committee on Infant Hearing, 2007). Early intervention, prior to 6 months of age, has been shown to afford children with hearing loss the opportunity to achieve language levels comparable to their hearing peers (Downs & Yoshinaga-Itano, 1999; Yoshinaga-Itano, Sedey, Coulter, & Mehl, 1998). Failure to provide infants with hearing loss the early auditory input necessary for the development of their auditory brain centers (and subsequent skills in listening, spoken language, and literacy) has been dubbed a "neurological emergency" by Dornan (2009).

Auditory input is best accessed during the years of the greatest neural plasticity. The detrimental effects of auditory deprivation due to hearing loss have been well documented. Hearing loss can have a negative effect on the development of the child's auditory system (Moore & Linthicum, 2007) and on the development of listening, speech, spoken language, literacy, and academic achievement (Blaiser & Culbertson, 2013; Ling, 2002; Paul & Whitelaw, 2011; Robertson, 2009).

Studies and intervention with children who have various levels of hearing loss can inform us about how hearing develops. Sharma and colleagues (2002a, 2002b, 2005, 2006) have studied severe to profoundly deaf children who received cochlear implants and confirmed that there is a critical period for auditory development. Children who received cochlear implants prior to 3 1/2 years of age developed "auditory brains" similar to those of hearing children; those older than 7 years of age did not.

Better speech perception and language skills have also been achieved by children who received cochlear implants early (Fryauf-Bertschy, Tyler, Kelsay, & Gantz, 1997; Kirk et al., 2002; Nicholas & Geers, 2006). The same type of improved outcome has been shown in studies of children who

Table 12.1 Auditory-Verbal Development in Typically Developing Children with Normal Hearing

Input: Auditory Development	Output: Speech Production/Spoken Language
Prenatal *Auditory Experiences in Utero:* • Typically developing child has 20 weeks of exposure to auditory stimuli prior to birth • Infant emerges literally wired for sound • Listens to mother's voice and environmental sounds (both from within and outside of the womb) • Born with a preference for mother's voice • Born with a preference for songs and stories heard in utero	

(continues)

Table 12.1 (*continued*)

Input: Auditory Development	Output: Speech Production/Spoken Language
Birth to 3 months *Reactions to Sounds:* Startle reflex, eye blink/eye widening, cessation of activity, limb movement, head turn toward or away, grimacing/crying, sucking, arousal, breathing change *Speech Perception Abilities:* • Can identify individual phonemes • Capable of detecting virtually every phoneme • Prefers vowels *Prosody/Suprasegmentals:* • Prefers human voice • Attentive to the rise and fall of intonation pattern • Attends to patterns of speech • Prefers native language to all others *Identification:* • Identifies mother's voice • Prefers songs heard prenatally	*Reflexive:* • Coos, gurgles, reflexive sounds *Physical Response to Sounds:* • Stilling, rhythmic movement, searching for sound's source *Vocalization:* • Goo sounds, laughter • Quasi-resonant nuclei (QRN), immature vowel-like sounds
3–4 months *Prosody/Suprasegmentals:* • Prefers utterances with intonation variation versus flat voice • Discriminates high and low sounds	
4–7 months **Early Auditory Feedback** *Auditory Tuning In:* • Listening to language for longer periods of time • Shows awareness of environmental sounds • Can be behaviorally pacified by music or song *Speech Perception:* • Recognition of mother's voice • Reacts to vocal mood differences *Localization:* • Localization to sound begins to emerge from eye gaze to head turn to localization to specific sound sources (directly related to motor development) *Auditory Memory:* • Beginning of auditory memory (distinguishes between voices of familiar people vs. strangers)	*Expanding Vocal Repertoire:* • Vocal play • Fully-resonant nuclei (FRN), vowel-like sounds, consonant-like sounds, consonant-vowel (CV) and vowel-consonant (VC) syllables emerge • Plays with streams of sounds, intonational patterns, raspberries, squeals, loudness play • Vocal turn-taking exchanges with parent
5 months *Early Auditory Comprehension:* • Responds to own name *Suprasegmentals/Prosody:* • Discriminates own language from others with same prosody	*Vocalization:* • CV syllable and some VC syllable vocalizations • Imitates pitch tone
6 months Correlation between achievements and speech perception and later word understanding, word production, and phrase production *Speech Perception:* • Preference for vowels ends *Early Auditory Feedback:* • Listens to self in vocal play *Auditory Identification:* • Begins to recognize own name and the names of family members *Reliable localization:* • Begins to respond to directives *Selective auditory attention:* • Will divert attention from one activity to a more desirable activity based on auditory input.	*Vocalization:* • May produce recognizable vowels: /u/a/i/

(*continues*)

Table 12.1 (*continued*)

Input: Auditory Development	Output: Speech Production/Spoken Language
The Sound with Meaning Connection: The "melody is the message." Child will interpret parents' intention by listening and reacting to tone of voice change. Happens prior to word comprehension.	

	Input: Auditory Development	Output: Speech Production/Spoken Language
8–10 months	*Synaptogenesis:* • Explosion of synaptic growth may be related to change in perception and production *Phonotactic Regularities and Prosody:* • Sensitive to regularities in word boundaries in infant-directed speech (IDS), even in another language • Begins storing sound patterns for words, although no meaning yet *Auditory Comprehension:* • Begins to comprehend words	*Vocalization: Canonical "Babble"* • Achieves strings of reduplicated and alternated syllable production; timing of syllable production sounds speech-like, stress patterns • Vowels, consonants becoming distinct *Increased Vocal Turn-Taking:* • Once true babble attained, parents expect more speech-like utterances. *Primitive Speech Acts (PSA):* • Expressing intentions nonverbally
8–14 months		*Protowords:* • Words invented by child, not adult, but have consistent meaning, such as "la-la" for blanket
9 months	*Speech Perception:* • Prefers nonwords composed of high phonotactic components *Auditory Attention:* • Sustained auditory attention • Will attend to auditory-based activities for increased periods of time *Phonotactic Probabilities* • Predicting likelihood of certain sound sequences, listening preference for nonwords with high phonotactic probability versus those with low probability	*Intentionality: "I Know What I Mean":* • Child attains cognitive/communication intents. • Achieves means–end concept • Uses vocal/verbal means to achieve ends in combination with visual and gestural mechanisms *Vocalization:* • Variegated babble: adjacent and following syllables are not identical
9–12 months		*9–12 months: Speech to Communicate* • Sound imitation of common household items and animals • Distinct word approximations and in some cases early single word utterances take place of crying to fulfill wants and needs • Verbal "nicknames" for distinct objects and people develop and remain consistent for that object or person
10 months	*Auditory Tuning In:* • Narrows auditory attention and speech perception: tunes in to mother language, loses universal interest in all speech sounds	
10–16 months		*Phonetically Consistent Forms (PCF):* • Speech sounds that have sound–meaning relationships, such as "puda" for the family cat *First Words:* • Context bound • Following the first word, during the next few months, children add an average of 8–11 words to their vocabularies each month
11 months	*Speech Perception:* • Identifies allophones and word boundaries	• Variegated babble • Word approximations
12 months	*Speech Perception:* • Hears word and consonant boundaries	

(*continues*)

Table 12.1   *(continued)*

Ages 12–24 months: Exploring and Expanding

	Listening: Auditory Comprehension	Speech Production and Spoken Language
12–18 months	*Early Auditory Comprehension:* • Odd mappings of words • Child attends to whole sentence • Is able to follow commands • Fully aware of the names for familiar objects and family members *Auditory Environment:* • Derives obvious pleasure from auditory activities like music, playing with friends, laughing, and being read to *Auditory Experience:* • Listening to speech for long periods of time is essential to the ultimate use of even single words	*Overextension and Underextension of Words:* • Language develops as a direct correlation of using that developing speech to ultimately gain a desired outcome through a communication interaction between the speaker and the listener *Gradual Decontextualization (to 18 months):* • Says first clear, distinct word and assigns that word to a single distinct object or person
16–20 months		*Fast Mapping:* • Ability to learn words in one or few exposures
18 months	*Auditory Vocabulary:* • Tremendous growth in vocabulary comprehension, 100–200 words understood	*First 50 Words Used: A First Language:* • Growth in expressive ability • Tremendous growth in one-word usage
18–24 months	*Auditory Localization:* • Will independently seek out a sound source in another room *Auditory Comprehension:* • Understands and follows verbal directions with two critical elements • Begins to respond appropriately to "What, where" questions	*Word Spurt: Vocabulary Spurt* • "Naming theory" seems to be a basis for noun usage, naming people, objects; occurs for most children when they hit the first 50 words mark • Will begin to sing along with songs or mimic the rhythm of a nursery rhyme

Ages 2–3

	Listening	Speaking
24–36 months	*Auditory Identification:* • Will identify a sound and share that identification with another person with exuberance • Desires to share auditory information with another person *Auditory Memory:* • Will share auditory experiences from memory (left brain) • Will sing complete or nearly complete songs from memory (right brain)	*Cognitive/Semantic:* • Two-word semantic relations, and three-word-plus utterances *Spoken Language and Play:* • Will hold a seemingly appropriate conversation with an inanimate object while playing *Presyntactic period*
26–32 months		*Phoneme repetition:* • Vocabulary size seems related to ability to repeat phoneme combinations, especially initial position in nonwords
By 36 months		*Early Syntactic:* • Recombination of two-plus-two word utterances • Early multiple word utterances, correct word order *Early Morphology:* • "ing"

Ages 3–4: Peers, Preschool

	Listening	Speaking
3–4 years	*Auditory Memory:* • Begins to show listening preferences for favorite stories or music and will follow simple aural commands *Auditory Attention:* • Development of sustained auditory attention for increasing periods of time *"Overhearing" or "Incidental" Learning Through Listening:* • Does not need to be involved in direct instruction or directly in a conversation to pick up on what is happening; uses words, expressions not directly taught	*Pragmatics:* • Able to hold an appropriate turn-taking conversation with a peer; continuing to develop conversational competence **Cognitive Semantic** *Phonology:* • Phonetic repertoire mastered for some phonemes • Phonological processes occurring

(continues)

Table 12.1   *(continued)*

	Listening	Speaking
	Auditory Feedback Mechanism: • Development of auditory feedback mechanism • Development of phonemic awareness and temporal processing *Distance Listening:* • Ability to search the auditory environment for information even if engaged in activity	*Preliteracy:* • Recitation by rhyme • Rhyme by pattern • Alliteration *Early Syntactic Child:* • Increased morphological use, correct sentence word order • Begins to produce increasingly complex sentences that adhere to spoken language rules
4–5 years	*Achieves Metalinguistic Ability Through Audition:* • Recognizes and can report when he or she hears someone make an error or slip of the tongue in spoken language • Uses auditory cues in conversations to recognize prosodic, pragmatics, semantic and syntactic errors in adult and peer speech	*Pragmatics/Discourse:* • Follows adult conventions for conversation mechanisms; able to take role as "conversational partner" *Preliteracy: Phonologic Awareness* • Syllable counting (50% of children by age 5)

Ages 5–6: Preacademic Readiness

	Auditory Developments	Speaking
5–6 years	*Auditory Attention:* • Development of an attention span for instruction, even if the topic is not of high interest *Auditory Memory:* • Stronger development for long-term auditory memory of linguistic information *Internal Auditory Feedback:* • Development of internal auditory feedback (reading voice in head); auditory self-correcting	*Pragmatics/Discourse:* • Oral narrative more developed *Early Literacy: Phonologic Awareness* • Initial consonant matching • Blending 2–3 phonemes • Counting phonemes: 70% of children by age 6 • Rhyme identification • Onset-rime division *Syntax* • Increasing mastery of complex language forms: relative clauses, coordination, subordination, use of the infinitive verbs • Increased mastery of language systems: tense marking, modals and semimodals, pronouns, determiners

Ages 7 and Up: Refining Auditory Skills

7 years	*Assessable Auditory Processing Function:* • Higher level auditory skills are mostly developed and intact: dichotic listening, auditory figure ground, selective auditory attention *Phonemic Awareness:* • Sound blending, sound symbol association *Prosody and Suprasegmentals* • Ability to sense vocal sarcasm • Ability to resist heavy accent and follow conversation (decoding and closure) *Auditory Lexicon:* • 14,000 words (approx.)	*Phonologic Awareness:* • Blending 3 phonemes • Segmentation of 3–4 phonemes (blends) • Phonetic spelling • Phoneme deletion *Syntax:* • Expressive vocabulary
8 years	*Auditory Processing Overload Strategies:* • Develops compensatory strategies when faced with the challenge of auditory processing overload • Uses volume independently to aid in focus and attention *Auditory Attention for Music* • Begins to have an "ear" for music, auditory attention for musical instruction	*Phonologic Awareness:* • Consonant cluster segmentation • Deletion with clusters

(continues)

Table 12.1 (*continued*)

	Auditory Developments	Speaking
9 years	*Auditory Input Primary for Instruction:* • Auditory begins to become the primary input system for classroom instruction • Higher level auditory visual integration skills for organization management like note taking • End of the right ear advantage	

Data from Owens, R.E. (2012), Language Development: An Introduction, Allyn and Bacon; Cole & Flexer (2011), Children with Hearing Loss: Developing Listening and Talking, Plural Publishing; and Oller (1986), Metaphonology and infant vocalizing, in Precursors of Early Speech, ed. Lindblom, B., and Zettersrom, R., Stockton Press.

received auditory–verbal therapy (Rhoades & Duncan, 2010) from an early age. These children achieved language levels commensurate with hearing peers (Dornan, Hickson, Murdoch, & Houston, 2007; Duncan, 1999; Rhoades & Chisolm, 2000) or went on to mainstream education and higher education (Goldberg & Flexer, 1993, 2001).

Rationale for Teaching Language Through Audition

How is it possible to achieve spoken language outcomes as described in the previous section with children who are deaf or hard of hearing? First, and most important, typically developing children learn speech and spoken language through audition, and it is the most effective way to acquire this competence and performance (Ling, 2002). Audition is so essential in this task that even a mild hearing loss can compromise spoken language learning (Flexer, 1995). It is possible for the child who is deaf or hard of hearing to acquire auditory spoken language because of the redundancy cues contained in spoken communication: communication context and intent, semantic content and noun–verb meanings, stress–time information, intonation patterns, word order regularity, phonotactic probability knowledge, reading body language, facial cues, tone of voice, and motivation to understand (Fry, 1978; Ling, 2002; Ling & Ling, 1978). We can give them access to the sounds of the speech input signal and, even if this not perfect, children with hearing loss can learn to fill in the gaps or "get the gist." Auditory comprehension improves as the child learns to use linguistic cues and the rules of language (Ling, 2002).

Second, the link between speech perception and production (as presented previously) is vital. Table 12.1 demonstrates how the infant increasingly tunes in to the cues for speech, initiates the process of development of control of motor speech, and uses vocal/speech behaviors to communicate in year one of life. The child's speech output in year one lags behind his or her auditory learning. First we listen, then we talk. Also, the infant's anatomy and physiology for speech production need to develop to enable more mature sound imitation. This is coupled with the increasing use of immature, then more mature vocalizations as a way to participate in communication with parents. There is evidence for a 15-month-old child with a severe hearing loss to **telescope vocal development**; within only 15 days of hearing aid wearing, she progressed from immature verbalizations to the production of the entire range of year one vocal behaviors (Paterson, 1992). This is evidence that a more biologically mature child was able to start catching up once her brain was able to access sound and spoken language input.

Audition assists speech acquisition. Children use hearing to help match their speech to adult models in their environment (Pollack, Goldberg, & Caleffe-Schenck, 1997). Children tend to talk the way they hear (Ling, 2002), so accurate input is needed for the child to develop appropriate speech and spoken language skills. The computer has been used as an analogy for this process; there is a saying from computer science: "garbage in, garbage out." In other words, if the child does not have **auditory access** to the complete speech signal, his or her ability to process that information and then produce accurate spoken language is compromised. In this type of scenario, acquiring adequate speech and spoken language skills becomes an arduous task (Cole & Flexer, 2011).

Third, most children with hearing loss can benefit from current hearing technologies. For children with profound losses, cochlear implants from an early age and appropriate auditory intervention have been shown to provide the auditory access needed for the development of listening and spoken language (Dornan et al., 2007; Nicholas & Geers, 2006).

Fourth, today the majority of children who are deaf or hard of hearing are using spoken language to communicate and are learning in regular education settings with typical hearing children (Gallaudet Research Institute, 2008; Luckner, 2010). We know that 92–96% of children with hearing loss have hearing parents; perhaps this is why most parents are choosing spoken language options (Mitchell & Karchmer, 2002). This trend means that many training programs are seeing the need to adjust their models and curriculum. Many deaf and hard of hearing students may be supported by professionals who do not have training in listening, speech, and spoken language development (Houston & Perigoe, 2010a, 2010b). In fact, there is federal awareness (Joint Committee on Infant Hearing, 2007) that there is a shortage of specially trained professionals who understand how to facilitate learning with advanced hearing technology with the birth to 5 years population. The same need exists to train flexible professionals who have a strong foundation of knowledge and skills in developing and maintaining development of listening and spoken language from birth through high school (Houston & Perigoe, 2010a, 2010b; Paterson & Cole, 2010).

What are some of the essential best practices and knowledge to ensure that each child with hearing loss can achieve optimal auditory development in the spoken language acquisition process? The following section will propose a framework for auditory skill development and suggest some tools for ongoing diagnostic assessment and auditory-based intervention.

A Framework for Auditory Skill Development

A model for auditory work originally suggested by Hirsh (1970) as a framework for adult aural habilitation and popularized by Erber (1982), Ling (2002), Ling and Ling (1978), and others still forms the starting point for current models and hierarchies used for younger children with hearing loss.

Although the levels in Table 12.2 are often presented as a hierarchy of development, they do, in fact, overlap. It is critical that the child who is deaf or hard of hearing develop awareness of sound and attention to auditory input as a foundational skill; however, it should be remembered that, like children with normal hearing, children with hearing loss do not necessarily develop these skills in a strictly hierarchical manner. In other words, they are developing all four levels of skill—detection, discrimination, identification, and comprehension—at the phoneme level, word level, sentence level, and discourse level concurrently. For example, the child may be working on *detection* of sound over distance, developing his or her ability to *identify* by imitating and alternating syllables that begin with various consonants (phoneme level), *discriminating* between words that differ in voicing of the initial consonant (word level), and demonstrating *comprehension* by recalling three critical elements in a message (sentence level) and by identifying an object from several descriptors (discourse level). This is because a child may be developing skills at more than one level simultaneously (Cole & Paterson, 1984; Paterson, 1982; Welling, 2010).

The expanded framework shown in Table 12.3 reflects this need for movement among all of the levels. We should not get stuck at the level of word discrimination, but move the child toward auditory comprehension of connected discourse. It can be used for assessment, goal setting, lesson planning, and intervention and incorporates the Hirsh (1970) and Erber (1982) levels with Ling's (2002) speech production model.

Typically developing children with normal hearing will develop listening skills within natural language contexts.

Table 12.2 Levels of Auditory Skill Development

Four Levels	Definition
Detection	The ability to perceive the presence (or absence) of sound. Detection tasks are often used when conditioning a child to sound when a child's verbal response is not required.
Discrimination	Involves the ability to determine whether two stimuli are the same or different. These can be two environmental sounds, two speech sounds, two words, two phrases, two sentences, or two songs/rhymes, for example.
Identification	Involves the child's ability to identify what has been labeled or named. This is sometimes called *recognition*.
Comprehension	The highest level of auditory processing. The term is generally used when talking about understanding the meaning of the auditory input and application to known information, experiences, and language. Anderson's (2004) checklist in Appendix B of this chapter provides further information on types of auditory comprehension.

Table 12.3   Framework for Developing Listening: Assessment, Goal Setting, Lesson Planning, and Intervention

	Sounds Nonspeech Speech	**Syllables** Nonsegmentals Segmentals	**Words** Content Function Semantics Morphology	**Phrases** Carrier Chunking Clauses	**Sentences** Increasing syntactic complexity Pragmatics	**Connected Discourse** Conversation Narration Explanation/ Directions Description Questions All aspects of language Songs/rhymes
Detection						
Discrimination						
Identification						
Comprehension						

Adapted from the following: Erber, N. (1982). Auditory training. Washington, DC: Alexander Graham Bell Association for the Deaf.; Ling, D. (2002). Speech and the hearing-impaired child: Theory and practice (2nd ed.). Washington, DC: Alexander Graham Bell Association for the Deaf.; Romanik, S. (2008). Auditory skills program for students with hearing impairment. Moorebank, Australia: New South Wales Department of Education and Training. Available from: http://www.schools.nsw.edu.au/media/downloads/schoolsweb/studentsupport/programs/disability/audskills.pdf

Children with hearing loss may need more structured listening settings for the practice of such skills. Generally, the older the child and the less well he or she uses his or her hearing, the more structured or formal the intervention will need to be (Ling, Perigoe, & Gruenwald, 1981).

Today, we have infant learners who may follow a more typical auditory–verbal learning trajectory, but we also still see children who are late starters. These may be children whose hearing losses were not detected until later, those with progressive hearing losses, those who develop hearing loss later, and those who (for whatever reason) start their auditory experience as toddlers or preschoolers. Auditory intervention may need to be more planned or structured for those who start later, while still being founded on a developmental, conversational model of spoken language acquisition (Paterson, 1982).

We have found the Auditory Learning Guide (ALG), which Walker (2009) adapted from work by Simser (1993), to be helpful in setting goals across several auditory skill levels. The ALG is reprinted in Appendix A at the end of this chapter, and should serve as a useful guide.

Conditions for Implementing the Model

What conditions are necessary for success in using this model of auditory skill development? Professionals working with the family need to ensure maximal auditory access with appropriate hearing technology, develop skill in using the Ling Six-Sound Test (Ling, 2006), provide an optimal auditory environment, and implement plans based on diagnostic information that incorporates the concept of hearing age or listening age.

Auditory Access

Ensuring that each child who is deaf or hard of hearing has optimal access to the speech signal through appropriate advanced hearing technology is a key principle of auditory-based learning approaches. What are the factors, protocols, assessment tools, and concepts involved in ensuring optimal auditory access? The factors include access to and consistent wearing of appropriate individual hearing instruments, monitoring of the child's auditory learning through the hearing device(s), appropriate ongoing audiologic management, and sufficient auditory input of language.

Current medical treatments and hearing technologies are now so sophisticated (with hearing aids, bone-anchored hearing aids, assistive listening devices, auditory training devices, sound field systems, cochlear implants, and brainstem implants) that the majority of children with hearing loss can be provided access to sounds across the entire spectrum of speech. Consistent use of appropriate hearing technology to provide this access is the critical first step in developing listening and spoken language in children with hearing loss. Cole and Flexer (2011) discuss this current availability of new hearing technologies as creating a new "acoustic conversation"—one in which children who are deaf or hard of hearing can function (with technology) as though they have only a mild or moderate hearing loss. Today, we can expect children who use cochlear implant(s) to achieve excellent vowel discrimination and to discriminate the high-frequency bursts that enable place discrimination among /p, t, k/, as well as the high-frequency turbulent noise for perception and discrimination of fricatives, such as "sh" and /s/. On the other hand, it is now the child who is wearing hearing aids who may have no or little access to high-frequency speech information and who may struggle to make those same discriminations. Because a greater amount of speech information is concentrated in the higher frequencies, access to speech sounds above 2000 Hz is needed to make the fine discriminations necessary for processing speech (Killion & Mueller, 2010).

Daily Perceptual Check of Detection and Discrimination: The Ling Six-Sound Test

It has become common practice for parents and professionals working with children with hearing loss to perform a daily morning listening check of the child's ability to detect or discriminate through their hearing instruments. The Ling Six-Sound Test (Ling, 2006) has become the established protocol. The sounds are arranged here in order, representing the lowest frequency of speech to the highest: /u/, /m /, /a/, /i/, "sh," and /s/. These six sounds represent the frequency range of the entire speech spectrum. Some professionals have added "silence" as another sound to check for false-positive responses (Cole & Flexer, 2011). This test has become popularized, and various versions and explanations of usage exist, both in print (Ling, 1989, 2002, 2006) and online (Advanced Bionics, 2012; Cochlear Corporation, 2012).

Each child who is deaf or hard of hearing is a unique listener. It is possible to identify speech perception problems by noting any auditory confusion while doing the test. One known phenomenon can be diagnosed as in the following example. In the administration of the Six-Sound Test, you say the /u/ vowel and the child repeats /u/. Then, you say the /i/ vowel and the child says /u/, not /i/. You repeat this several times and the child still cannot discriminate the /i/ from the /u/. Why does this happen? The child is able to perceive both the low-frequency, first formant (F1) and the mid-frequency second formant (F2) of /u/. However, /u/ and /i/ have a similar, low-frequency first formant (F1), which is created by resonance in the pharynx. The second formant (F2) resonates in front of the tongue. The /i/ vowel is a high, front vowel and the tongue constriction creates a high F2 at about 2700 Hz. A child who cannot hear at this higher frequency will not be able to tell /u/ and /i/ apart; therefore, these two vowels will sound the same. This is an example of how knowledge of speech acoustics is essential for working with the child who is deaf or hard of hearing.

Understanding Acoustic Cues for Prosody and Redundancy in the Speech Signal

As we saw earlier in Table 12.1, infants tune in to the prosodic features of parent talk and begin to deduce meaning in context before they are developmentally able to focus on word boundaries. Auditory development in the earliest stages seems based on the "melody of the message" (Fernald, 1989). This is why babies like songs, rhythm, repetition, sing-song voices, and all the vocal variations that adults use in infant-directed speech (Cole & Flexer, 2011; Owens, 2012). Infants do not start by listening for phonemes or suprasegmental features in isolation. In fact, it seems easier for them and for us as adults to tune in to the spoken message if there is more acoustic information to work from. The child with hearing loss needs the same opportunity to learn to deduce meaning from spoken input that is sufficiently long enough to convey essential prosodic information. As you can see in Table 12.4, prosody carries an enormous meaning load in English (Cole & Paterson, 1984), from the intonation contours that are created when we produce different sentence modalities, to the crucial stress-timing features that are a hallmark of English. The table indicates that acoustic cues for prosody are in the low- and mid-frequency range, where almost every child who is deaf or hard of hearing has auditory access. In fact, these prosodic cues are *only* available to us through auditory perception (Ling, 2002), and it is almost impossible to speech-read them. It is crucial that professionals working with all ages of children who are deaf and hard of hearing understand how prosody occurs and the important role it plays in auditory comprehension of connected discourse (Paterson, 1986).

Here is a quick exercise to help with the concept. The difference in meaning in the identical utterances listed in Table 12.5 is comprehended by the listener through attention to the redundant prosodic and linguistic cues. The meanings are:

1. *Possession:* Tell me who owns the object.
2. *Modify the noun:* Tell me which object.
3. *Identify the object:* Tell me what you own.

Linguistic cues: the word order creates the sentence pattern for transitive sentence and statement and helps the listener predict what information will follow. The pronoun *I* signals who (subject) and signals that a verb is coming; the verb *have* signals possession and that an object is coming; the adjective *blue* signals that a noun is coming. However, additional suprasegmental changes are produced that we listen to as prosodic cues: Stress marking of the key word in the

Table 12.4 Prosodic Feature Comparison: The Acoustic Cues for Perception and Production

Suprasegmentals of Speech in Isolation	Prosodic Features as They Appear in Spoken Language	Acoustic Terms and Measurement	Acoustic Information Required to Perceive and Discriminate Speech Sounds/Prosody, Related to Audiogram	Anatomy and Physiology: Part(s) of the Speech System Involved in Production
Vocalization	Overall vocal quality, timbre • Oral vs. nasal sounding • Not harsh	Fundamental frequency, Fo: Measured in cycles per second (cps) or Hertz (Hz)	Male voice: 100–120 Hz Female voice: 160–200 Hz Child voice: 300 Hz	• Vocal folds • Phonation
Duration	Timing changes: • Rhythm • Rate of speech • Pause patterns • Juncture	Duration: Measured in milliseconds (msec)	Voicing: 250 Hz 500 Hz	• Vocal folds, phonation • Breath/air flow • Dynamic force in lungs
Intensity	Stress marking: • Marking primary stress in words Voice loudness variations: • Whisper • Soft voice • Normal conversational voice • Loud voice • Outdoor voice	Amplitude: Measured in decibels (dB)	Voicing: 250 Hz 500 Hz 1000 Hz	• Vocal folds, phonation • Breath/air flow • Subglottal pressure variations

Pitch	Intonational contour variations:
	• Appears across utterances and sentences, and between sentences
	• Each sentence modality has a unique intonation pattern:
	  • Statement pattern
	  • Question pattern
	  • Command pattern
	  • Negative pattern
	Tone of voice:
	• Affect: joy, sadness, sarcasm, etc.
	Habitual vocal pitch:
	• Appropriate for age
		Frequency: Measured in Hertz (Hz)	Voicing:
			250 Hz
			500 Hz
			1000 Hz
				• Vocal folds, phonation
				• Breath/air flow
				• Vocal fold tension
				• Vocal fold mass changes

Adapted from the following: Cole, E. B., & Paterson, M. M. (1984). Assessment and treatment of phonologic disorders in the hearing impaired. In J. Costello (Ed.), Recent advances in speech disorders in children (pp. 93–127). San Diego, CA: College-Hill Press.; Ling, D. (2002). Speech and the hearing-impaired child: Theory and practice (2nd ed.). Washington, DC: Alexander Graham Bell Association for the Deaf.; Ling, D., & Ling, A. H. (1978). Aural habilitation: The foundations of verbal learning. Washington, DC: Alexander Graham Bell Association for the Deaf.; Paterson, M. M. (1986). Maximizing the use of residual hearing with school-aged hearing impaired children. Volta Review Monograph, 88(5), 93–106.

Table 12.5 Prosody: The Importance of Suprasegmental Changes for Understanding Language

Phrase	Meaning	Word Class
1. I have a blue <u>car</u>.	Tells me the object	Noun
2. I have a <u>blue</u> car.	Tells me which object	Adjective
3. <u>I</u> have a blue car.	Tells me who owns the object	Personal pronoun

Underline indicates primary stress marking.

utterance (mostly a rapid intensity change with duration); intonation contour across the utterance, which signals sentence pattern as a statement; and interaction of duration and intonation pattern, which carries the tone of voice or attitude of the speaker (boasting, happiness, etc.). Try producing these utterances with a flat voice and then with appropriate prosodic features. See how much you rely on the acoustic cues to quickly identify, discriminate, and comprehend.

Auditory Environment and Auditory Input

The term **auditory environment** has come into recent use to describe the child's listening situation, both in the home and, later, at school. Once the family and child with hearing loss have gone through screening, diagnostic audiology, and fitting of amplification or cochlear implant, long-term habilitation or intervention provides the regularity of support for parent and child (Cole, Carroll, Coyne, Gill, & Paterson, 2004). One of the first goals is to help the parent understand the importance of creating an optimal auditory environment. This means more than just having the parent assess the noise in the environment. In addition to reducing background noise by turning off televisions, radios, and other electronic devices and machines, the parent can improve the child's auditory access by moving closer to the child. Reducing the distance from 6 feet to 3 feet increases the sound input to the child by 6 decibels (dB). Halving the distance again to 1 1/2 feet adds an additional 6 dB. Thus, sitting close to the child and being on the same level, perhaps side-by-side, can help improve auditory access. Ling refers to this as keeping the child "within earshot" (Ling, 1980).

Overhearing or Incidental Learning

Children with hearing loss should first learn to listen in optimal conditions where the signal-to-noise ratio is good and the distance from the adult's voice to the microphones of the child's hearing technology is fairly close. Once the child begins to learn to listen and attach linguistic meaning to the speech signal, listening confidence grows. Then, the child who is deaf or hard of hearing can perceive, discriminate, localize, and comprehend from greater distances than earshot (Ling, 1980). The goal is to help the child learn how to acquire spoken language through listening. To do this effectively, the child needs to learn the cues for redundancy: prosodic patterns, phonotactic probabilities, context of the conversation, word and world knowledge, and knowledge of the rules of syntax. Today, we expect many of these children to also demonstrate spontaneous learning without direct instruction. The typical child with normal hearing develops the ability to learn through overhearing. In fact, it is suggested that overhearing or incidental learning accounts for a substantial amount of world knowledge, vocabulary development, and social awareness. Learning through distance listening and overhearing is a desirable goal for the child who is deaf or hard of hearing to achieve (Beck & Flexer, 2011; Cole & Flexer, 2011).

Talk Time: Amount and Quality of Input

The most important sensory input that the child receives is spoken language. This helps to establish skills for entry into the social world of communication. Abundant spoken language input is needed for the child to develop adequate spoken language skills. This was demonstrated in a landmark study by Hart and Risley (1995), who did frequency counts of words heard by children. They found that children who heard more words spoken by adults in their environment had better vocabularies and IQ scores. This research has been corroborated by more recent studies using electronic recording and analysis devices (Oller et al., 2010; Zimmerman et al., 2009) and was the basis for the development of the LENA technology (LENA Foundation, http://www.lenafoundation.org).

LENA stands for Language Environment Analysis. The LENA system uses an automatic electronic recording device and computer analysis software to analyze the child's listening language environment. The software package provides reports on frequency of adult talk, frequency of conversational turns, child vocalizations, and amount of background noise in the child's language learning environment. It has been used in both home and school settings.

Because a child spends more time with the family than at intervention sessions, it is vital to encourage parents or caregivers to become knowledgeable and confident in how they talk, how much they talk, and what they talk about to their child. The LENA has become a clinical research tool that can provide information to parents about how much time they spend talking to their child, how many conversational turns the child takes, and their child's vocalizations. It can also report the amount of background noise, such as television or radio sound. Recent studies using the LENA system with young children with hearing loss indicate that the technology holds great promise for guiding parents in these key areas, so that the quality and quantity of auditory language input to the child can be increased (Morrison & Lew, 2012; Yoshinaga-Itano et al., 2011).

Hearing Age: Tracking Auditory Learning

A concept of **hearing age** or *listening age* is useful when working with children with hearing loss (Cole & Flexer, 2011; Cole & Paterson, 1984; Pollack et al., 1997). Hearing age is calculated from the date the child begins to consistently wear appropriate hearing technology. For example, if a child is 2 years old and began wearing hearing aids consistently at 3 months of age, then his functional hearing age would be 21 months. This child is not far behind and has a good chance of closing the gap between his or her hearing/listening age and his or her chronological age. A child of 3 years whose hearing loss was detected late and who did not start wearing hearing aids until 2 years old would have a hearing age of 1 year. At 2 years behind his chronological age, this child will have a more challenging time closing the gap between his or her hearing/listening age and chronological age. This calculation process can become complex if there are periods when the child does not have good auditory access to spoken language. This might be due to damaged or lost technology, poor earmolds, ear infections, deteriorating hearing thresholds, or reluctance of the child to wear the hearing technology (or the parent to put it on the child). In addition, if the child becomes a cochlear implant candidate, it is useful to calculate the amount of time of successful implant use with appropriately mapped implant(s), especially if the child did not have good access to the complete speech signal prior to receiving the implant.

The use of hearing age helps put into perspective the child's length of listening and how he or she is progressing. A child with normal hearing usually listens for about a year before first words emerge, so we need to give the child with hearing loss a sufficient amount of time to learn to listen. However, an older child (say 3 years old) with sufficient cognitive experience can accelerate learning once he or she knows how to listen and learning happens.

Auditory Hierarchies, Checklists, and Developmental Scales

In the past 20 years, universal newborn hearing screening with early detection of hearing loss, improved hearing technologies, the lowering of the age of cochlear implantation, and expectations of parents in choosing auditory–oral education options have all had an impact on the requisite knowledge and skills needed by professionals. Cochlear implants in particular have led to a surge in interest in using audition to develop spoken language. More and more professionals, cochlear implant and hearing aid manufacturers, and professional organizations have produced information related to auditory-based learning for children with hearing loss. Jointly written textbooks on auditory–verbal therapy (Estabrooks, 2012; Rhoades & Duncan, 2010), auditory models, hierarchies of auditory skills, checklists, and scales of development have appeared. Some focus purely on auditory skills, whereas others have information on additional areas of development. Although both types are helpful, it is essential for the professional who is providing intervention to be aware of the holistic development of each child and see how auditory skills are being acquired in relation to other areas of development. As we observe and document the progress of a child with hearing loss, it is important to view the whole child—not a set of ears in isolation (Boothroyd & Gatty, 2012).

A list of useful resources, including auditory hierarchies, checklists, and developmental scales, can be found in Appendix C at the end of this chapter. It is by no means an exhaustive list, but will give the reader some resources. The Auditory Skills Checklist by Anderson (2004) is available online and also printed by permission at the end of this chapter. Also available online is the Integrated Scales of Development by Cochlear Corporation (2009). In conjunction with other auditory measures, these can be useful when observing the child's listening behaviors to help guide both assessment and intervention.

Functional Auditory Assessment

The term **functional auditory assessment** has been used to describe a variety of parent and teacher reporting tools. Good summaries of these are available in Cole and Flexer (2011, pp. 164–165), from Tharpe & Flynn (2012, available from the Oticon website: www.oticon.com/~asset/cache.ashx?id=10835&type=14&format=web), and on Anderson's website (http://successforkidswithhearingloss.com/tests). For our purposes, we consider functional assessments of listening to encompass not only observational reports, but also diagnostic assessments of the child's listening skills on a variety of tasks.

Why do a functional listening assessment? Assessment is the basis for setting long- and short-term goals. It gives a baseline of performance and, when readministered, measures growth and the effectiveness of our intervention. It determines what we teach and, often, the order in which we teach it. An audiogram is limited in what it can tell us about how a child hears. It gives us information about the frequency and intensity of the child's hearing thresholds (both unaided and aided), but does not tell us anything about durational cues or how sound is processed and interpreted. Two children with similar audiograms may differ greatly in their listening and speaking skills.

Many factors can impact listening and spoken language outcomes. Some of these are intrinsic to the child, such as cognitive ability, the presence of other disabilities, learning style, and ability of the brain to process speech and spoken language input. Extrinsic factors may include age at identification and intervention, appropriateness of hearing technology, consistent wearing of hearing technology, type and amount of intervention, and parental support. It is therefore often difficult to predict functional listening abilities from audiograms. We need to go beyond the audiogram to find out what the child can do in real-life situations outside of the audiology booth. Functional assessment of listening does not replace traditional audiological assessment, but can complement and help us determine the amount of carryover (Robbins, Svirsky, Osberger, & Pisoni, 1998). By evaluating how the child uses his or her hearing, we get a more complete picture of the child's abilities.

As with any type of assessment, professionals need to have a basic understanding of what we are assessing and why we are assessing it. Are we using the results to set goals, measure the effectiveness of our intervention, or establish eligibility for services? We need to be able to assess clients of different ages and abilities. We need to adapt assessments as needed and to select goals, teach, and then reassess. We also need to be able to interpret our assessment results and explain them to the family.

Assessments may be formal or informal. Most formal tests are available commercially, but do not underestimate the value of teacher-made assessments. Tests may be normed or criterion referenced. Due to the lack of current normed data for children with hearing loss, we are primarily using criterion-referenced tests, which assess the child's level of performance against his or her earlier scores. Tests may be subjective (such as parent reports) or objective, such as those based on observation or on having the child demonstrate specific tasks. It is usually instructive to have a variety of assessments and not base all information on one kind of assessment. For example, questionnaires are helpful, but we suggest that you confirm these impressions by observing what the child does and perhaps developing some informal diagnostic activities to assess his or her listening skills.

Rather than give an exhaustive list of tests, we will talk about types of tests and suggest some assessments we have used with success. Then we will provide some guidelines for creating your own assessments.

Questionnaires

Several questionnaires are available that fall into two categories: those for parents and those for teachers. Although parent reports are subjective, they can be an excellent starting point when assessing infants and very young children. They can also be useful with hard to test children. Teacher reports can give good insight into how the child functions in the classroom. The professional should be familiar with a few of these tools and how they can be used.

Two parent interview tools that we have found helpful are the Meaningful Auditory Integration Scale (MAIS; Robbins, Renshaw, & Berry, 1991) and the Infant–Toddler Meaningful Auditory Integration Scale (IT-MAIS; Zimmerman-Phillips, Osberger, & Robbins, 1997). These scales consist of 10 probe items designed to assess the young child's use of hearing, hearing technology, and early auditory skills. The MAIS was designed for children ages 3 and up and the IT-MAIS was later developed for children ages 0–3 years. The IT-MAIS is now available from Advanced Bionics online (http://c324175.r75.cf1.rackcdn.com/IT-MAS_20brochure_20_2.pdf). We have found that, because companies sometimes change where particular pages are located on their websites, it is often more efficient to find items by using a web search engine.

Another useful tool is *LittlEARS: Auditory Questionnaire Manual: Parent Questionnaire to Assess Auditory Behavior in Young Children* (Coninx, Weichbold, & Tsiakpini, 2003), which is available through Med-El.

A parent tool that guides the parent through observation of listening activities is the test of Early Listening Function (ELF, Anderson, 2002). This has the added advantage of assessing the young child's ability to hear a variety of speech and environmental sounds at different distances. It also looks at listening in quiet versus listening in noise, thus sensitizing the parent to the importance of the auditory environment.

Two tools useful for classroom teachers are the Screening Instrument for Targeting Educational Risk (SIFTER, Anderson, 1989) and the Preschool SIFTER (Anderson & Matkin, 1996). These each have 15 items that help the teacher identify which children may be at risk for educational failure. These and other assessment tools by Anderson are available for free from her website (http://successforkidswithhearingloss.com/tests).

Closed-Set Auditory Assessments

Closed-set assessments have a fixed number of stimuli from which the child chooses the correct answer. For example, the child may have a set of four objects or picture cards from which to choose—a ball, a cookie, a hotdog, and a hamburger. The examiner presents the word through audition only, such as "cookie," and the child must select the correct item. In our experience, it is highly advantageous to have the child repeat the word (or an approximation) before selecting the item. This helps the tester to determine whether the child is selecting what he or she actually heard or is just picking a favored item. Two well-known assessments used in closed-set tasks are the Early Speech Perception Test (ESP), which uses pictures, and the Low-Verbal ESP, which uses objects (Moog & Geers, 1990). These are both word-level tests, but phrase- and sentence-level assessments can be constructed for using written sentences (for students who are readers) or pictures.

Open-Set Auditory Assessments

Open-set assessments are tests for which there are no materials—the items on the test are unknown to the child. This is a more difficult assessment, because the child does not have a group of items from which to choose. The set can be limitless; however, it is important to remember that the items need to be within the child's receptive language vocabulary. The Glendonald Auditory Screening Procedure (GASP) has a word-level test of 12 words and a sentence-level series of 10 questions (Erber, 1982). Both the GASP words and GASP sentences are straightforward and do not take very long to administer or score. They may need to be adapted for young children.

A useful assessment for older students is *Auditory Rehabilitation: Memory, Language, Comprehension Test Probes* (Stefanakos & Prater, 1982). Originally designed for hearing individuals, we find this a very good assessment for children ages 10 and older who are placed in regular education classrooms. It begins with having the evaluator read one sentence and assessing the child's ability to answer one fact-based question based on the information provided in the sentence. The probes increase in length and complexity until the examiner is reading a short paragraph and asking five fact-based and two inference questions. Many of the passages contain new or unknown information/vocabulary, so it is a worthwhile assessment of whether the child can process (and remember) new information.

Comprehensive Assessments

A test that assesses a wide range of auditory abilities is the Auditory Perception Test for the Hearing-Impaired (APT/HI-R) (Allen, 2008). Designed for ages 3 and older, the test begins at a basic level of sound detection and progresses

through 16 skill areas of discrimination tasks, identification, comprehension with a picture prompt, and, finally, open-set auditory comprehension (similar to the GASP sentences). Skills are assessed in auditory plus visual versus auditory-only presentations, and results are reported on a student profile. This profile is a visual representation of the student's auditory functioning on each of the auditory skills assessed. Comparison of the auditory plus visual and the auditory-only profiles over time are useful for documenting student progress (Rosa-Lugo & Allen, 2011).

Practical Application: Developing Your Own Assessments

Auditory learning is a dynamic process, and therefore assessment at various levels is needed. Children who are deaf or hard of hearing are a heterogeneous population; in other words, no two children are alike. It is necessary to gear your selection of assessments toward the individual child and his or her particular abilities. Once a professional understands the rationale behind the various assessments, it is possible to construct assessments that meet the needs of each child. This can be particularly useful when assessments need to be adapted or constructed for students with hearing loss and additional challenges or those with linguistic or cultural differences.

For example, if you were working with a 2 1/2-year-old child with limited vocabulary, you would need to select items that would be in the child's listening vocabulary. Your instinct might be to use picture cards and have the child point, but it would be better to use three-dimensional objects or toys, because they will be more engaging and can be used in a more informal way. Table 12.6 provides an example of words that differ in number of syllables (pattern perception), two-syllable spondee words with equal stress, and three-syllable words that you might use in such an auditory task.

For a young child with very little vocabulary, you might use sound–object or sound–action associations, often called the "learning to listen" sounds (Estabrooks & Birkenshaw-Fleming, 2006; Rhoades, 2000). These usually include animal and vehicle sounds and emphasize different suprasegmental features of speech. They should be done with toys in an informal play situation to see what the child can select from a small set of choices. Table 12.7 provides an example of how these might be organized for an informal auditory-only assessment.

For an open-set word test, again, you should be guided by the child's vocabulary. Table 12.8 lists some words you might use with a young preschool-aged child with hearing

Table 12.6   A Closed-Set Auditory Task

Pattern Perception	Spondees	Monosyllables
Ball	Hotdog	Ball
Cookie	Airplane	Book
Hotdog	Toothbrush	Bird
Hamburger	Bathtub	Boat
Total Correct		

Vary order of presentation within each column.

Table 12.7   A Closed-Set Auditory Task Using Learning to Listen Sounds

Pattern Perception	Two Syllables	Single, Extended Sounds
moo	quack-quack	mmm >>>
oink-oink	oink-oink	ah >>>>
hop-hop-hop	beep-beep	oo >>>
Total Correct		

Vary order of presentation within each column.

Table 12.8   Open-Set Auditory Tasks for a Young Child with Hearing Loss

GASP WORDS
(vary order of presentation)

One Syllable	Two-Syllable Trochees (Unequal Stress)	Two-Syllable Spondees (Equal Stress)	Three Syllables
Shoe	Water	Airplane	Butterfly
Fish	Table	Popcorn	Elephant
Ball	Pencil	Toothbrush	Santa Claus
Total Correct:_____ /12			

Sample Auditory Assessment for Open-Set Words

Child's Name _____ C.A. _____ H.A. _____ Date _____

(vary order of presentation)

One Syllable	Two-Syllable Trochees (Unequal Stress)	Two-Syllable Spondees (Equal Stress)	Three Syllables
Shoe	Cookie	Backpack	Hamburger
Fish	Baby	Hotdog	Elephant
Ball	Pencil	Bathtub	Santa Claus
Total Correct:_____ /12			

Blank Table for My Own Words

Child's Name _____ C.A. _____ H.A. _____ Date _____

(vary order of presentation)

One Syllable	Two-Syllable Trochees (Unequal Stress)	Two-Syllable Spondees (Equal Stress)	Three Syllables
Total Correct:_____ /12			

Adapted from Erber, N. (1982). Auditory Training. Washington DC: Alexander Graham Bell Association.

loss. First, we have presented Erber's word list from the GASP (1982), then our own words (based on a fictitious child), and, finally, left a blank table for you to use for creating your own words. Remember to vary the order of presentation of the words (don't just read down or across the list) and to give the assessment through audition alone with no visual or context cues.

This has been only a sampling of functional listening assessments and how you might also develop your own auditory assessments. Ongoing diagnostic assessment and intervention is an integral part of listening and spoken language programs.

Summary

Speech pathologists and teachers of the deaf/hard of hearing play a critical role on the team with audiologists and other professionals. They need to be able to interpret results from the audiologist and be able to explain these results to parents. In addition, they should assess the functional listening skills of the child and see how these results fit with the child's test results from the audiologist. An understanding of how auditory skills develop, how they are related to the development of spoken language, and how to observe and assess these skills is critical in order to lay the foundation for intervention. In conjunction with the parents, professionals should design an integrated program that incorporates acquisition of listening skills into the development of speech and spoken language.

When consistently using appropriate, current hearing technology, children with hearing loss have the opportunity to process spoken language through hearing. However, intensive auditory stimulation may be necessary for them to attain the listening and speaking skills commensurate with typically developing peers. Much depends on the ability of professionals and support personnel to monitor hearing technology, report any changes in hearing or suspected technology issues to the audiologist, optimize the child's auditory access to the speech signal, and provide effective assessment and intervention that supports use and carry-over of listening and spoken language skills to everyday, real-life communication.

As speech and hearing professionals, we are part of a collaborative team approach, seeking to develop the most effective interventions possible. The coordination of assessment and intervention among team members is critical to the child's progress and the success of his or her educational program. Our goals for intervention need to be grounded in our understanding of how typical children develop and founded on our assessments and observations of individual child behaviors. Intervention must be based on the most current information available on the child's performance—in other words, it is goal driven. In this process, we need to be asking the right questions.

Assessment and intervention that puts the emphasis on speech production, without addressing underlying auditory abilities, reduces our effectiveness as professionals and compromises the abilities of our students to succeed. An approach that answers these questions and puts appropriate emphasis on optimal auditory access for the development of listening and spoken language development makes our intervention evidence-based and yields the most likely path to success for the child. In addition, approaches that focus on the integration of listening, speech, and spoken language, rather than on isolated auditory training, will be more beneficial in the long-term.

In this chapter, we have given an overview of auditory development in typically developing children and discussed some important issues relative to the child who is deaf or hard of hearing. We have presented a framework for assessment and intervention and discussed various functional listening assessments. The next crucial step is how to plan and implement intervention for the child who is deaf or hard of hearing. The reader is encouraged to use more than just this resource when providing auditory interventions in a therapeutic setting. There are several tools and resources available, including curricula and free online materials designed for children with hearing loss, which are presented in the appendixes at the end of the chapter. We hope that these can guide you toward acquiring the knowledge and skills necessary to support children in developing listening and spoken language skills for meaningful communication.

Discussion Questions

1. Why is it important to understand how auditory skills develop in typically developing children with normal hearing?
2. What is the relationship between listening and spoken language?
3. What elements need to be in place for a child with hearing loss to learn language through audition?
4. What is the concept of "hearing/listening age," and why is it important?
5. Discuss ways to ensure a beneficial auditory environment for learning through listening.
6. Discuss the four levels of auditory skill development proposed by Hirsh. How might they guide assessment and intervention?
7. What is the rationale for conducting a diagnostic, functional listening assessment with a child who is deaf or hard of hearing?

References

Advanced Bionics. (2012). *The Ling six sound check*. Available from http://www.advancedbionics.com/content/dam/ab/Global/en_ce/documents/recipient/Ling_Six_Sound_Check-6.pdf.

Allen, S. G. (2008). *Auditory perception test for the hearing impaired–revised (APT/HI-R)*. San Diego, CA: Plural.

Anderson. K. L. (1989). *Screening instrument for targeting educational risk (SIFTER)*. Tampa, FL. Educational Audiology Association. Available from https://successforkidswithhearingloss.com/uploads/SIFTER.pdf.

Anderson, K. L. (2002). *Early listening function (ELF): Discovery tool for parents and caregivers of infants and toddlers*. Available from https://successforkidswithhearingloss.com/uploads/ELF_Questionnaire.pdf.

Anderson, K. L. (2004). *Auditory skills checklist*. Available from https://successforkidswithhearingloss.com/resources-for-professionals/early-intervention-for-children-with-hearing-loss.

Anderson, K. L., & Matkin, N. (1996). *Screening instrument for targeting educational risk in preschool children (age 3–kindergarten) (Preschool SIFTER)*. Available from https://successforkidswithhearingloss.com/uploads/Preschool_SIFTER.pdf.

Beck, D. L., & Flexer, C. (2011). Listening is where hearing meets brain . . . in children and adults. *Hearing Review*, 18(2): 30, 32–35.

Blaiser, K. M., & Culbertson, D. S. (2013). Language and speech of the deaf and hard of hearing. In R. L. Schow & M. A. Nerbonne (Eds.), *Introduction to audiologic rehabilitation* (6th ed., pp. 211–242). Boston, MA: Pearson.

Boothroyd, A. (1997). Auditory development of the hearing child. *Scandinavian Audiology*, 26(Suppl. 46): 9–16.

Boothroyd, A., & Gatty, N. (2012). *The deaf child in a hearing family: Nurturing development*. San Diego, CA: Plural.

Cochlear Corporation. (2009). *The integrated scales of development*. Listen, learn and talk. Available from http://hope.cochlearamericas.com/reading-room/listen-learn-talk.

Cochlear Corporation. (2012). *The Ling-6 sounds*. Available from http://www.cochlear.com/files/assets/Ling-6%20sound%20test%20-%20how%20to.pdf.

Cole, E. B., Carroll, N., Coyne, J., Gill, E., & Paterson, M. M. (2004). Early spoken language through audition. In S. Watkins (Ed.), *Ski-HI curriculum: Family-centered programming for infants and young children with hearing loss (Revised)* (Vol. I, pp. 137–141; Vol. II, pp. 1279–1394). Logan, UT: Hope.

Cole, E. B., & Flexer, C. (2011). *Children with hearing loss: Developing listening and talking* (2nd ed.). San Diego, CA: Plural.

Cole, E. B., & Paterson, M. M. (1984). Assessment and treatment of phonologic disorders in the hearing impaired. In J. Costello (Ed.), *Recent advances in speech disorders in children* (pp. 93–127). San Diego, CA: College-Hill Press.

Coninx, F., Weichbold, V., & Tsiakpini, L. (2003). *LittlEARS auditory questionnaire*. Available from http://www.medel.com/support-rehabilitation/.

Dornan, D. (2009). *Hearing loss in babies is a neurological emergency*. Washington, DC: Alexander Graham Bell Association for the Deaf and Hard of Hearing.

Dornan, D., Hickson, L., Murdoch, B., & Houston, T. (2007). Outcomes of an auditory-verbal program for children with hearing loss: A comparative study with a matched group of children with normal hearing. *Volta Review*, 107(1): 37–54.

Downs. M., & Yoshinaga-Itano, C. (1999). The efficacy of early identification and intervention for children with hearing impairment. *Pediatric Clinics of North America*, 46(1): 79–87.

Duncan, J. (1999). Conversational skills of children with hearing loss and children with normal hearing in an integrated setting. *Volta Review*, 101: 193–211.

Erber, N. (1982). *Auditory training*. Washington, DC: Alexander Graham Bell Association for the Deaf.

Estabrooks, W. (Ed.). (2012). *101 frequently asked questions about auditory-verbal practice: Promoting listening and spoken language for children who are deaf and hard of hearing and their families*. Washington, DC: Alexander Graham Bell Association for the Deaf and Hard of Hearing.

Estabrooks, W., & Birkenshaw-Fleming, L. (2006). *Hear & listen! Talk & sing!* Washington, DC: Alexander Graham Bell Association for the Deaf and Hard of Hearing.

Fernald, A. (1989). Intonation and communication intent in mothers' speech to infants: Is the melody the message? *Child Development*, 60: 1497–1510.

Flexer, C. (1995). FAQ on classroom management of children with minimal hearing loss. *Hearing Journal*, 48(9): 10.

Fry, D. (1978). The role and primacy of the auditory channel in speech and language development. In M. Ross & T. G. Giolas (Eds.), *Auditory management of hearing impaired children: Principles and prerequisites for intervention* (pp. 15-43). Baltimore, MD: University Park Press.

Fryauf-Bertschy, H., Tyler, R. S., Kelsay, D. M. R., & Gantz, B. J. (1997). Cochlear implant use by prelingually deafened children: The influences of age at implant and length of device use. *Journal of Speech, Language, and Hearing Research*, 40: 183–199.

Gallaudet Research Institute. (2008, Nov.). *Regional and national summary report of data from the 2007–08 annual survey of deaf and hard of hearing children and youth*. Washington, DC: GRI, Gallaudet University.

Goldberg, D. M., & Flexer, C. (1993). Outcome survey of auditory-verbal graduates: Study of clinical efficacy. *Journal of the American Academy of Audiology,* 4: 189–200.

Goldberg, D. M., & Flexer, C. (2001). Auditory-verbal graduates. An updated outcome survey of clinical efficacy. *Journal of American Academy of Audiology,* 12(8): 406–414.

Hall, S. L., & Moats, L. C. (1998). *Straight talk about reading: How parents can make a difference in the early years*. Chicago, IL: Contemporary Books

Hart, B., & Risley, T. R. (1995). *Meaningful differences in the everyday experience of young American children*. Baltimore, MD: Paul H. Brookes.

Hirsh, I. J. (1970). Auditory training. In H. Davis & S. Silverman (Eds.), *Hearing and deafness* (pp. 346–359). New York: Holt, Rinehart & Winston.

Houston, K. T., & Perigoe, C. B. (Eds.). (2010a). Professional preparation for listening and spoken language practitioners. *Volta Review* (monograph).

Houston, K. T., & Perigoe. C. (2010b). Speech-language pathologists: Vital listening and spoken language professionals. *Volta Review,* 110(2): 219–230.

Joint Committee on Infant Hearing. (2007). Year 2007 position statement: Principles and guidelines for early hearing detection and intervention programs. *Pediatrics,* 120(4): 898–921. Available from http://pediatrics.aappublications.org/content/120/4/898.full?ijkey=oj9BAleq21OlA&keytype=ref&siteid=aapjournals.

Killion, M. C., & Mueller, H. G. (2010). Twenty years later: The new count-the-dots method. *Hearing Journal,* 63(1): 10–15.

Kirk, K. I., Miyamoto, R. T., Lento, C. L., Ying, E., O'Neill, T., & Fears, B. (2002). Effects of age at implantation in young children. *Annals of Otology, Rhinology and Laryngology,* 189: 69–73.

LENA Research Foundation. Available from http://www.lenafoundation.org.

Ling, D. (1980). Keep your hearing-impaired child within earshot. *Newsounds,* 6: 5–6.

Ling, D. (1989). *Foundations of spoken language for hearing-impaired children*. Washington, DC: Alexander Graham Bell Association for the Deaf.

Ling, D. (2002). *Speech and the hearing-impaired child: Theory and practice* (2nd ed.). Washington, DC: Alexander Graham Bell Association for the Deaf.

Ling, D. (2006). The six-sound test. In W. Estabrooks (Ed.), *Auditory-verbal therapy and practice* (pp. 307–310). Washington, DC: Alexander Graham Bell Association for the Deaf and Hard of Hearing.

Ling, D., & Ling, A. H. (1978). *Aural habilitation: The foundations of verbal learning*. Washington, DC: Alexander Graham Bell Association for the Deaf.

Ling, D., Perigoe, C., & Gruenwald, A. (1981). *Phonetic level speech teaching*. Educational videotape series. Montreal, Quebec: McGill University.

Luckner, J. (2010, Feb.). *Suggestions for preparing itinerant teachers*. Presentation at the national conference of the Association of College Educators for the Deaf and Hard of Hearing (ACE-DHH), Lexington, KY.

Mitchell, R. E., & Karchmer, M. A. (2002). Chasing the mythical ten percent: Parental hearing status of deaf and hard of hearing students in the United States. *Sign Language Studies,* 4(2): 138–163.

Moog, J. S., & Geers, A. E. (1990). *Early speech perception (ESP) test*. St. Louis, MO: Central Institute for the Deaf.

Moore, J., & Linthicum, F. R. (2007). The human auditory system: A timeline of development. *International Journal of Audiology,* 46(9): 460–478.

Morrison, H., & Lew, V. (2012). *An analysis of the natural language environment of children with hearing loss: The impact of home language and maternal education level*. Poster session, Alexander Graham Bell Association for the Deaf and Hard of Hearing, Orlando, FL.

Nicholas, J. G., & Geers, A. E. (2006). Effects of early auditory experience on the spoken language of deaf children at 3 years of age. *Ear and Hearing,* 27(3): 286–298.

Oller, D. K. (1986). Metaphonology and infant vocalizations. In B. Lindblom & R. Zetterstrom (Eds.), *Precursors of early speech* (pp. 21-35). New York: Stockton Press.

Oller, D. K., Nigogi, S., Gray, S., Richards, J. A., Gilkerson, D., Xu, D., et al. (2010). Automated vocal analysis of naturalistic recordings from children with autism, language delay, and typical development. *Proceedings from the National Academy of Natural Sciences of the United States of America,* 107(30),13354-13359.

Owens, R. E. (2012). *Language development: An introduction* (8th ed.). Needham Heights, MA: Allyn and Bacon.

Paterson, M. M. (1982). Integration of auditory training with speech and language for severely hearing-impaired children. In D. G. Sims, G. G. Walter, & R. L. Whitehead (Eds.), *Deafness and communication: Assessment and training* (pp. 261–270). Baltimore, MD: Williams and Wilkins.

Paterson, M. M. (1986). Maximizing the use of residual hearing with school-aged hearing impaired children. *Volta Review Monograph,* 88(5), 93–106.

Paterson, M. M. (1992). *Vocalization behaviours of a severely hearing-impaired infant in the first fifteen days of hearing aid wearing*. Poster session, Alexander Graham Bell Association for the Deaf International Convention. San Diego, CA.

Paterson, M. M., & Cole, E. B. (2010). The University of Hartford and CREC Soundbridge: A new master's of education in aural habilitation and education of hearing impaired children. *Volta Review,* 110(2): 279–291.

Paul, P. V., & Whitelaw, G. M. (2001). *Hearing and deafness: An introduction for health and education professionals*. Sudbury, MA: Jones and Bartlett.

Pollack, D., Goldberg, D., & Caleffe-Schenck, N. (1997). *Educational audiology for the limited-hearing infant and preschooler: An auditory-verbal program* (3rd ed.). Springfield, IL: Charles C. Thomas.

Rhoades, E. (2000). *Sound-object associations (the learning to listen sounds)*. Available from http://www.listen-up.org/dnload/listen.pdf.

Rhoades, E. A., & Chisolm, T. H. (2000). Global language progress with an auditory-verbal approach. *Volta Review,* 102: 5–25.

Rhoades, E. A., & Duncan, J. (2010). *Auditory-verbal practice: Toward a family-centered approach*. Springfield, IL: Charles C. Thomas.

Robbins, A. M., Renshaw, J. J., & Berry, S. W. (1991). Evaluating meaningful integration in profoundly hearing impaired children (MAIS). *American Journal of Otolaryngology,* 12(Suppl.): 144–150.

Robbins, A. M, Svirsky, M. A., Osberger, M. J., & Pisoni, D. B. (1998). Beyond the audiogram: The role of functional assessments. In F. H. Bess (Ed.), *Children with hearing impairment: contemporary trends* (pp. 105–124). Nashville, TN: Vanderbilt Bill Wilkerson Center Press.

Robertson, L. (2009). *Literacy and deafness: Listening and spoken language*. San Diego, CA: Plural.

Rosa-Lugo, L. I., & Allen, S. G. (2011, March 15). Assessing listening skills in children with cochlear implants: Guidance for speech-language pathologists. *ASHA Leader.*

Saffran, J. R., Werker, J. F., & Werner, L. A. (2006). The infant's auditory world: Hearing, speech and the beginnings of language. In D. Kuhn, R. S. Siegler, D. William, & R. M. Lerner (Eds.), *Handbook of child psychology* (6th ed., Vol 2., pp. 58–108). Hoboken, NJ: John Wiley and Sons.

Sharma, A., & Dorman, M. (2006). Central auditory development in children with cochlear implants: Clinical implications. *Recent Advances in Otorhinolaryngology,* 64: 66–68.

Sharma, A., Dorman, M., & Kral, A. (2005). The influence of a sensitive period on central auditory development in children with bilateral and unilateral cochlear implants. *Hearing Research,* 203: 134–143.

Sharma, A., Dorman, M. F., & Spahr, A. J. (2002a). Rapid development of cortical auditory evoked potentials after early cochlear implantation. *Neuroreport,* 13: 1365–1368.

Sharma, A., Dorman, M. F., & Spahr, A. J. (2002b). A sensitive period for the development of the central auditory system in children

with cochlear implants: Implications for age of implantation. *Ear and Hearing,* 23: 532–539.

Simser, J. I. (1993). Auditory-verbal intervention: Infants and toddlers. *Volta Review,* 95(3): 217–229.

Stefanakos, K., & Prater, R. (1982). *Auditory rehabilitation: Memory, language, comprehension test probes*. Austin, TX: Pro-Ed.

Tharpe, A. M., & Flynn, T. S. (2012). *Incorporating functional auditory measures into pediatric practice: An introductory guide for pediatric hearing professionals*. Available from http://www.oticon.com/~asset/cache.ashx?id=10835&type=14&format=web.

Walker, B. (2009). *Auditory learning guide (ALG)*. Available from http://www.firstyears.org/c4/alg/alg.pdf

Welling, D. (2010). Hearing and language development. In B. Shulman & N. C. Capone (Eds.), *Language development: Foundations, processes and clinical applications* (pp. 95–134). Sudbury, MA: Jones and Bartlett.

Yoshinaga-Itano, C., Gilkerson, J., Baca, R., Beams, D., & Wiggins, M. (2011, Feb. 21–22). *Adding the missing link to language assessment: LENA*. Paper presented at the EHDI conference, Atlanta, GA.

Yoshinaga-Itano, C., Sedey, A. L., Coulter, D. K., & Mehl, A. L. (1998). Language of early- and later-identified children with hearing loss. *Pediatrics,* 102: 1161–1171.

Zimmerman, F. J., Gilkerson, J., Richards, J. A., Christakis, D. A., Xu, D., Gray, S., et al. (2009). Teaching by listening: The importance of adult-child conversations to language development. *Pediatrics,* 124(1): 342–349.

Zimmerman-Phillips, S., Osberger, M. F., & Robbins, A. M. (1997). *Infant-toddler meaningful auditory integration scale (IT-MAIS)*. Sylmar, CA: Advanced Bionics. Available from http://www.advancedbionics.com/content/dam/ab/Global/en_ce/documents/libraries/AssessmentTools/3-01015_ITMAIS%20brochure%20Dec12%20FINAL.pdf.

Appendix 12-A: Auditory Learning Guide

Introduction

The ALG is a *guide*- a hierarchical list of auditory behaviors, intended to provide professionals with:

- a **"roadmap"** through the development of a listening function
- a tool to help the child achieve an **optimal** rate of auditory learning
- a tool to help the child become a **confident** listener
- a tool that can help a child function with greater ease in a hearing environment.

It is *not* an exhaustive list of skills a child must master, step-by-step, in order to develop a complete listening function. Some of the behaviors are self-explanatory and some require further information, typically obtained when the ALG is presented in a workshop.

The ALG is in "all in one" chart form, rather than in a series of lists, so the professional (and parents) can see each auditory behavior as part of the "big picture" in auditory learning rather than focus on each separate auditory skill. The color-coding gives a "ball-park" idea about timelines for auditory learning. As professionals become more skilled, children are likely to move faster through timelines. Children with more hearing may move faster. Children who are implanted at later ages may move faster through some steps due to increased attention span.

The guide includes five areas, or *levels,* listed across the top of the page (Sound Awareness, Phoneme Level, Discourse Level, etc.). Each level has one or more *steps*. Having all the levels on one chart rather than as separate lists, helps to communicate visually that several **areas of auditory development occur concurrently** for children who are deaf/hh, in the same way as they do for hearing children. The layout also reinforces the need to plan for auditory learning at several different levels, rather than to master one level before going onto the next.

Auditory Learning Guide

SOUND AWARENESS (Speech and Environmental Sounds)	PHONEME LEVEL** (Speech Babble)	DISCOURSE LEVEL (Auditory Processing of Connected Speech)	SENTENCE LEVEL	WORD LEVEL
Step 1 - Detect * the presence of any speech syllable.	**Step 1** - Imitate physical actions (before speech imitations).	**Step 1a** - Imitate motions of nursery rhymes/songs with accompanying vocalization.	**Step 1** - Identify familiar stereotypic phrases or sentences.	**Step 1a** - Identify and imitate approximations of "Learning To Listen" sounds varying in suprasegmentals and vowel content, e.g., (a-a-a)/airplane, (u-)(u)/train, (oi) (oi) pig in isolation, at the end, and then in the middle of a sentence.
Step 2 - Detect* vowel variety, [u] [a] [l] and raspberries [b-r-r]	**Step 2** - Imitate any phoneme that child produces spontaneously when given hand cue (or other cue).	**Step 1b** - Identify nursery rhymes or songs.	**Step 2** - Recall two critical elements in a message.	**Step 1b** - Identify one, two, and three syllable words in isolation, e.g., cat vs. chicken vs. kangaroo.
Step 3 - Detect* consonant variety, e.g., [m-m-m], [b^] [b^] [b^] and [wa] [wa]	**Step 3** - Imitate varying suprasegmental qualities in phonemes (vary intensity, duration, and pitch) aeee (long) vs [ae ae] (pulsed); [ae-ae] loud/quiet/whispered; [ae] high/mid/low pitch.	**Step 2** - Answer common questions with abundant contextual support, e.g., "What's that?," "Where's mama?," "What is _____ doing?"	**Step 3** - Recall three critical elements in a message.	**Step 2** - Identify words having the same number of syllables but different vowels/diphthongs and consonants, e.g., horse vs. cow vs. sheep.
Step 4 - Detect* the presence of environmental sounds at loud, medium, and soft levels at close range, at a distance of 6–12 ft. and at a distance of greater than 12 ft.	**Step 4** - Imitate vowel and diphthong variety, e.g., [u], [ae], [au], [i], etc.	**Step 3** - Identify a picture that corresponds to a story phrase in a three or four scene-story.	**Step 4** - Complete known linguistic messages from a closed set (ex: nursery rhymes, songs, familiar stories).	**Step 3a** - Identify words in which the *initial* consonants are the same but the vowels and final consonants are different, e.g., ball vs. bike.
Step 5 - Detect* whispered [hae] [hae] and [p] [p] [p]	**Step 5** - Imitate alternated vowels and diphthongs, e.g., [a-u] [e-I] [a-I]	**Step 4** - Identify an object from several related descriptors (closed set).	**Step 5** - Answer common questions about a disclosed and familiar topic: a) without pictorial cues; (b) over the telephone c) on audio/videorecording.	**Step 3b** - Identify words in which the *final* consonants are the same but the vowels and initial consonants are different, e.g., food vs. card.
Step 6 - Detect* the sounds of the Six SounJ Test.	**Step 6** - Imitate consonants varying in manner (fricatives, nasals, and plosives). Use phonemes previously produced, e.g., /h/ vs. /m-m-m/ vs. /p/.	**Step 5** - Follow a conversation with the topic disclosed.	**Step 6** - Recall four or more critical elements in a message to follow multiple element directions.	**Step 4** - Identify words in which the initial and final consonants are identical but the vowels/diphthongs are different, e.g., book vs. back.
Step 7 - Detect* the sounds of the Six Sound Test at various distances.	**Step 7** - Imitate consonants differing in voiced vs. unvoiced cues, e.g., [b^] [b^] vs. [p] [p] and then with vowel variety, [bobo] [pae-pae]	**Step 6a** - Answer questions about a story with the topic disclosed.	**Step 7** - Complete known linguistic messages (open set).	**Step 5a** - Identify words in which the vowels & final consonants are identical but the *initial* consonants differ by three features - manner, place of articulation, and voicing, e.g., mouse vs. house.
Step 8 - Locate the direction of sound if amplified binaurally.	**Step 8** - Alternate consonants varying in place cues, first with varying vowels, e.g., /ma-ma/ /no-no/; /go-go/ bi-bi/ etc.	**Step 6b** - Answer questions about a story with the topic disclosed; story is teacher-recorded.	**Step 8** - Follow open set directions and instructions (disclosed).	**Step 5b** - Identify words in which the vowels & initial consonants are identical but the *final* consonants differ by three features - manner, place of articulation, and voicing, e.g., comb vs. coat.

Step 9 - Alternate syllables with varying consonants and same vowel, e.g., [bi], [di], [hi], [go]

Step 7 - Recall details of a story (topic disclosed).

Step 8 - Sequence the events of a story (topic disclosed).

Step 9 - Retell a story with the topic disclosed, recalling all the details in sequence.

Step 10 - Make identification based on several related descriptors (open set).

Step 11 - Follow a conversation of an undisclosed topic.

Step 12 - Retell a story about an undisclosed topic, recalling as many details as possible.

Step 13 - Process information in noise and at various distances.

Step 14 - Process group conversations.

Step 9 - Recall specific elements in a sentence by answering questions about an undisclosed but familiar topic.

Step 10 - Repeat each word in a sentence exactly.
a.) predictable sentences "I'm going to the grocery store to buy cereal and milk."
b.) less predictable sentences "A woman hit me so I told her to calm down."

Step 11 - Recall specific elements in a sentence by answering questions on an undisclosed topic.

Step 6 - Identify words in which the vowels and the final/initial consonants are identical but the initial/final consonants differ by two features: (a) manner and place (voicing in common), *moat* vs. *goat*; (b) manner and voicing (place in common), *man* vs. *pan*; (c) place and voicing (manner in common), *boat* vs. *coat*.

Step 7a - Identify words in which the vowels and final consonants are identical but the *initial* consonants differ by only one feature - manner of articulation, e.g., *ball* vs. *mall*.

Step 7b - Identify words in which the vowels and initial consonants are identical but the *final* consonants differ by only one feature - manner of articulation, e.g., *cloud* vs. *clown*.

Step 8a - Identify words in which the vowels and final consonants are identical but the *initial* consonants differ by only one feature - voicing, e.g., *coat* vs. *goat*.

Step 8b - Identify words in which the vowels and initial consonants are identical but the *final* consonants differ by only one feature - voicing, e.g., *bag* vs. *back*.

Step 9a - Identify words in which the vowels and final consonants are identical but the initial consonants differ by only one feature - place of articulation, e.g., *bun* vs. *gun*.

Step 9b - Identify words in which the vowels and initial consonants are identical but the *final* consonants differ by only one feature - place of articulation, e.g., *sheep* vs. *sheet*.

KEY

YEAR 1
YEAR 2
YEAR 3
YEAR 4

The color codes in the chart designate auditory behaviors to be mastered by the end of the specified year, given optimally fitted hearing devices.

This guide is intended to aid professionals in the *beginning* stages of learning an auditory-based approach. As professionals acquire more experience in auditory teaching, children should progress more rapidly. The information on this chart was adapted from Judy Simser's article in the *Volta Review* (1993) (** items), from the Auditory Skills Program, New South Wales Department of School Education, from the Foreworks Auditory Skills Curriculum (1976, North Hollywood, CA), and from teacher input.

Notes:

* A detection response could include turning head, pointing to ear, clapping, dropping a toy in a container, etc.

Reference:

Simser, J.I. (1993). Auditory-verbal intervention: Infants and toddlers. *Volta Review* 95(3): 217–229.

Appendix 12-B: Auditory Skills Checklist

Child's Name:_____ Birth Date:_____ Person Reviewing Skills:_____

Dates Auditory Skills Reviewed:_____

Directions: Skills should be checked-off only if the child responds or has responded using auditory-only clues, without any visual information available. Although these skills are listed in a relatively typical order of development, it is common for children to increase in the depth of their development in previously acquired skills while learning skills at more advanced levels. Work on skills from one or two levels at a time. A child's rate of progression can depend on cognitive ability, the ability to attend for periods of time, vocabulary size, ability to point, etc. Every time you monitor auditory skill development, check off changes in the child's ability to respond or perform each skill that is being worked on. Estimates of percent of the time the child is seen to respond are approximations only based on the observation of the parents and others who regularly interact with the child. In subsequent reviews of the child's auditory skill development check off progress made (e.g., add check to E column if child is seen to begin to respond or demonstrate skill).

NOT PRESENT (0–10%)   E = EMERGING (11–35%)   I = INCONSISTENT (36–79%)   A = ACQUIRED (80–100%)

E √	I √	A √	AUDITORY SKILL	EXAMPLE	APPROX DATE ACQUIRED
			LEVEL ONE		
			Child wears hearing aids or implant all waking hours	Hearing aids worn at all times except for naps and bathing.	
			Awareness to sound: Child nonverbally or verbally indicates the presence or absence of sound.	Child's eyes widen when she hears her mother's voice.	
			Attention to sound: Child listens to what he hears for at least a few seconds or longer.	Child pauses to listen to father's voice.	
			Searching for the source of sound: Child looks around, but does not necessarily find sound source.	Child glances or moves in search of the sound.	
			Auditory localization: Child turns to the source of sound.	Child turns to Mom when she calls her.	
			LEVEL TWO		
			Auditory feedback: Child uses what he hears of his own voice to modify his speech, so that it more closely matches a speech model.	Parent says ee-oh-ee and child imitates. Parent says woof-woof and child imitates	
			Auditory discrimination of nonlinguistic sounds and suprasegmental aspects of speech: Child perceives differences between sounds or sound qualities, such as loudness, long/short, pitch.	Child indicates which toys from 2 available made a loud sound;	
			Distance hearing: Child responds at increasing distances from the source of the sound.	Mother calls child from another room, and she hears her.	
			Auditory association of environmental, animal or vehicle sounds, and/or familiar person's voices.	Child identifies dog barking, points to the dog. Child hears Dad's car and smiles because she knows Dad is now home.	

E √	I √	A √	AUDITORY SKILL	EXAMPLE	APPROX DATE ACQUIRED
			LEVEL THREE		
			Auditory identification or association of different-sounding and familiar words and phrases – OBJECTS – closed set	Child has 3 favorite toys on the floor and gives one to the parent when it is named.	
			Auditory identification or association of different-sounding and familiar words and phrases – OBJECTS – open set	In the grocery store parent asks child to help find the apples.	
			Auditory identification or association of different-sounding and familiar words and phrases – COMMON PHRASES – closed set	Child responds by clapping when parent says "Patty Cake" (no motions) or raises arms when parent says "So Big!"	
			Auditory identification or association of different-sounding and familiar words and phrases - SIMPLE DIRECTIONS – closed set	Child is in getting dressed with clothes laid out; parent asks child to give her the socks.	
			LEVEL FOUR		
			Auditory identification or association of different-sounding and familiar words and phrases – COMMON PHRASES OR SIMPLE DIRECTIONS – open set	"Where's Daddy?" "Ow! My finger hurts!" "Give mommy a kiss!" Upon entering the bedroom, parent asks child to get his socks.	
			Discrimination of words on the basis of segmental features: indicate words with different vowels but the same initial or final consonants	Child can hear the difference between words like bat, bite, boat, bee	
			Conditional response to sound (if 18 month or older): Child conditions to respond to the presence of sound.	Child claps when he perceives any or all of Ling's sounds (oo, ah, ee, sh, s, m)	
			Discrimination of words on the basis of segmental features: indicate different manner of consonants but same vowels	Child can tell difference between words like see, knee, bee	
			LEVEL FIVE		
			Discrimination of words on the basis of segmental features: indicate same vowels, but consonants differ in voicing	Child can tell difference between sue-zoo; cap-cab; curl-girl	
			Discrimination of words on the basis of segmental features: indicate words with different manner and place of consonants but same vowel sound	Child can tell difference between words like hill, still, pill	
			Auditory recall: Child remembers groups of words that contain TWO CRITICAL ELEMENTS	Child is 'helping' to set the table and has big and little spoons and forks. Child can bring a big spoon to the parent.	
			Auditory recall: Child remembers groups of words that contain THREE CRITICAL ELEMENTS	Big red ball, little blue car, big red car, little blue ball	
			LEVEL SIX		
			Discrimination of words on the basis of segmental features: indicate same manner of consonants but different place of consonants	Child can tell difference between words like tea, pea, key	
			Auditory recall: Child remembers groups of words that contain FOUR CRITICAL ELEMENTS	Big dog with long black hair, little cat with short brown hair	
			Auditory sequencing digits: Child repeats several numbers or letters in correct order	Child repeats the model "3-6-2-4"	
			Auditory sequencing directions: Child carries out multipart directions	Put the kitty under the chair, the mommy in the car, and the bike by the tree	
			LEVEL SEVEN		
			Figure-ground discrimination: Child identifies and comprehends primary speaker from a background of noise or competing voices	Child hears and understands mom talking while music is playing	

E √	I √	A √	AUDITORY SKILL	EXAMPLE	APPROX DATE ACQUIRED
			Auditory recall: Child remembers groups of words that contain >FOUR CRITICAL ELEMENTS	Parent describes items in kitchen utensil drawer and child picks correct one	
			Auditory sequencing a story: Child retells story in correct sequence	Retell 3 Little Pigs or any other favorite story	
			Auditory blending: Child synthesizes isolated phonemes into words, or single words into sentences	Child blends the sounds h-a-t to produce the word 'hat'	
			LEVEL EIGHT		
			Auditory sequencing rhymes and songs: Child acts out and memorizes rhymes and songs	I'm a Little Teapot; Itsy Bitsy Spider	
			Identification based on several related descriptions and contextual clues, including expansion of vocabulary	Child participates in "description games" such as "I'm thinking of something that is red. It's a fragrant flower which grows on a bush. Its stem has thorns on it. People give them for Valentine's Day."	
			Auditory closure: Child understands and supplies the whole word or message when a part is missing	Child completes the statement: "Triangle, square, and rectangle are all _____". Or "snow is white, grass is _____"	
			Processing questions: Child answers thinking process questions	"What do you do when you're hungry?"	
			LEVEL NINE		
			Auditory analysis: Child processes phonemes, morphemes, and syntactic or semantic structures embedded in words and sentences.	Child related "-ed" to past tense in words. Child responds appropriately when an adult says, "Give me the shoe or the sock"	
			Auditory tracking: Child follows text as an adult reads aloud	Child moves finger over the pictures in a storybook as an adult reads the book.	
			Processing main ideas of stories and discussions	Child understands the main idea of a story. Child understands and participates in word, card, and board games. Child understands and participates in conversations.	
			Auditory comprehension: Listens and comprehends while engaged in another activity	Child listens to and understands a story while brushing his/her hair	
			LEVEL TEN		
			Auditory comprehension: Child understands relationship between verbal language and children's literature (story grammar)	Child relates to "Once upon a time," "lived happily every after," etc.	
			Auditory comprehension: Child carries on a conversation using auditory-only cues	Child carries on a conversation in the car or in the dark	
			Auditory comprehension: Child understands messages from electrical sound sources, such as tape recorders, videos/DVD, radio, etc	Child understands the words to a song on a tape recorder. Child understands the message from a school loudspeaker	
			Auditory comprehension: Child understands conversations on the telephone	Child talks to grandmother and is able to answer questions and discuss with her	

Appendix 12-C: Resources

Christina Perigoe, PhD
Marietta M. Paterson, EdD

The following is a list of selected readings, auditory resources, CDs, videotapes/DVDs, and websites. This is not an exhaustive list, but it is a good starting place for parents and professionals interested in learning more about auditory development and about using listening to develop spoken language in children with hearing loss. It includes some older resources, so the reader may want to look at what has been incorporated into newer resources—especially those that are child- and family-centered. We have put an asterisk (*) next to those that are available for free on the Internet. Internet resources sometimes change their URL addresses, so it is a good practice to use a search engine to find the item.

Suggested Readings

Estabrooks, W. (1994). *Auditory-verbal therapy for parents and professionals*. Washington, DC: Alexander Graham Bell Association for the Deaf.

Estabrooks, W. (1998). *Cochlear implants for kids*. Washington, DC: Alexander Graham Bell Association for the Deaf.

Estabrooks, W. (Ed.). (2006). *Auditory-verbal therapy and practice*. Washington, DC: Alexander Graham Bell Association for the Deaf and Hard of Hearing.

Estabrooks, W., & Marlowe, J. (2002). *The baby is listening*. Washington, DC: Alexander Graham Bell Association for the Deaf and Hard of Hearing.

Ling, D. (1984). *Early intervention for hearing impaired children: Oral options*. Boston, MA: College-Hill Press.

*National Center for Hearing Assessment and Management & The Alexander Graham Bell Association for the Deaf and Hard of Hearing. (2012). *Early hearing detection and intervention programs: A blueprint for success*. Available from http://nc.agbell.org/Document.Doc?id=817.

Rossetti, L .M. (2001). *Communication intervention: Birth to three*. Albany, NY: Delmar.

Srinivasan, P. (1996). *Practical aural habilitation for speech-language pathologists and educators of hearing-impaired children*. Springfield, IL: Charles C. Thomas.

Talbot, P. (2002). *Topics in AV therapy: A selection of handouts*. Available from Acoustic Achievements, 16 Victory Street, Ronkonkoma, NY 11779. Also available from the First Years website: http://firstyears.org/c4/u3/talbotflyer.pdf.

Resource Guides and Teaching Materials

Alberg, J. (2010). *Understanding your child's hearing loss: A guide for parents*. Raleigh, NC: Beginnings. Available from https://www.ncbegin.org/index.php?option=com_rokquickcart&view=rokquickcart&Itemid=251.

Estabrooks, W. *Hear & listen! Talk & sing!* Washington, DC: Alexander Graham Bell Association for the Deaf and Hard of Hearing. Book and music CD. Available from the AG Bell bookstore: http://www.agbell.org.

Estabrooks, W. *Songs for listening, Songs for life*. Washington, DC: Alexander Graham Bell Association for the Deaf and Hard of Hearing. Book and music CD. Available from the AG Bell bookstore: http://www.agbell.org.

Hackett, L., & Rodriguez, L. (2004). *Comfort level checklist for auditory-verbal families*. San Antonio, TX: Sunshine Cottage for Deaf Children. Available from http://www.sunshinecottage.org/index.php/educational_products/our_products/comfort_level_checklist/.

Pepper, J., & Weitzman, E. (2004). *It takes two to talk: A practical guide for parents of children with language delays* (3rd ed.). Toronto, Canada: The Hanen Centre. Available from http://www.hanen.org/Guidebooks---DVDs/SLPs.aspx.

Sindrey, D. (1997). *Cochlear implants auditory training guidebook*. London, Ontario, Canada: Wordplay.

Sindrey, D. (1997). *Listening games for littles*. London, Ontario, Canada: Wordplay.

Sisson, M. (2008). *Workbook for parents of children who are newly identified as hard of hearing*. Available from Oticon Pediatrics, 580 Howard Avenue, Somerset, NJ 08873.

Auditory Assessments/Assessment Information

American Speech-Language Hearing Association (ASHA). *Directory of speech-language pathology assessment instruments*. Available from http://www.asha.org/assessments.aspx.

*Anderson, K. L. *Supporting success for children with hearing loss*. Available from https://successforkidswithhearingloss.com/resources-for-professionals/early-intervention-for-children-with-hearing-loss.

For assessments see http://successforkidswithhearingloss.com/tests.

Gallaudet University. *Suggested scales of development and assessment tools*. http://www.gallaudet.edu/Clerc_Center/Information_and_Resources/Cochlear_Implant_Education_Center/Resources/Suggested_Scales_of_Development_and_Assessment_Tools.html.

Auditory Checklists, Hierarchies, and Developmental Scales

*Alexander Graham Bell Association for the Deaf and Hard of Hearing. *Listening and spoken language knowledge center*. Available from http://www.listeningandspokenlanguage.org/Tertiary.aspx?id=1215.

*Cochlear Corporation. (2009). *The integrated scales of development. Listen, learn and talk*. Available from http://hope.cochlearamericas.com/reading-room/listen-learn-talk.

Estabrooks, W., & Marlowe, J. (2000). In *The baby is listening*. Washington, DC: Alexander Graham Bell Association for the Deaf and Hard of Hearing.

*Rhoades, E. *Auditory development scale: 0–6 years*. Available from http://www.auditoryverbaltraining.com/scale.htm.

*Simser, J. *Auditory-verbal techniques and hierarchies*. Available from http://auditory-verbalcommunicationcenter.blogspot.com/2011/06/auditory-verbal-techniques-and.html.

Sunshine Cottage School for Deaf Children. *Cottage acquisition scales for listening, language & speech (CASLLS)*. San Antonio, TX: Sunshine Cottage School for Deaf Children. Available from http://www.sunshinecottage.org/index.php/educational_products/our_products/caslls/.

*Walker, B. (2009). *Auditory learning guide (ALG)*. First Years: Professional Development Through Distance Education. Available from http://www.firstyears.org/c4/alg/alg.pdf.

Auditory Curriculum Guides

Auditory Skills Curriculum
Romanik, S. Moorebank, Australia: New South Wales Department of Education and Training. Originally developed in 1990, the revised edition (2008) includes placement test, manual, DVD, and CD with resource material. Available from http://www.schools.nsw.edu.au/media/downloads/schoolsweb/studentsupport/programs/disability/audskills.pdf.

Auditory Skills Curriculum, Auditory Skills Instructional Planning System (ASIPS)
Stein, D., Benner, G., Hoverstein, G., McGinnis, M., & Theis, T. (1976). Portland, OR: Foreworks. Available from http://www.foreworks.com/fore.html.

AuSpLan: Auditory Speech and Language: A Manual for Professionals Working with Children Who Have Cochlear Implants or Amplification
McClatchie, A., & Therres, M. (2003). Oakland, CA: Children's Hospital & Research Center. *Ausplan summary guide available from Advanced Bionics: http://www.advancedbionics.com/content/dam/ab/Global/en_ce/documents/libraries/AssessmentTools/3-01066-D-2_AuSPLan%20Supplement-FNL.pdf.

Learn to Talk Around the Clock—A Professional's Early Intervention Toolbox
Rossi, K. Washington, DC: Alexander Graham Bell Association for the Deaf and Hard of Hearing. Available from http://www.LearnToTalkAroundTheClock.com.

Listen Little Star: Family Activity Kit
Dornan, D. (2003). Brisbane, Australia. Available from Hear and Say: http://www.hearandsaycentre.com.au/ListenLittleStar.html.
Format: Year 1 activity book, program guide, and DVD

My Baby and Me: A Book About Teaching Your Child to Talk
Brooks, B. M. St. Louis, MO: Moog Center for Deaf Education. Available from http://www.moogcenter.org/Bookstorenbspnbspnbspnbspnbsp/tabid/149/Default.aspx.
Format: binder

Ski-HI Curriculum: Family-Centered Programming for Infants and Young Children with Hearing Loss (Revised)
Watkins, S. (Ed.). (2004). Logan, UT: Hope, SKI-HI Institute Utah State University. Available from http://hopepubl.com/products.php?cat=5.

Sound Foundation for Babies
Cochlear Corporation. Available from http://hope.cochlearamericas.com/node/2256.
Format: 40 online weekly lessons, songs, and rhymes
Sound Foundations for Toddlers
Cochlear Corporation. Available from http://hope.cochlearamericas.com/node/4410.
Format: 40 online weekly lessons, songs, and rhymes
Speech Perception Instructional Curriculum and Evaluation (SPICE)
Biedenstein, J., Davidson, L., & Moog, J. (1995). Available from http://www.cid.edu/ProfOutreachIntro/EducationalMaterials.aspx.

Format: Manual, rating forms, toys, cards, video, acoustic hoop *SPICE for Life*
West, J., & Manley, J. Available from: http://www.cid.edu/ProfOutreachIntro/EducationalMaterials.aspx. Format: Manual, resource book, CD, cards, tracking form
St. Gabriel's Curriculum for the Development of Audition, Language Speech, Cognition
Tuohy, J., Brown, J., & Mercer-Moseley, C. (2001). New South Wales, Australia: St. Gabriel's School for Hearing Impaired Children.
St. Gabriel's Curriculum and IEP Goal Writer. Available from http://www.hearandsaycentre.com.au/Cart/Professional_Education_and_Development/Training_Resources.aspx.

Videotapes/DVDs

ABCs of AVT. (Estabrooks, W.).Washington, DC: Alexander Graham Bell Association for the Deaf and Hard of Hearing.
The Baby Is Listening. (Estabrooks, W., & Marlowe, J.). Washington, DC: Alexander Graham Bell Association for the Deaf and Hard of Hearing.
Listen, Learn and Talk. Sydney, Australia: Cochlear Corporation.
Listen to This I & II. (Estabrooks, W.). Washington, DC: Alexander Graham Bell Association for the Deaf and Hard of Hearing.
What Professionals Need to Know for Cochlear Implant Rehabilitation. (Bader, J., Biever, A., & Tyabji, A. H.) 2006. Washington, DC:

Alexander Graham Bell Association for the Deaf and Hard of Hearing.
* The following DVDs are all free for download or ordering from http://www.oraldeafed.org:
   Hear the Difference
   Make a Difference
   Dreams Made Real
   Dreams Spoken Here
   Speaking for Myself

Internet Resources (Most are Free)

Advanced Bionics:

IT-MAIS: http://www.nationaldb.org/documents/IT-MAS_20brochure_20_2.pdf
Learning to Listen Sounds: http://www.hearingjourney.com/userfiles/File/1_05instr.pdf
Ling Six Sound Test: http://www.advancedbionics.com/us/en/support/tools_for_schools.html
The Listening Room (Hearing Journey): http://www.hearingjourney.com/index.cfm?langid=1

Alexander Graham Bell Association for the Deaf and Hard of Hearing: Listening and Spoken Language Knowledge Center: http://www.agbell.org
Auditory-Verbal Center (Atlanta): http://www.avchears.org
Auditory-Verbal Training (Ellen Rhoades): http://www.auditoryverbal-training.com
Beginnings (North Carolina): http://www.ncbegin.org

Cochlear Corporation:

HOPE online courses (free) http://hope.cochlearamericas.com/online-courses
Ling-6 Sounds: http://www.cochlear.com/files/assets/Ling-6%20sound%20test%20-%20how%20to.pdf
Ling-6 Sounds Flash Cards: http://www.cochlear.com/files/assets/Ling%20cards.pdf

Speech Sounds Guide: Consonants: http://professionals.cochlearamericas.com/sites/default/files/resources/Speech%20Sound%20Rehab._0.pdf
Speech Sounds: Vowels: http://hope.cochlearamericas.com/sites/default/files/resources/Speech-Sounds-Vowels.pdf
Sound Foundation for Babies: 40 online weekly lessons, songs and rhymes: http://hope.cochlearamericas.com/node/2256
Sound Foundations for Toddlers: 40 online weekly lessons, songs and rhymes: http://hope.cochlearamericas.com/node/4410

Deaf Children Can Speak: http://www.deafchildrencanspeak.com
Hear and Say (Brisbane, Australia): http://www.hearandsaycentre.com.au
Hear in Dallas: http://www.hearindallas.com
John Tracy Clinic (including parent support and resources in Spanish): http://www.johntracyclinic.org

Ling Six-Sound Test: http://www.jtc.org/uploads/docs/The-Ling-Six-Sound-Test.PDF
Ling Speech Cards: http://www.jtc.org/professionals/purchase-ling-speech-cards

Life Is Bliss (blog): http://ardinger.typepad.com/bliss/audio_verbal_therapy/
Listen and Talk: http://www.listentalk.org
Listen-Up Web: http://www.listen-up.org
Listening for Life (Joanna Stith): http://www.listeningforlife.com

Net Communications for Communication Disorders and Sciences (Judith Kuster): http://www.mnsu.edu/comdis/kuster2/welcome.html

Med-El: http://www.medel.com/us/index/index/id/1/title/HOME

Online comic book: Will Wonder and his Robot Ears: http://www.medel.com/data/willwonder/?PHPSESSID=v0u91v2cujk7fvt9334vk8pq80

My Baby's Hearing: Boys Town National Research Hospital: http://babyhearing.org

National Center for Hearing Assessment and Management (NCHAM): http://www.infanthearing.org

Natural Communication, Inc.: http://www.nciohio.com

Oral Deaf Education: http://www.oraldeafed.org

Sound-Object Associations (The Learning to Listen Sounds): http://www.listen-up.org/dnload/listen.pdf

Voice for Hearing Impaired Children (Canada): http://www.voic-efordeafkids.com

WE Listen International: http://welisteninternational.com

Chapter 13

Hearing Issues in the Early Intervention Years

Nancy G. Schneider, MA, CCC-A, FAAA
Audiologist

Key Terms

Automated auditory
  brainstem response
  (AABR) screening
Early hearing detection and
  intervention (EHDI)
External auditory canal
  atresia

Functional auditory
  assessments
Individuals with Disabilities
  Education Act (IDEA)
Medical home
Microtia

Minimal hearing loss
Otoacoustic emission (OAE)
  screening
Universal newborn hearing
  screening (UNHS)

Objectives

- Illustrate the deleterious effects that hearing loss of any type, degree, and configuration in one or both ears can have on the development of infants and toddlers
- Explain recommended protocols for infants requiring audiologic follow-up as a result of all possible newborn hearing screening outcomes
- List risk indicators for possible late onset hearing loss as defined by the current Joint Committee on Infant Hearing position statement and the importance of ongoing audiologic monitoring

- Describe the purpose of utilizing functional auditory assessment tools for all children under the age of 3 years who have been identified with hearing loss
- Explain the various roles that speech-language pathologists play in the Early Hearing Detection and Intervention process for children diagnosed with hearing loss as well as for those awaiting confirmation of their current auditory status

Introduction

"The goal of early hearing detection and intervention (EHDI) is to maximize linguistic competence and literacy development for children who are Deaf or hard of hearing. Without appropriate opportunities to learn language, these children will fall behind their hearing peers in communication, cognition, reading and social-emotional development." (Joint Committee on Infant Hearing, 2007) Over the span of the last 75 years, early identification of hearing loss in young children has evolved from the subjective observation of the auditory response behaviors of toddlers to bells and rattles to the current administration of objective electroacoustic/electrophysiologic hearing screening measures performed on infants less than 24 hrs old. With the advent of user-friendly hearing screening technology, passage of national and state legislation supporting **universal newborn hearing screening (UNHS)**, and the endorsement of professional organizations on the importance of early hearing loss detection in infants and toddlers, more than 97% of children born in the United States are receiving their very first hearing screening prior to nursery discharge, compared with less than 3% in 1989 (White, Forsman, Eichwald, & Munoz, 2012). The effectiveness of universal newborn hearing screening has also resulted in a significant decrease in the age at which children are diagnosed with hearing loss and, subsequently, when they receive medical intervention, initial hearing aid fitting, cochlear implantation, connection to parent support services, and enrollment in early intervention. In addition, advancements in the development of evidence-based protocols for hearing screening, pediatric audiologic evaluation, and audiologic monitoring have resulted in not only earlier identification of bilateral peripheral hearing loss of varying types, degrees, and configurations, but also the early diagnosis of unilateral hearing loss and central forms of auditory pathology such as auditory neuropathy/auditory dyssynchrony (AN/AD).

As shown in **Figure 13.1**, hearing loss has been found to be the most common congenital health condition screened for in the neonatal period (White, 2002). The incidence of hearing loss is estimated to range from 1 to 6 per 1,000 live births; however, these figures increase if transient conductive and late-onset hearing losses are also included (White & Behrens, 1993). Depending on the electroacoustic/electrophysiologic method used, initial hearing screening can be effectively administered as early as 6–14 hrs after birth, with repeat screening often being performed prior to an infant's discharge from the nursery. Diagnostic audiologic evaluation, administered by audiologists with expertise in working with infants and toddlers, can also be performed as early as prenursery discharge, though it is typically conducted on an outpatient basis within the first 2–3 months of life. Even at such a young age, objective electroacoustic/electrophysiologic testing can yield accurate information regarding the hearing status of each ear and, in the cases where hearing loss is present, provide comprehensive information on its type, degree, and configuration.

Current newborn hearing screening and pediatric audiologic assessment timelines are in sharp contrast to those

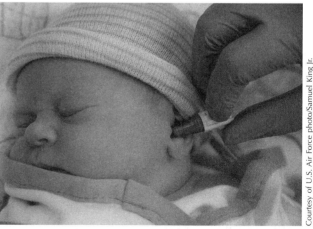

Figure 13.1 Objective hearing screening measures can be performed mere hours following birth.

referenced in the Commission on Education of the Deaf's 1988 report, "Toward Equality: Education of the Deaf," which revealed that the average age of identification of profound hearing loss in the United States was 2.5 years (Commission on Education of the Deaf, 1988), with mild or unilateral hearing losses not identified until entry into kindergarten. Delays in the identification of pediatric hearing loss in one or both ears not only adversely affect the developing auditory nervous system of a young child, but also can have deleterious consequences for social, emotional, cognitive, and academic development, and subsequently, for the vocational and economic potential of children as they age into adulthood (Northern & Downs, 2002; National Institutes of Health Consensus Statement, 1993). Research has shown that the earlier pediatric hearing loss is identified and treatment begun, the greater the likelihood of preventing or reducing the disabling effects that can result (Apuzo & Yoshinaga-Itano, 1995). Because the most critical period for speech and language acquisition is during the first 3 years of life, it has become a national goal to reduce the age of hearing loss identification to within the first few months of life (Joint Committee on Infant Hearing, 1994).

The successful coordination and administration of effective newborn hearing screening and follow-up services can only be accomplished through the collaborative efforts of all stakeholders involved in the UNHS process, including, but not limited to, birthing facilities, parents, physicians, nurses, audiologists, speech-language pathologists, healthcare providers, early interventionists, hearing aid dispensers, parent support organizations, community and state agencies that provide family-centered services, and state and federal legislators. Full participation of each stakeholder ensures that the goals of early hearing loss identification and the provision of appropriate habilitative services are being met in a timely manner for very young children and that these services include a seamless transition from screening to diagnosis to a habilitation plan leading from early intervention to preschool.

What Is EHDI?

Early hearing detection and intervention, or, as it is better known, EHDI (pronounced "Eddie"), is a national public health initiative that has become part of the gold standard of neonatal hearing health care. Hospital-based newborn hearing screening programs began as far back as the 1960s; however, technological advancements in the field of audiology coupled with widespread acceptance of the need for

early hearing loss identification in inf evolution of the current EHDI process.

Almost immediately after the Commis of the Deaf published its 1988 report (....... previously), C. Everett Koop, the Surgeon General of the United States, issued the following statement: "By the year 2000, 90% of children with significant hearing loss be identified by 12 months of age" (Mauk & Behrens, 1993). The U.S. Department of Health and Human Services' *Healthy People 2000* national healthcare report included Dr. Koop's recommended timeline as part of its public health goals (National Center for Health Statistics, 2001). As a result, the Newborn and Infant Hearing Screening and Intervention Act (also known as the Walsh Bill, named for New York Congressman James Walsh) was passed in 1999 (National Center for Hearing Assessment and Management [NCHAM], n.d.), leading to improved hearing healthcare services for infants, toddlers, and their families. As a result of this landmark legislation, funding was provided to all states from both the Centers for Disease Control and Prevention (CDC) and the Health Resources Services Administration (HRSA) to support the development, planning, implementation, and monitoring of EHDI programs throughout the country.

EHDI programs support the early identification of hearing loss through universal newborn hearing screening (UNHS), timely audiologic and medical evaluations and monitoring, enrollment in early intervention (EI), and ongoing connections to family support services. EHDI programs, established in all 50 states and the U.S. territories, strive to achieve the nationally recognized 1-3-6 Rule, which includes screening all infants for hearing loss prior to 1 month of age (preferably prior to nursery discharge); conducting a complete, ear-specific, pediatric audiologic evaluation on infants who do not pass their newborn hearing screening by no later than 3 months of age; and enrolling children who have been identified with hearing loss of any degree into an appropriate, family-centered, culturally competent early intervention program before 6 months of age. In addition to the 1-3-6 Rule, national EHDI goals also include appropriate audiologic monitoring for children presenting with risk indicators for late onset hearing loss, ensuring that all children with hearing loss are established with a **medical home**, creation of a state-specific EHDI tracking and surveillance system to minimize the possibility of children being lost to follow-up, and establishment of a system that monitors and evaluates a state's progress toward meeting the national EHDI goals and objectives.

The gold standard for each step of the EHDI process is outlined in a regularly published set of guidelines developed by the Joint Committee on Infant Hearing (JCIH). JCIH is represented by a variety of different professional organizations, all of whom share a common interest in the early identification of hearing loss in infants and toddlers. Organizations currently represented in JCIH include the American Speech-Language-Hearing Association, American Academy of Audiology, American Academy of Otolaryngology—Head and Neck Surgery, American Academy of Pediatrics, Directors of Speech and Hearing Programs in State Health and Welfare Agencies, and the Council on Education of the Deaf, including the American Society for Deaf Children, Alexander Graham Bell Association for the Deaf and Hard of Hearing, Conference of Educational Administrators of Schools and Programs for the Deaf, Convention of American Instructors of the Deaf, National Association of the Deaf, and Association of College Educators of the Deaf and Hard of Hearing. Since 1971, JCIH has regularly published position statements that outline recent research and recommended practices for UNHS, diagnostic audiologic evaluation, audiologic monitoring, and appropriate intervention for infants and toddlers at risk for, or diagnosed with, all degrees of hearing loss (JCIH, 2007).

Personnel involved in the hands-on provision of hearing screening services as well as those responsible for the administrative oversight of hospital-based UNHS programs often vary from state to state and even from hospital to hospital. Hearing screeners may be nurses, audiologists, physicians, speech-language pathologists, technicians, and, in some cases, trained volunteers. Administrative management of UNHS programs typically is limited to audiologists or neonatologists, who are responsible for providing training and supervision to screeners, ensuring that hearing screening equipment is functioning in accordance with manufacturers' specifications and developing quality assurance policies and procedures to monitor the performance of their facility's UNHS program.

The mission of all EHDI programs is to meet all national EHDI goals, but there can be great variability in the legislative requirements in place for each state and territory to ensure that these goals are being met. EHDI programs throughout the United States typically are funded with federal grants and are supported by evidence-based practice guidelines from professional organizations, recommendations by a variety of advocacy groups, and legislative directives on both federal and state levels. Although all 50 states have EHDI programs in place, as of December 2009, laws and/or regulations related to UNHS have been passed in only 43 (NCHAM, 2011). State-specific UNHS and follow-up legislation typically indicates the minimum expectations of state policy makers, but does not necessarily define all aspects of what state newborn hearing screening programs are doing. An excellent resource for locating individual state/territory EHDI program guidelines and requirements, as well as legislative mandates, can be found at the National Center for Hearing Assessment and Management (NCHAM) website at www.infanthearing.com.

EHDI Rule #1: Screening by 1 Month of Age

Because behavioral observation screening procedures do not provide accurate predictions of hearing impairment for newborns, the presence of hearing loss can be inferred through the use of electrophysiologic and electroacoustic screening tools such as **automated auditory brainstem response (AABR)** and/or evoked **otoacoustic emission (OAE) screening**. An important caveat regarding these screening tools is that they are not, technically, direct measures of hearing; rather, they are measures of auditory nerve integrity and cochlea integrity, respectively. We can, however, make an estimate of hearing sensitivity based on these procedures. Although the objective hearing screening tools of the past focused on identification of infants with severe to profound degrees of hearing loss, current newborn screening methodologies for infants allow reliable detection of hearing loss of greater than 30 decibels hearing level (dB HL) in the frequency region important for speech recognition in one or both ears. The development of these portable, user-friendly, and affordable hearing screening technologies has allowed for cost-effective, mass hearing screening of newborns by a variety of healthcare personnel (including the SLP on occasion) in birthing facilities, pediatric practices, and health clinics throughout the world (**Figure 13.2**).

As noted in Figure 13.2, evoked OAE screening is performed by placing a small probe at the entrance to the infant's ear canal while the infant is lying in a quiet state. The probe assembly generates a series of quiet clicks or tones that travel through the ear canal to the middle ear and through to the inner ear. In a normally functioning cochlea, a small echo is generated by the outer hair cells within the cochlear structure, which then travels back through the middle and outer ear to be picked up by a sensitive microphone within the OAE probe. The echo response (or OAE)

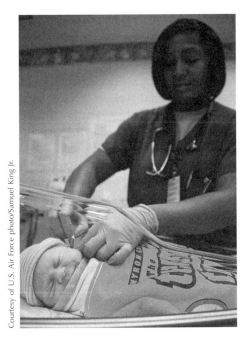

Courtesy of U.S. Air Force photo/Samuel King Jr.

Figure 13.2 An otoacoustic emissions screening being performed on a newborn infant.

is then analyzed by a computer, which generates a pass response if the OAE is present and a refer result if the OAE is absent or too small to measure. Although a pass result on an OAE screening does not definitely confirm the presence of normal hearing for all frequencies, it does rule out the presence of a peripheral handicapping hearing loss. OAEs are absent in individuals who present with hearing loss greater than approximately 30 dB HL (depending on type of OAE screening performed); however, an OAE refer result may also be the screening outcome when transmission of the OAE is compromised by the presence of middle or outer ear pathology or by high levels of myogenic or environmental noise during the screening procedure. Children who refer on OAE screening for one or both ears will require hearing rescreening no later than 1 month of age to determine if abnormal screening results persist in the weeks after birth when vernix is no longer present in the ear canal and amniotic fluid has been absorbed in the middle ear cavity.

To review, there are two types of evoked OAE technology available for use in newborn hearing screening programs: transient evoked otoacoustic emission (TEOAE) screening and distortion product otoacoustic emission (DPOAE) screening. Both OAE technologies are administered in a similar fashion, and can usually take less than 5 minutes to perform on a child in a quiet state; however, they differ in the types of auditory stimuli used to generate an echo

response; TEOAE screening utilizes a click stimulus and DPOAE screening uses two simultaneous pure tones. Passing either a TEOAE or DPOAE screening does not provide any information about the auditory system beyond the level of the cochlea; it offers information only about peripheral auditory functioning (up to and including the cochlea in each ear). Use of evoked OAE technology is an appropriate screening tool for infants in the term nursery or those who have been in the neonatal intensive care nursery for fewer than 5 days. For children who have had longer than a 5-day NICU stay, the screening measure of choice is the automated auditory brainstem response (AABR) screener.

AABR screening is performed by introducing soft, high-pitched clicking sounds to the ear canal via a probe placed at the opening of the infant's ear or through a small adhesive earphone coupled to the area surrounding the external ear. Figure 13.3 illustrates electrode placement used with AABR screening. Electrodes are placed on the infant's head that are designed to pick up the presence of ongoing EEG activity as well as the changes in that activity as a result of the introduction of sound. The auditory stimulus generated by the AABR unit passes through the external, middle, and inner ear; however, unlike the evoked OAE screening tools, the AABR signal also makes its way to the auditory portion of the eighth cranial nerve (VIII) up to where the auditory nerve meets the brainstem. Like OAE screening, it is especially crucial that the infant is in a calm, settled state and in a quiet screening environment throughout the screening process because patient movement and/or vocalizations can adversely affect the administration of the screening. A complex filtering system within the AABR unit digitally removes the random EEG signals and transmits the averaged auditory response to a computer that compares the infant's response pattern to a template of a normal AABR response. If the responses match, the AABR will generate a pass result; if a match does not occur, a refer result is offered.

Like OAE screening methodology, an AABR response will be absent in individuals presenting with hearing loss greater than 30 dB HL, but may also be absent in the ears of infants with outer and/or middle ear pathology or in those infants who present with immature brainstem function or brainstem pathology. In keeping with the Year 2007 JCIH Position Statement, any infants who do not pass AABR screening must be rescreened with AABR technology and not rescreened solely with OAE technology. A passing OAE outcome will not completely address the refer result that occurred in AABR screening, because the OAE response is generated by the cochlea and will therefore not be able to rule out the possibility of hearing loss originating from higher levels in the auditory system that are screened for in an AABR.

Some birthing hospitals will opt to utilize a two-tiered approach to newborn hearing screening, using both OAE and AABR technologies when screening for peripheral hearing loss for newborns that don't pass an initial OAE screening. Hearing screening refer rates tend to be somewhat higher with the isolated use of evoked OAE screening than those noted for AABR screening in isolation. Use of a two-tiered approach to screening (i.e., rescreening infants who refer on OAE screening with AABR) yields the lowest refer rate of all. Another benefit to the utilization of both OAE and AABR is to also be able to screen for more central forms of hearing loss, specifically in identifying the condition known as auditory neuropathy/auditory dyssynchrony (AN/AD). Should the outcome of this screening yield a robust passing outcome during OAE screening and a refer on AABR screening, the results are highly suggestive of AN/AD and require immediate referral for a comprehensive pediatric audiologic evaluation for further assessment for this auditory condition.

Prior to the release of the Year 2007 JCIH Position Statement, birthing facilities could choose to utilize either OAE or AABR screening technology because the focus of UNHS at that time was to rule out peripheral hearing loss. In 2007, JCIH expanded the focus of newborn hearing screening so that it is no longer the norm to screen only for unilateral or bilateral peripheral hearing loss (e.g., sensory hearing loss originating in the cochlea, permanent conductive hearing loss, and/or mixed hearing loss), but also to screen for neural hearing loss (particularly in children who are considered at risk for this condition, such as infants with a prolonged NICU stay of greater than 5 days).

The type of screening tool selected for use in a birthing facility is dictated in part by the administrator who oversees the UNHS program, but is more related to the type of nursery population to be screened. As such, JCIH now requires hospitals to screen infants with AABR if a child has had a greater than 5-day stay in the NICU. If an infant is screened with AABR and doesn't pass for one or both ears, they are to be rescreened with AABR within 1 month of life or referred for a diagnostic auditory brainstem response evaluation by an audiologist with expertise in working with a pediatric population. Some birthing hospitals without NICUs have opted to purchase and utilize AABR screening on all their newborns; however, the

requirement for AABR rescreening or referral for diagnostic ABR testing remains the same, whether the infant has stayed in the NICU for more than 5 days or not.

Regardless of the screening tool used, a refer result prior to nursery discharge can prompt either a referral for an outpatient rescreening within the first month of life or a direct referral for a complete pediatric audiologic evaluation well before 3 months of age. Other Year 2007 JCIH Position Statement recommendations include rescreening both ears of children who present with a unilateral refer result on their initial hearing screening as opposed to rescreening only the affected ear. The rationale for bilateral rescreening is related to possible errors in the documentation of a nursery-based unilateral refer result. Results of inpatient hearing screening outcomes are often recorded in the child's electronic birth certificate and/or may be documented in a written hospital nursery discharge summary. Although it is uncommon, the potential for documenting the wrong ear as the refer ear on a child with a unilateral hearing screening refer result is always a possibility; therefore, rescreening of both ears ensures that no child is discharged from an inpatient or outpatient hearing screening program without assurance of accurate ear-specific screening results.

If a child passes their hearing screening prior to nursery discharge but is readmitted to the hospital within 1 month of life due to presentation of a healthcare issue associated with potential hearing loss, JCIH recommends rescreening of each ear prior to hospital discharge. Birthing hospitals must ensure that all screening results and recommendations (e.g., pass, refer, pass with recommendation for audiologic monitoring due to the presence of risk indicators) be presented to parents and the medical home provider who has been identified in the birth record as the child's future source of medical care. The **medical home** refers to a healthcare provider (pediatrician, nurse practitioner) who oversees coordination of comprehensive, family-centered, and accessible health care throughout a child's lifetime. A comprehensive resource for the concept of a medical home can be found at the American Academy of Pediatrics website: www.aap.org. In addition to sharing objective hearing screening results with the medical home, the results of a child's hearing screening and follow-up recommendation need to be offered to parents in an understandable and culturally sensitive manner with regard to the implications of screening outcomes and recommendations, including information as to where the child can receive follow-up services for rescreening, diagnostic audiologic evaluation, or audiologic monitoring, if necessary.

Barriers to Newborn Hearing Screening

There are circumstances in which hearing screening cannot be performed, either because the infant is considered medically fragile and there are medical contraindications to screening administration or because the child presents with unilateral or bilateral **microtia** with **external auditory canal atresia**. For infants considered too medically fragile to undergo hearing screening in the nursery, the screener must obtain clearance from the child's physician prior to attempting to conduct the screening. Infants born with external auditory canal (EAC) atresia cannot undergo hearing screening of their affected ear(s) because they do not possess an entrance to the external auditory canal. The appropriate course of action for infants with EAC atresia (also known as aural atresia) is a direct referral for diagnostic auditory brainstem response evaluation via both air and bone conduction prior to 3 months of age in order to determine cochlear function in the atretic ear(s), as well as to obtain a baseline measure of auditory functioning in the unaffected ear in cases of unilateral EAC atresia. Infants with microtia (with or without EAC atresia) or any other type of facial differences are best served by a referral to a craniofacial center for multidisciplinary team assessment along with regular monitoring of audiologic, speech-language, medical, developmental, and psychosocial status, as well as for parent support services.

Although JCIH encourages newborn hearing screening, along with appropriate follow-up and resource information, to be provided to families in an understandable and culturally sensitive manner, there may still be a variety of reasons why families of children requiring follow-up do not comply. Parents typically receive a wealth of information in their discharge plan paperwork and may feel overwhelmed with the volume of documents received, all while trying to adjust to the changes in lifestyle that occur with the addition of a newborn to the family. Insurance impediments may also make locating a pediatric audiologist who participates in a family's insurance plan challenging and lead to a child being lost to follow-up. Terms and vocabulary used in the UNHS process may be unfamiliar to families and to hospital staff who provide general scheduling for outpatient appointments. As a result, a child may inadvertently be scheduled for an OAE screening, when in fact, they may actually be in need of an AABR screening. Similarly, an appointment for a 15-minute rescreening may be scheduled when the child should instead receive a one and a half (1 ½) hour diagnostic auditory brainstem response evaluation. This may result in the child being turned away from

the appointment without the proper follow-up appointment being rescheduled. In addition, families often rely on medical referral for outpatient rescreening or audiologic evaluation via the support of their pediatrician, who may have to provide necessary written referral in accordance with insurance provider guidelines. Another scenario may be if the family's medical home provider is unfamiliar with national EHDI guidelines, or if they choose to advocate the antiquated and nonevidence-based "wait and see" approach regarding referral for audiologic evaluation, then parents may not feel comfortable pursuing recommended follow-up without their pediatrician's support. JCIH, state-based EHDI programs, and the American Academy of Pediatrics have all developed a wealth of materials for the pediatric community to highlight the importance of early hearing loss detection as well as outline guidelines for timely referral for infants and toddlers regarding rescreening, diagnostic audiologic evaluation, and audiologic monitoring for late onset hearing loss.

EHDI Rule #2: Pediatric Audiologic Evaluation by 3 Months of Age

JCIH's second rule in the 1-3-6 trilogy involves prompt referral of infants who do not pass their hearing screening for one or both ears (or who are not able to be screened because of medical contraindications or the presence of external auditory canal atresia) for comprehensive, ear-specific, pediatric audiologic evaluation no later than 3 months of age. The American Speech-Language-Hearing Association and JCIH (ASHA, 2004; JCIH, 2007) both recommend an evidence-based pediatric audiologic evaluation that comprises specific test protocols for children between birth and 36 months of age. For children under the age of 6 months, pediatric audiologic evaluation should include comprehensive child and family case histories; frequency-specific, tone-burst diagnostic ABR studies by both air and bone conduction; click-evoked ABR testing using both condensation and rarefaction stimuli (particularly if there are concerns regarding the possible presence of auditory neuropathy/auditory dyssynchrony); OAE screening; high-frequency tympanometry (with a 1,000 Hz probe tone); and a review of the family's observations of the infant's responses to sound, including use of a **functional auditory assessment** tool. Because ABR studies require the child to be in a quiet state, the goal is for infants who are referred on their hearing screenings to receive their audiologic evaluations as soon as possible so that the evaluations can be performed under natural sleep conditions rather than with the use of sedation.

Children undergoing comprehensive audiologic evaluation from 6 to 36 months of age would undergo many of the same tests noted in the previous section for the hearing status of each ear to be determined. Unlike infants, toddlers are capable of offering reliable and repeatable behavioral responses to tonal and speech stimuli, and JCIH endorses the use of either visual reinforcement audiometry (VRA) or conditioned play audiometry (CPA) based on the child's level of development, along with a comprehensive child and family case history, speech detection and recognition measures, replacement of the use of high-frequency tympanometry with standard probe tone frequency tympanometry studies, acoustic reflex testing, functional auditory assessment, and parental reports of both auditory and visual behaviors along with a review of communication milestones. If results of this diagnostic audiologic test battery reveal the presence of hearing loss in one or both ears, or if test results are inconclusive, referral for diagnostic auditory brainstem response studies is advised. Infants and toddlers diagnosed with unilateral or bilateral sensorineural, permanent conductive, or mixed forms of hearing loss or auditory neuropathy/auditory dyssynchrony should be referred for early intervention services within 2 days of the diagnosis. In addition, the child will need to undergo a series of medical evaluations including, but not limited to, examination by an otolaryngologist, ophthalmologist, and geneticist. Coordination of these evaluations, as well as any other referrals to other medical specialists, are to be coordinated by the medical home, with all medical assessments preferably performed by physicians with experience and expertise in working with a pediatric population. It is noteworthy to mention that part of this medical "work-up" may include a comprehensive evaluation of the renal system. The SLP need not be surprised at this recommendation. In utero, both the auditory and renal systems develop at approximately the same time. Should a complication occur during this time frame, damage to both systems may result.

As physicians with expertise in identifying medical conditions of the ears, nose, throat, and related head and neck structures, otolaryngologists will serve as the medical professionals charged with diagnosis, treatment, and otologic management of the child with hearing loss. In addition to obtaining a prenatal and perinatal history (to investigate the possible presence of risk indicators to hearing loss), otolaryngologists will also conduct an overall head and neck examination with special attention to the auditory structures (e.g., presence of stigmata, ear tags/pits, external auditory canal atresia, or stenosis) as well as craniofacial disorders (e.g., cleft lip, cleft palate, facial asymmetry,

craniosynostosis, micrognathia, etc.). Based on physical exam, case history information, and results of audiologic evaluation, the otolaryngologist may refer the child for imaging studies such as computed tomography (CT) scans or magnetic resonance imaging (MRI) of the temporal bones to obtain a clearer view of internal auditory structures and possible malformation. In addition, referral will be made for laboratory studies including, but not limited to, EEG, blood work, and urinalysis to aid in the diagnostic process of determining the etiology of the hearing loss. Results of these evaluations may prompt referral to other medical specialists for further evaluation and monitoring. In keeping with JCIH recommendations, any child diagnosed with hearing loss who is considered a candidate for amplification in one or both ears should be fit with appropriate hearing aid(s) within 1 month of diagnosis, for families who elect to pursue this option. The otolaryngologist is the physician who will provide otologic clearance for hearing aid fitting and will also continue to provide services to children with hearing loss for evaluation and treatment of middle ear pathology, candidacy for pressure equalization (PE) tubes, removal of impacted cerumen, and evaluation for cochlear implantation.

A Word About Genetics

Approximately 40% of hearing loss diagnoses are thought to be due to infectious agents or environmental factors (for example, bacterial or viral infections, ototoxic drug exposure, and acoustic trauma), with the remaining 60% attributed to genetic causes. Thirty percent of genetic hearing loss is considered syndromic in nature, and 70% is deemed nonsyndromic (Pletcher, 2012). Genetic evaluation for children with hearing loss includes an investigation of hearing loss etiology as well as forming a determination regarding the probability of recurrence risk of hearing loss in the affected child's siblings or their future children. A typical genetics evaluation for children identified with hearing loss would include a thorough three- to four-generation family history (with special attention to hearing status of family members) and a physical examination of the child, including otologic, ophthalmologic, endocrine, cardiac, nephrology, and craniofacial evaluations. Today, genetic evaluation and testing for children identified with hearing loss is an established step in the etiologic diagnosis of hearing loss (JCIH, 2007). Both families and physicians gain valuable information from a genetics evaluation that can guide both medical management of and intervention for babies with hearing loss. Parents and physicians need to be aware of the findings of genetic testing to understand whether the child's hearing loss may be part of a syndrome in which other health conditions that require medical evaluation, treatment, and monitoring may be present. An understanding of the etiology of the hearing loss may also help to guide families in making decisions regarding their child's habilitation plan. Genetic counseling can be especially useful in relieving a parent's sense of confusion as to the cause of an unexpected hearing loss diagnosis for the child. The information provided by the genetics team can assure parents that their child's hearing loss was not a result of a nonrelated event during pregnancy, thereby allaying the possible guilt a parent may feel, and assist in their acceptance of their child's needs so they may move forward in their habilitative process.

Ninety percent of children with hearing loss are born to hearing parents who may not have any experience with hearing health care or hearing loss. Culturally deaf parents may react quite differently to the news that their child has been diagnosed with a hearing loss and embrace the diagnosis without the communication concerns expressed by parents who are unfamiliar with the richness and pride inherent in the Deaf Community. JCIH therefore advocates that discussions with all parents regarding their child's hearing status and communication options be handled with sensitivity to cultural attitudes and beliefs and be presented in an unbiased manner.

Functional Auditory Assessment Tools: Looking Beyond the Audiogram

In addition to obtaining pediatric audiologic evaluation information regarding the type, degree, configuration, and laterality of a child's hearing loss, **functional auditory assessment** tools can offer useful information to parents regarding the impact hearing loss has on their child's day-to-day communicative functioning; provide validation of hearing aid fitting, cochlear implantation, and use of assistive listening technology; assist in the process of determining a child's eligibility for enrollment into EI; and serve as measurement tools for evaluating the efficacy of therapeutic intervention (Anderson, 2006). In addition, questioning parents and caregivers with regard to personal observations of their child's auditory response behaviors in real-world settings through the administration of functional auditory assessments can provide information about how a child uses his or her hearing in a variety of real-world listening environments, both in quiet settings and when speech is presented in background noise. The *Guidelines for the Audiologic Assessment of*

Children from Birth to 5 Years of Age (ASHA, 2004) includes the following recommendation:

> . . . in addition to the assessment of peripheral hearing status, it is essential for audiologists working with infants and young children to consider the functional implications of hearing loss. As it is feasible within the time constraints of clinical practice, assessments of speech perception ability and screening for communication skills, cognitive development and social-emotional status should be included as part of the pediatric test battery.

Speech-language pathologists have a variety of standardized tools available to assess both expressive and receptive speech-language development; however, use of functional auditory assessment tools with infants and toddlers with hearing loss will yield additional useful information in developing a habilitation plan that best meets a child's needs, regardless of the severity of their hearing loss. The following functional auditory assessment tools are considered appropriate for use with children presenting with hearing loss under the age of 3 years and can evaluate a child's listening skills in meaningful, real-world situations as well as encourage parent participation in the hearing loss discovery, monitoring, and intervention process:

> *Developmental Index of Audition and Listening (DIAL):* The DIAL (Palmer & Mormer, 1999 is a functional auditory assessment tool that is based on the types of listening behaviors one would expect to observe in children at specific developmental ages. The DIAL was constructed on the basis of human development with a specific focus on auditory skill development for children from birth to 22 years of age. Valente, Hosford-Dunn, and Roeser (2000) describe the DIAL as a tool that provides audiologists with a "systematic way of evaluating the current abilities and needs of the child as related to the range of auditory signals that are used in a day-to-day life."

> *Early Listening Function (ELF):* The ELF (Anderson, 2002) is designed to assist parents in systematically observing and rating their child's auditory awareness skills in response to stimuli presented during a variety of listening environments, including variations in distance from the sound source relative to the child's location (e.g., 6 inches, 3 feet, 6 feet, 10 feet, and 15+ feet) and with stimuli presented at different intensity levels (e.g., observing the child's responses to quiet, typical, and loud listening activities). The ELF not only assists families in the

observation of their child's auditory behaviors, but also provides a mechanism to track improvement in auditory development over time. Families can use this tool with children from 5 months to 3 years of age to measure improvements in auditory skills under aided listening conditions; audiologists, in turn, can use the ELF as a validation measure for determining the functional benefit of amplification. Furthermore, the ELF is useful not only in providing feedback to parents, but also in helping them to understand the ramifications distance and noise effects have on their child's hearing.

Functional Auditory Performance Indicators (FAPI): The FAPI (Stredler, Brown & Johnson, 2010) is designed to assess children's auditory skills by examining seven categories of auditory development (sound awareness, sound is meaningful, auditory feedback, localization, auditory discrimination, short-term memory, and linguistic auditory processing). The FAPI uses a hierarchical sequence of development, opposed to limiting observation to "detection only," as in the ELF. The results of these assessments are combined to formulate a functional auditory skill profile that describes a child's use of auditory stimuli in natural settings and their ability to generalize these skills to different listening environments. There are no age limits on the use of this tool, and it allows for several different skills to be evaluated over time. There are also no age norms because the protocol is used to monitor progress of the development of auditory skills.

Auditory Behavior in Everyday Life (ABEL): Purdy and colleagues (2002) developed the Auditory Behavior in Everyday Life (ABEL) questionnaire to assess parental perceptions of their children's auditory behavior. The original 49-item questionnaire was intended to assess auditory communication, environmental awareness, functional independence, and social/communication skills. The goal was to capture some of the changes in children's everyday auditory behavior in a reliable and easily quantifiable manner. The 24-item ABEL questionnaire has an excellent overall reliability of 0.95. The items fall within three factors: Aural–Oral, Auditory Awareness, and Social/Conversational Skills. Children's auditory behavior can be assessed using an overall rating, or separately for each of the three factors.

LittlEARS Auditory Questionnaire: The questionnaire portion of the LittleEARS battery (Kühn-Inacker, Weichboldt, Tsiakpini, Conninx, & D'Haese, 2003) is designed to assess the auditory behaviors of children with hearing loss up to the age of 24 months after cochlear implantation or hearing aid fitting. This parent questionnaire consists of 35 age-related questions that require a yes/no response from parents/caregivers and provides information on preverbal auditory development in the child's first 2 years of hearing in their natural environment. This tool has been validated in normally hearing children, and assesses auditory development and early speech production in a child's natural environment.

Parents' Evaluation of Aural/Oral Performance of Children (PEACH): The PEACH questionnaire (Ching & Hill, 2007) was designed to assess the effectiveness of amplification in real-world situations through systematic use of parent observations. The PEACH, which can be used with children as young as 1 month old and up to 7 years old, includes 15 probe questions, administered by any professional trained to work with families of children with hearing loss, and is scored on the basis of how frequently relevant auditory behaviors occur. Subscale scores can also be calculated for elements such as "hearing aid usage, loudness discomfort, functional performance in quiet and noise, awareness of environmental sounds and use of the telephone."

Infant-Toddler Meaningful Auditory Integration Scale (IT MAIS): Zimmerman-Phillips and colleagues (1998) modified the Meaningful Auditory Integration Scale (Robbins, Renshaw, & Berry, 1991) to be used with children from birth to 3 years of age. This functional auditory assessment tool was developed for children who have a profound hearing loss and have been fit with hearing aids or a cochlear implant. Like the PEACH, the IT MAIS is administered to parents by an audiologist. It examines three primary areas: vocalization behavior, alerting to sounds, and deriving meaning from sound. Scoring is based on the percentages of time that a child demonstrates specific auditory abilities. Detailed documentation of parent responses to structured interview questions is required, as are parental reports on specific areas of behaviors observed.

FM Listening Evaluation: The FM Listening Evaluation (Johnson, 2004) evaluates the use and benefits for children of amplification and FM systems after initial fitting, and quarterly thereafter. This functional auditory assessment tool can be completed by a parent or professional working with the child. Not only does this tool provide outcome measures of benefit and is a suitable tool for comparing performance with various types of FM systems, but it also can be used to assess the counseling and technical support needs of parents.

Having access to the results of these assessments may offer critical information to the EI community in determining a child's candidacy for enrollment in therapy services by providing information beyond what a typical audiogram might suggest.

EHDI Rule #3: Enrollment in Early Intervention by 6 Months of Age

Successfully identifying infants with hearing loss at birth through newborn screening without effective follow-up services that include rescreening, diagnostic evaluation, and appropriate intervention defeats the very purpose of the screening. Ideally, all children under the age of 3 years presenting with any degree of unilateral or bilateral hearing loss should be referred to EI within 2 days of diagnosis. JCIH (2007) indicates that children with hearing loss be considered eligible for EI with a provider who is knowledgeable about hearing loss as soon as possible after diagnosis, or no later than 6 months of age. The goal of timely enrollment in a culturally sensitive, community-based, collaborative, and developmentally appropriate EI program is to prevent the significant negative effects that even a **minimal hearing loss** can have on a child's overall development. Studies reveal that children with hearing loss, without other disabilities, who receive EI before 6 months of age have language development similar to their normally hearing peers and, when compared with children who do not have early access to EI services, show significantly improved social-emotional development as well as communication outcomes in the areas of vocabulary development, receptive and expressive language, syntax, and speech production (Moeller, 2000; Yoshinaga-Itano, 2000).

JCIH (2007) describes the "Quality of Care" for infants and toddlers with hearing loss. These guidelines are designed to highlight components of early intervention that are unique to children who have confirmed hearing loss in one or both ears. EI services should:

- Be family centered
- Provide families with unbiased information on all options regarding approaches to communication

- Monitor development at 6-month intervals with norm-referenced instruments
- Include individuals who are Deaf or hard of hearing
- Provide services in a natural environment in the home or in the center
- Offer high-quality service regardless of where the family lives
- Obtain informed consent
- Be sensitive to cultural and language differences and provide accommodations as needed
- Conduct annual surveys of parent satisfaction

Intervention for children with hearing loss requires a close-knit team that includes the family and both individuals working within the child's EI program and professionals working outside the perimeters of the EI system of care, including but not limited to physicians, speech-language pathologists, and audiologists. Complete medical and audiologic records as well as other diagnostic information are essential and invaluable in the understanding of the child's unique needs. All of the individuals involved in a child's care in the EI system need to work together to ensure all necessary data are collected and assimilated into the planning for the child. The early intervention system "should be family centered with infant and family rights and privacy guaranteed through informed choice, shared decision-making, and parental consent in accordance with state and federal guidelines. Families should have access to information about all intervention and treatment options and counseling regarding hearing loss" (JCIH, 2007). The JCIH 2007 Position Statement also indicates that, "The Child and family should have immediate access to high-quality technology including hearing aids, cochlear implant(s) and other assistive devices when appropriate."

Part C of the **Individuals with Disabilities Education Act (IDEA)** indicates that EI services should be provided in ". . . natural environments, including the home and community settings in children without disabilities participate" (IDEA, 2004). Although natural environments may include the home or child care venue, the key consideration is that it be a location that employs the mode of communication used by the child with hearing loss and that the child be exposed to peers and adults who are fluent in this communication methodology, thereby allowing them to serve as models to the child in how to communicate effectively. In keeping with the spirit of defining a natural environment for a child with hearing loss, EI services need to consider use of home-based and center-based intervention options that offer a language-rich environment. A language-rich environment needs to include EI personnel who are able to communicate with the child in whichever mode has been defined by the parents in conjunction with the EI team. Similarly, children with hearing loss need to be surrounded by children who share similar communication methodologies so that even activities of play will foster an environment where all children with hearing loss can communicate freely with their peers. This language-rich environment defines the context of least restrictive environments and natural environments for infants and toddlers who are deaf or hard of hearing (DesGeorges, DeConde Johnson, & Stredler Brown, 2005).

As part of the EI process, in addition to assessing the child, the family's concerns, available resources, and priorities for a comprehensive habilitation plan are explored. Information from assessment is then used to identify child and family outcomes, and the services and supports that will be needed to meet these outcomes are written into the Individualized Family Service Plan (IFSP). As new information regarding the child's communication status is brought to the attention of the IFSP team, the IFSP plan is reviewed and revised on a regular basis, typically every 3 months. The progress of a child with permanent hearing loss and/or auditory neuropathy/dyssynchrony should be reviewed at least every 3 months, particularly if the child has recently received a hearing aid(s), or a cochlear implant(s). Six-month intervals are appropriate after 2 years of implantation or device use, provided that the child is progressing. The child's progress toward expected milestones postimplant or postamplification should be evaluated to determine if the child is meeting target listening and verbal skills. Communication abilities should be evaluated to determine if the child is developing in a manner commensurate with methodology and age expectations; however, if there is limited or no progress, or if the child's unaided thresholds or aided performance has deteriorated, audiologic monitoring should occur at 1- to 3-month intervals to determine if any changes in hearing or middle ear status have occurred or if amplification or assistive technology needs to be modified to meet the child's current listening needs. Recommendations for the IFSP should be based on evaluation recommendations and on a comprehensive assessment of the child and the family's priorities, resources, and concerns. Families should be provided with unbiased and comprehensive information regarding all EI options in order to support families in selecting the programs, providers, settings, and services that best meet the needs of the child.

Beyond Newborn Hearing Screening: Risk Indicator Monitoring

Up until this point in this chapter, discussion has focused on either children who passed their newborn hearing screening or those who referred on screening and were ultimately diagnosed with hearing loss. It is important to consider that passing a newborn hearing screening prior to 1 month of age does not necessarily mean that a family's journey through the EHDI process has come to an end. Hearing screening for infants and toddlers may extend throughout early childhood, particularly for those infants who require ongoing audiologic monitoring due to the presence of a risk indicator for late onset hearing loss.

Implementation of UNHS ensures that *all* infants have equal access to early hearing loss identification, as opposed to earlier risk-based approaches to hearing screening in which only those children who were identified as having one or more risk indicators to hearing loss were targeted for screening. Although previous risk-based approaches to screening identified many children who went on to receive a diagnosis of permanent hearing loss, retrospective studies ultimately revealed that 50% of children who are identified with hearing loss present with no risk indicators at all (JCIH, 2000). Even with the advent of UNHS, infants presenting with risk indicators to possible late onset hearing loss continue to hold a special place in the UNHS process because currently accepted national guidelines extend the need for rescreening and pediatric audiologic monitoring throughout early childhood to detect hearing loss that may occur post-nursery discharge. With each publication of the JCIH Position Statement, updates are made to the list of risk indicator conditions that warrant ongoing audiologic monitoring as well as the recommended time frames for follow-up. The current list of risk indicators included in the Year 2007 Position Statement is as follows:[1]

- *Caregiver concern* regarding hearing, speech, language, or developmental delay
- *Family history* of permanent childhood hearing loss
- All infants with or without risk factors requiring a NICU stay for more than 5 days, including any of the following: *ECMO*, assisted ventilation, exposure to ototoxic medications (gentamycin and tobramycin) or loop diuretics (furosemide/lasix); in addition,

---

[1]Risk indicators highlighted with italicized text require more frequent audiologic monitoring because they are conditions of greater concern in terms of development of delayed onset hearing loss.

regardless of length of stay, hyperbilirubinemia requiring exchange transfusion
- Intrauterine TORCH infections, particularly *CMV*, herpes, rubella, syphilis, and toxoplasmosis
- Craniofacial anomalies, especially those involving the temporal bone, the pinna, the ear canal, ear tags, or preauricular pits
- Physical findings associated with a syndrome known to include hearing loss
- *Syndromes associated with progressive hearing loss*
- *Neurodegenerative disorders*
- *Culture-positive postnatal infections associated with sensorineural hearing loss*
- Head trauma, especially *basal skull/temporal bone fractures* requiring hospitalization
- *Chemotherapy*

Previous JCIH Position Statements made recommendations for uniform audiologic monitoring of children presenting with risk indicators every 6 months until the age of 3 years. Although the general 6-month audiologic reevaluation timeline recommendation was an easy guideline to remember for birthing hospitals and physicians, it proved to be an unrealistic healthcare goal given the large volume of children presenting with risk indicators for late onset hearing loss who would require, at a minimum, six separate pediatric audiologic evaluations from birth to the age of 3 years. Families of newborns presenting with risk indicators struggled to locate the limited number of qualified pediatric audiologists available in their geographic region who could provide audiologic assessments on children from 6 to 36 months of age. Available pediatric audiology facilities were overwhelmed with the number of referrals for risk factor monitoring evaluations, and appointment wait times increased exponentially. Many health insurance companies rejected bills for audiologic monitoring services, particularly in circumstances where challenges in obtaining ear-specific test results due to patient fatigue or higher than acceptable levels of activity resulted in more than one clinical encounter for a 6-month recall appointment. It became an impossible undertaking for EHDI programs to effectively track the timeliness and outcomes of audiologic monitoring, unless 6-month recall appointments were strictly adhered to and a complete assessment was obtained for each visit. Most challenging of all became the increasing difficulty in advocating for a globally used 6-month recall schedule in children who either required far more frequent monitoring (e.g., children diagnosed with meningitis or CMV, or those treated with chemotherapy) or who may not have required as much monitoring over as long a period of

time (e.g., children who were referred for audiologic evaluation due to caregiver concern, but who were found to present with normal hearing bilaterally with no evidence of retrocochlear pathology, or children referred for audiologic evaluation as a result of sustaining head trauma in the absence of a skull fracture who were found to have normal hearing). This made it difficult to justify recall every 6 months until the age of 3 years. The conservative recommendations of 6-month recall for all in the Year 2000 JCIH Position Statement was modified to a more specific set of recommendations in the Year 2007 Statement, which stated that children with risk indicators should continue to receive periodic audiologic monitoring; however, the time frames were to be determined based on the specific risk indicator and the child's needs. At a minimum, all children with risk indicators to late onset hearing loss must undergo a complete audiologic evaluation by 24 and 30 months of age, with certain risk indicators requiring more frequent assessments throughout the birth to age 3 time frame.

According to the National Institutes of Health Consensus Conference on Early Identification of Hearing Impairment (1993), as many as 70% of infants and children with hearing impairment are identified because of parental concerns about their child's hearing. Therefore, it is important to educate parents about signs of hearing impairment and familiarize them with normal developmental milestones for expressive and receptive speech and language development. Ongoing parental counseling is advised for those babies who present with risk indicators for late onset hearing loss, but who passed their initial hearing screening.

The Year 2007 JCIH Position Statement incorporated a special safety net to ensure that all children receive ongoing surveillance of developmental milestones and communication skills, and provision of regular inquiries regarding parent concerns on these issues during well baby visits to the medical home. The American Academy of Pediatrics developed the Pediatric Periodicity Schedule, which stipulates that all children, regardless of whether they present with any risk indicators to hearing loss, receive global developmental screening with validated measurement tools at specific ages (9, 18, and 24–30 months of age), or at any time if concerns are raised by parents, caregivers, or healthcare professionals regarding the child's communication ability. If the child does not pass the communicative screening measures conducted in the medical home, or if any concerns regarding hearing or speech-language development are raised by the family to the medical home provider, they are to be immediately referred to a speech-language pathologist and audiologist for comprehensive assessments. In addition, pediatricians are advised to assess middle ear status at all well child visits and refer for otologic evaluation if persistent middle ear effusion lasts for beyond 3 months. In addition to adhering to the JCIH 1-3-6 Rules, the AAP supports referring for audiologic evaluation the siblings of the pediatric family member who sustains a hearing loss.

A Word About Children with Multiple Disabilities

It is estimated that 30–40% of children with permanent childhood hearing loss will present with at least one additional disability (Gallaudet Research Institute 2003; Laurent Clerc Deaf Education Center, n.d.), including but not limited to developmental delays; cleft palate; vision loss; transient middle ear disorders resulting in fluctuating conductive overlay to the permanent hearing loss; cerebral palsy; balance difficulties; seizure disorders; cardiac, renal, or orthopedic problems; craniofacial anomalies; autism; and an array of syndromes that include hearing loss. Approximately 70% of children with vision loss have an additional disability (Chen, 2000), and up to 80% of children with a dual sensory loss (vision loss and hearing loss) also present with other disabilities (Minnesota Deaf-Blind Technical Assistance Project, n.d.). These data emphasize the importance of assessing sensory status through audiologic and ophthalmologic evaluations for infants with developmental delays or disabilities, and highlights the need for an interdisciplinary approach to EI assessment and services. Although many of these disabilities accompanying hearing loss may be apparent at birth, the extent and nature of others may not be recognized until considerably later, making comprehensive follow-up a necessity. Members of the EI team who work with infants and toddlers with hearing loss must be aware of the significant number of additional healthcare issues and learning problems that potentially coexist in these children. It is vital for all EI professionals to provide sensitive, well-coordinated care for these families because caring for these children's diverse and frequent needs is demanding for both families and providers of EI services. Medical and habilitative care professionals should be mindful of changes in hearing and vision status and ensure that audiologic and ophthalmologic statuses are monitored regularly. Early intervention services must be carefully designed to take into account the unique learning needs of a child with multiple disabilities, with thoughtful consideration about how to make information accessible to the child and how to establish language and communication.

The SKI-HI Institute (www.skihi.org) is an organization based at Utah State University whose goal is to enhance the lives of young children with special needs, their families, and caregivers to ensure that children with special needs become able participants in society. SKI-HI provides technical assistance and ongoing support to the states implementing Institute programs through the use of newsletters, additional on-site visits, phone calls, and regional conferences. Founded in 1972, its training and services focus on early intervention and early childhood programming for infants and young children, ages birth to 5 years, with hearing and vision impairments and other disabilities.

The Speech-Language Pathologist's Role in the EHDI Process

In addition to offering the expected evaluation and treatment therapy for children who exhibit speech-language delays as a consequence of pediatric hearing loss, speech-language pathologists play a vital role throughout the EHDI process, from administration of newborn hearing screening in the nursery to developing the communication abilities of infants and toddlers who are diagnosed with hearing loss as a result of early hearing loss identification. To be effective in this role, speech-language pathologists must be aware of the historical trends in universal newborn hearing screening and how these programs are being implemented around the country (Houston, 2009). In addition, as per ASHA's document entitled *Roles and Responsibilities of Speech-Language Pathologists in Early Intervention: Guidelines* (ASHA, 2008), appropriate roles for speech-language pathologists serving infants and toddlers include, but are not limited to, awareness of "federal, state, agency, and professional policies and procedures pertaining to screening (including hearing), evaluating, and assessing infants and toddlers with, or at risk for, disabilities; standardized measures for screening, evaluation, and assessment and their psychometric properties that are available and appropriate for infants and toddlers." Speech-language pathologists who work in a birthing hospital setting may be called upon to provide hearing screening services to infants in the nursery. In addition, the expertise of a speech-language pathologist will also play a role in collaboration with other health professionals by identifying neonates at risk for hearing loss.

Speech-language pathologists are in the ideal position to explain to parents the variety of effects that an unidentified pediatric hearing loss can have on their child's speech and language development. As such, the speech-language pathologist can reinforce the need for audiologic evaluation for families of children who did not pass their newborn hearing screening and who have not complied with this recommendation for audiologic follow-up or for those children for whom a potential late-onset hearing loss is of concern. The speech-language pathologist's ongoing review of communication and developmental milestones paired with discussion on how pediatric hearing loss of any degree in one or both ears can impede a child's ability to achieve these milestones can empower families to recognize potential gaps in their child's communicative skills. Even children presenting with **minimal hearing loss** (e.g., mild bilateral hearing loss or unilateral hearing loss of any degree) may exhibit communication difficulties that may not be obvious in the neonatal period, but, through the watchful eyes of both their speech-language pathologist and parents, will become obvious during the early years of life. Studies have demonstrated that children with minimal hearing loss can exhibit a myriad of communication difficulties, including phonological, vocabulary, and language delays; present with difficulty understanding speech presented in background noise; experience difficulty localizing the source of a sound; encounter problems with reading comprehension and additional educational difficulties resulting in grade retention and resource room assistance; and experience social-emotional dysfunction, including low self-esteem, low energy, high stress, and short-term memory deficits (Bess, Dodd-Murphy, & Parker, 1998; Bess & Tharpe, 1984; Oyler & Matkin, 1988; Oyler, Oyler, & Matkin, 1987). Because there is no clear way to predict which children with minimal hearing loss will experience difficulties, and consequently which children will benefit from early intervention and early amplification, the speech-language pathologist and audiologist caring for a child with this diagnosis should both be responsible for regular reevaluation of hearing status, monitoring of communication development, and educating families and early interventionists on how to help give these children the best chance for success (McKay, Gravel, & Tharpe, 2008).

Given the collaboration evident between the speech-language pathology and audiology communities, sharing a comprehensive list of local diagnostic audiology facilities that provide services to pediatric patients would help expedite referral for audiologic evaluation if questions arise regarding the current state of a child's hearing or middle ear status. Reinforcement of the purpose of hearing screening, diagnostic audiologic testing, and ongoing monitoring, as well as reviewing the rationale behind audiologic recommendations for follow-up services, can help empower families to be able to advocate for the hearing healthcare needs of their children. Families should be provided with written materials and pertinent websites to use as reference materials between appointments and throughout the habilitation process.

Although audiologists and otolaryngologists are the primary professionals involved in diagnosing hearing loss in children, speech-language pathologists play a significant role in supporting parents through the adjustment process. Parents of a child with hearing loss may encounter a speech-language pathologist at any stage of their hearing loss discovery process (e.g., shock, denial, anger, grief, and acceptance). Until more information is known about where the family is in this process, it is especially helpful for parents to take the lead in expressing their needs at any given time, and to do so with professionals who are keenly aware of the impact hearing loss can have on a child. Allowing parents to ask questions and express their concerns and feelings about their child's diagnosis in an accepting and empathetic environment will allow them to move toward making informed decisions regarding their child's habilitation plan.

Reinforcing the Option of Speaking with a Trained Support Parent

Trained support parents have experienced firsthand the emotions and challenges related to having a child with special needs and are able to support other parents. In addition, they have participated in specific and ongoing skill building and training sessions in preparation for their role of offering emotional and informational support to families who would like to talk to another parent who has had similar experiences. They have gone through a parent-to-parent support orientation to familiarize themselves with communication skills, listening skills, and peer-support skills Trained support parents do not provide counseling but offer encouragement, emotional support, and information on an informal and personal basis. Trained support parents do not give advice; they offer suggestions or outline options, but leave the decision making to the parent.

With each appointment, the speech-language pathologist can continue to engage parents in a series of conversations that will allow them time to digest information regarding test results/recommendations, communication options (if applicable), and short- and long-term habilitation plans so that they can more fully participate in the decision-making process that best suits the unique needs of their child. Parents should be encouraged to bring additional family members to audiology and/or speech therapy appointments for support and have the option of contacting the clinician (telephone, email and so on) inbetween appointments should questions or concerns arise.

Summary

The EHDI process is a multidisciplinary team approach to the hearing health care of infants and toddlers. It is a public health initiative with strong support from medical professionals, parents, JCIH members, advocacy agencies for children with hearing loss, and federal and state government policy makers. Although the ultimate goals of early hearing loss identification and timely intervention and habilitation are simple and straightforward, the success of this process is dependent on the awareness and action of all the stakeholders involved. EHDI has been and continues to be a work in progress on both national and state levels as new, evidence-based practices become available in the screening, diagnostic, and habilitative process and as greater numbers of healthcare providers and parents become advocates for ensuring that EHDI goals are being met. Although challenges in funding, insurance impediments to care, and availability of healthcare providers with expertise in working with very young children with hearing loss still exist, EHDI programs throughout the United States continue to work toward finding solutions that will allow the achievement of all EHDI goals in a timely and seamless manner.

Speech-language pathologists will always play a vital role in the EHDI process. Speech-language pathology services can be found embedded into:

- Provision of hearing screening services,
- Identification of children presenting with risk indicators for late onset hearing loss,
- Making timely referrals for audiologic evaluation and monitoring,
- Assisting families in navigating their child's hearing loss journey from hearing loss diagnosis to entry into early intervention,
- Transitioning from early intervention to pre-K,
- Connecting families to resources and agencies that serve as a bridge to the Deaf and hard of hearing communities, and
- Providing speech-language therapeutic services to children identified with all types and degrees of hearing loss.

In the early intervention process, it is the ultimate goal of the speech-language pathologist to ensure that each child has the best access to early communication skill development as a foundation for optimal social, academic, and vocational outcomes.

Discussion Questions

1. You recently received a referral requesting a speech-language evaluation for a 20-month-old male who presents with delays in both cognitive skills and speech-language development. Case history information reveals that he passed his newborn hearing screening prior to nursery discharge. Medical history since that time has been unremarkable with the exception of a brief stay in the hospital at 15 months of age, following a fall from a high chair that resulted in a skull fracture. Should additional pediatric audiologic assessment have been performed? If so, why? What further recommendations should you consider regarding this child's hearing health care?

2. In reviewing medical records of a premature 10-month-old female (31 weeks gestational age) in your care, you learn that she referred bilaterally on two automated auditory brainstem response (AABR) screenings prior to discharge from the NICU, where she was a patient for 3 weeks. Her parents present documentation that shows she has since passed a transient evoked otoacoustic emission (TEOAE) screening of each ear during a well-baby visit with her pediatrician at 3 months of age. Has this child received appropriate follow-up related to her abnormal hospital hearing screening result? If not, why not? Is additional testing warranted? If so, what type of testing?

3. Describe each of the goals of the nationally recognized 1-3-6 Rule in regards to early hearing detection and intervention, and discuss the adverse consequences on a child's development of not adhering to these timelines.

4. Discuss the newborn hearing screening protocols for infants in the term (or well-baby) nursery as compared to those children who have had a NICU stay of greater than 5 days. What is the rationale behind these differences, and what is the appropriate follow-up for children in either nursery who do not pass their hearing screening prior to nursery discharge?

5. Describe which medical specialists need to be consulted for children who have been diagnosed with permanent hearing loss of any degree/configuration in one or both ears and what the rationale is for referral to each of these professionals.

6. Discuss the role that functional auditory assessments have on developing a full understanding of the impact a unilateral or bilateral hearing loss of any degree, type, or configuration can have on a child's day-to-day communication.

7. What are the benefits of ensuring that children who are diagnosed with hearing loss are enrolled in early intervention prior to 6 months of age? Describe how provision of a natural environment for early intervention services (Part C of the Individuals with Disabilities Education Act services takes on a different meaning for children with hearing loss than for children with normal hearing who receive early intervention services).

8. Describe the various roles speech-language pathologists play in the early hearing detection and intervention process. In what ways can a speech-language pathologist empower families of children from birth to age 3 to ensure their optimal hearing health care?

9. After several years of working as a speech-language pathologist in your state's early intervention (EI) system, you have decided to relocate to a bordering state to take a similar EI position. Should you assume that the regulatory requirements for each state regarding universal newborn hearing screening are identical in meeting national EHDI goals? If not, what resources should you review to address your new state's EHDI program requirements?

References

American Speech-Language-Hearing Association. (2004). *Guidelines for the audiologic assessment of children from birth to 5 years of age.* Available from http://www.asha.org/policy/GL2004-00002/

American Speech-Language-Hearing Association. (2008). *Roles and responsibilities of speech-language pathologists in early intervention: Guidelines.* Available from http://www.asha.org/policy/GL2008-00293/

Anderson, K. (2002). *Early listening function (ELF) instrument for infants and toddlers with hearing loss.* Available from http://www.karenandersonconsulting.com. https://successforkidswith-hearingloss.com/uploads/ELF_Questionnaire.pdf

Anderson, K. (2006). *Determining the need and benefit of FM use: Measurement of outcomes* [PowerPoint slides]. Available from www.kandersonaudconsulting.com/.../Determining_Need_and_Benefit_of_FM_Use_HANDOUT.ppt. http://www.slideserve.com/Ava/determining-need-and-benefit-of-fm-use-measurement-of-outcomes

Apuzo, M., & Yoshinaga-Itano, C. (1995). Early identification of infants with significant hearing loss and the Minnesota child development inventory. *Seminars in Hearing,* 16: 124–139.

Bess, F. H., Dodd-Murphy, J., & Parker, R. A. (1998). Children with minimal sensorineural hearing loss: Prevalence, educational performance, and functional status. *Ear and Hearing,* 19(5): 339–354.

Bess, F. H., & Tharpe, A. M. (1984). Unilateral hearing impairment in children. *Pediatrics,* 74(2): 206–216.

Chen, D. (2000). Identifying vision and hearing problems in infants with disabilities. *IDA News,* 27(3): 1–3.

Ching, T. Y. C., & Hill, M. (2007). The parents' evaluation of aural/oral performance of children (PEACH) scale: Normative data. *Journal of the American Academy of Audiology,* 18: 221–237.

Commission on Education of the Deaf. (1988). *Toward equality education of the deaf: A report to the President and Congress of the United States.* Washington, DC: U.S. Government Printing Office.

DesGeorges, J., DeConde Johnson, C., & Stredler Brown, A. (2005). *Natural environments: A call for policy guidance.* Available from http://www.handsandvoices.org/articles/early_intervention/V10-4_policyGuidance.htm.

Gallaudet Research Institute, Gallaudet University. (2003). *Regional and national summary.* Available from http://research.gallaudet.edu/Demographics/2003_National_Summary.pdf.

Houston, K. T. (2009). *Trends in early identification and early intervention in infant identified with hearing loss.* Available from http://www.speechpathology.com/articles/trends-in-early-identification-and-1168.

Individuals with Disabilities Education Act. (2004). PL 108-446, 20 USC 1400 note. 118. Stat. 2647. Available at http://www.ed.gov/policy.

Johnson, C. D., & Von Almen, P. (2004). Functional listening evaluation. In C. D. Johnson, P. V. Benson, & J. B. Seaton (Eds.), *Educational audiology handbook* (pp. 336–339). San Diego, CA: Singular.

Joint Committee on Infant Hearing. (1994). 1994 position statement. *ASHA*, 36(12): 38–41.

Joint Committee on Infant Hearing. (2000). Year 2000 position statement: principles and guidelines for early hearing detection and intervention programs. *Pediatrics*, 106(4): 808–809.

Joint Committee on Infant Hearing. (2007). Year 2007 position statement: Principles and guidelines for early hearing detection and intervention programs. *Pediatrics*, 120(4): 898–921.

Kühn-Inacker, H., Weichboldt, V., Tsiakpini, L., Conninx, F., & D'Haese, P. (2003). *LittleEARS auditory questionnaire (LEAQ): Parent questions to assess auditory behavior*. Innsbruck, Austria: MED-EL.

Laurent Clerc Deaf Education Center, Gallaudet University. (n.d.). *Deaf students with disabilities*. Available from http://www.gallaudet.edu/clerc_center/information_and_resources/info_to_go/educate_children_(3_to_21)/students_with_disabilities.html.

Mauk, G. W., & Behrens, T. R. (1993). Historical, political and technological context associated with early identification of hearing loss. *Seminars in Hearing*, 14: 1–17.

McKay, S., Gravel, J. S., & Tharpe, A. M. (2008). Amplification considerations for children with minimal or mild bilateral hearing loss and unilateral hearing loss. *Trends in Amplification*, 12(1): 43–54.

Minnesota Deaf Blind Technical Assistance Project. (n.d.). *Overview of deafblindness and implications*. Available from http://www.dbproject.mn.org/overview.html.

Moeller, M. P. (2000). Early intervention and language development in children who are deaf and hard of hearing. *Pediatrics*, 106(3): e43.

National Center for Health Statistics. (2001). *Healthy people 2000 final review*. Hyattsville, MD: Public Health Service. Library of Congress Catalog Card Number 76-641496.

National Center for Hearing Assessment and Management. (n.d.). *EHDI legislation: Overview*. Available from http://www.infanthearing.org/legislation/.

National Institutes of Health. (1993, March 1–3). Early identification of hearing impairment in infants and young children. *NIH Consensus Statement*, 11(1): 1–24.

Northern, J. L., & Downs, M. P. (2002). *Hearing in children* (5th ed.). Baltimore, MD: Lippincott, Williams & Wilkins.

Oyler, R. F., & Matkin, N. D. (1988). Unilateral hearing loss: Demographics and educational impact. *Language, Speech, Hearing Services in Schools*, 19: 191–210.

Oyler, R. F., Oyler, A. L., & Matkin, N. D. (1987). Warning: A unilateral hearing loss may be detrimental to a child's academic career. *Hearing Journal*, 9: 18–22.

Palmer, C., & Mormer, E. (1999). Goals and expectations of the hearing aid fitting. *Trends in Amplification*, 4(2): 61–71.

Pletcher, B. A. (2012, Jan. 2). *Genetics of childhood hearing loss: Non-syndromic and syndromic deafness* [PowerPoint slides]. Invited presentation, New Jersey Early Hearing Detection and Intervention Pediatric Hearing Healthcare Teleconference, Trenton, NJ.

Purdy, S. C., Farrington, D. R., Moran, C. A., Chard, L. L., & Hodgson, S. A. (2002). ABEL: Auditory behavior in everyday life. *American Journal of Audiology*, 11: 72–82.

Robbins, A. M., Renshaw, J. J., & Berry, S. W. (1991). Evaluating meaningful integration in profoundly hearing impaired children. *American Journal of Otolaryngology*, 12(Suppl): 144–150.

Stredler Brown, A., & Johnson, C. D. (2010). *Functional auditory performance indicators: An integrated approach to auditory skill development (FAPI)*. Available from http://www.arlenestredlerbrown.com. http://www.tsbvi.edu/attachments/FunctionalAuditoryPerformanceIndicators.pdf

Valente, M., Hosford-Dunn, H., & Roeser, R. J. (2000). *Audiology treatment*. In M. Valente, H. Hosford-Dunn, & R. J. Roeser (Eds.), *Audiology: Treatment*. New York: Thieme Medical.

White, K. R. (2002, Aug.). *The status of early hearing detection and intervention in the US* [PowerPoint slides]. Invited presentation, National Symposium for Infant Hearing, Breckenridge, CO. Available from http://www.infanthearing.org/slideshows/index.html.

White, K. R., & Behrens, T. R. (Eds.). (1993). The Rhode Island Hearing assessment project: Implication for universal newborn hearing screening. *Seminars in Hearing*, 14: 1–119.

White, K. R., Forsman, I., Eichwald, J., & Munoz, K. (2012). *The foundations and evolution of early hearing detection and intervention*. Available from The NCHAM eBook: A Resource Guide for Early Hearing Detection & Intervention, http://www.infanthearing.org/ehdi-ebook/2012_ebook/.

Yoshinaga-Itano, C. (2000). Successful outcomes for deaf and hard-of-hearing children. *Seminars in Hearing*, 21(4): 309–326.

Zimmerman-Philips, S., Osberger, M. J., & Robbins, A. M. (1998). Infant-toddler meaningful auditory integration scale (IT-MAIS). In W. Estabrooks, (Ed.), *Cochlear implants for kids* (pp. 376–386). Washington, DC: Alexander Graham Bell Association for the Deaf.

Appendix 13-A: Websites: Pediatric Hearing Healthcare and Related Resource Information for Families of Children with Hearing Loss

Beginnings: For Parents of Children Who Are Deaf or Hard of Hearing, Inc.*
http://www.ncbegin.org

My Baby's Hearing*
http://www.babyhearing.org

Raising Deaf Kids*
http://www.raisingdeafkids.org/about.php

Hands and Voices
http://www.handsandvoices.org

Centers for Disease Control and Prevention: Hearing Loss in Children*
http://www.cdc.gov/ncbddd/hearingloss/index.html

Listen-up
http://www.listen-up.org

National Institute on Deafness and Other Communication Disorders: Health Information*
http://www.nidcd.nih.gov/health/

National Center for Hearing Assessment and Management
http://www.infanthearing.org

Laurent Clerc National Deaf Education Center: Info to Go
http://clerccenter.gallaudet.edu/InfoToGo

U.S. Department of Education, Office of Special Education and Rehabilitation Services: Opening Doors: Technology and Communication Options for Children with Hearing Loss*
http://www2.ed.gov/about/offices/list/osers/products/opening_doors/index.html

American Academy of Audiology
http://www.howsyourhearing.org

American Speech-Language-Hearing Association
http://www.asha.org/public

American Academy of Otolaryngology—Head and Neck Surgery: Pediatric*
http://www.entnet.org/healthinformation/Pediatric.cfm

Cleft Palate Foundation[1]
http://www.cleftline.org

American Society for Deaf Children
http://www.deafchildren.org

---

*Indicates website information is available in English and Spanish.

Alexander Graham Bell Association for the Deaf and Hard of Hearing
http://www.agbell.org

National Cued Speech Association
http://www.cuedspeech.org

John Tracy Clinic*
http://www.jtc.org

National Association of the Deaf
http://www.nad.org

Parent2Parent USA
http://www.p2pusa.org

Appendix 13-B: Hearing Healthcare Infant/ Toddler Case History Questionnaire (HHITCH-Q)

The following set of questions may be helpful in obtaining a comprehensive hearing healthcare history on children in your caseload ranging in age from birth to 3 years. The questions will serve as guidelines to pertinent aspects within the entire early hearing detection and intervention (EHDI) continuum of care, though some questions may not be applicable for all children. Regardless of the answers provided by parents and/or caregivers, it is especially important to obtain written parental consent through a signed and dated Release of Information form to allow you access to formal documentation of a particular child's newborn hearing screening, rescreening results, audiologic evaluations, hearing aid verification or cochlear implant mapping information, pertinent medical reports, early intervention information, and other tests that may have been performed (if applicable). Of interest will be verifying that a clear picture emerges regarding the hearing (and, if applicable, hearing aid or cochlear implant) status of each child for whom you provide speech-language pathology services. If hearing status is unknown, the speech-language pathologist will play a truly vital role in encouraging family compliance in securing pediatric audiologic assessment to determine comprehensive information regarding this child's auditory functioning.

Newborn Hearing Screening Inquiries

- Did the child undergo a newborn hearing screening? ☐ Yes ☐ No ☐ Unknown
  - If so, how old was the child when the screening was performed? _____ ☐ ?
  - Where was the screening performed? _____ ☐ ?
  - What type of screening was conducted? ☐ OAE ☐ AABR ☐ Both ☐ ?
  - What was the result of the screening?
    OAE: Right Ear: ☐ Pass   ☐ Refer   ☐ Did Not Test ☐ ?
    OAE: Left Ear: ☐ Pass   ☐ Refer   ☐ Did Not Test ☐ ?
    AABR: Right Ear: ☐ Pass   ☐ Refer   ☐ Did Not Test ☐ ?
    AABR: Left Ear: ☐ Pass   ☐ Refer   ☐ Did Not Test ☐ ?
  - What follow-up recommendations were given as a result of the screening?
    _____ ☐ ?
  - Does the family have any questions regarding the results of their child's hearing screening? ☐ Yes ☐ No
  - If yes, what questions or concerns do they have?
    _____

Newborn Hearing Rescreening Inquiries

- Did this child undergo a hearing rescreening (if applicable)? ☐ Yes ☐ No ☐?
  - If so, how old was this child when the rescreening was performed? _____ ☐ ?
  - Where was the rescreening performed? _____ ☐ ?
  - What was the result of the rescreening?
    OAE: Right Ear: ☐ Pass   ☐ Refer   ☐ Did Not Test ☐ ?
    OAE: Left Ear: ☐ Pass   ☐ Refer   ☐ Did Not Test ☐ ?
    AABR: Right Ear: ☐ Pass   ☐ Refer   ☐ Did Not Test ☐ ?
    AABR: Left Ear: ☐ Pass   ☐ Refer   ☐ Did Not Test ☐ ?
  - What follow-up recommendations were given as a result of the rescreening? _____ ☐ ?

- If this child initially referred on AABR screening, were they rescreened with AABR technology?   ☐ Yes ☐ No ☐?
- Does the family have any questions regarding the recommendation for rescreening with AABR and not OAE? ☐ Yes ☐ No ☐?
- Does the family have any questions regarding their rescreening results/recommendations?   ☐ Yes ☐ No ☐?

Children Who Passed Their Newborn Hearing Screening, but Who Present with Risk Indicators to Possible Late Onset Hearing Loss Inquiries

- Do you or your family have any concerns regarding this child's hearing or any possible speech, language, or developmental delays?   ☐ Yes ☐ No
- Is there a history of permanent childhood hearing loss in this family (including parents, siblings, grandparents, great-grandparents, cousins, aunts, or uncles)?   ☐ Yes ☐ No ☐?
  - If so, do you know the etiology of the hearing loss?   ☐ Yes ☐ No ☐?
  - Specify their relationship to the child _____ and, if known, the etiology of the loss _____
- Did this child spend more than 5 days in the neonatal intensive care unit (NICU) prior to nursery discharge? ☐ Yes ☐ No ☐?
- While in the NICU for over 5 days, did this child receive (check all that apply):
  ☐ *Extracorporeal membrane oxygenation (ECMO)* ☐ Assisted ventilation ☐ Ototoxic medications (gentamycin and tobramycin) or loop diuretics (furosemide/lasix)? ☐?
- Has this child ever undergone an exchange transfusion to treat hyperbilirubinemia?   ☐ Yes ☐ No ☐?
- Has this child been diagnosed with intra-uterine infections or TORCH infections (check all that apply):
  ☐ *CMV* ☐ Herpes ☐ Rubella ☐ Syphilis ☐ Toxoplasmosis ☐ None ☐?
- Does this child present with any craniofacial anomalies such as, but not limited to (check all that apply):
  ☐ Malformation of the external ear (microtia) ☐ External auditory canal atresia ☐ Ear tags
  ☐ Pre-auricular pits ☐ Malformation of the temporal bone ☐ Cleft palate ☐ Other not listed here
  (please specify: _____) ☐ None ☐?
  - If the observed facial difference is related to the ear, which ear(s) is affected?   ☐ Right ear ☐ Left ear ☐ Both ears
  - Does this child receive services from a craniofacial or cleft palate team?   ☐ Yes ☐ No ☐?
    If so, where is the team located? _____
    When was the last visit with the team? _____
    When does this child return to the team? _____
    What recommendations were made at the most recent team meeting? _____
    _____
    _____
- Does this child present with any physical findings that may be associated with a syndrome known to include a sensorineural or conductive hearing loss?   ☐ Yes ☐ No ☐? If yes, specify findings:
  _____
- Does this child present with a syndrome known to include (check all that apply):   ☐ Hearing loss ☐ *Progressive* hearing loss ☐ *Late onset* hearing loss? ☐ None ☐?
- Has this child been identified with a *neurodegenerative disorder*?   ☐ Yes ☐ No ☐? If yes, specify findings:
  _____
- Has this child been diagnosed with a *culture-positive postnatal infection associated with sensorineural hearing loss,* including, but not limited to, bacterial and viral meningitis?   ☐ Yes ☐ No ☐? If yes, specify findings:
  _____

- Has this child ever sustained a head trauma?   ☐ Yes   ☐ No   ☐?
  - If so, when did the incident occur? _____
  - If so, what were the circumstances of the trauma and when did it occur? _____
  - Were they diagnosed with either *a basal skull* or *temporal bone fracture* that required hospitalization?   ☐ Yes   ☐ No   ☐?
- Has this child ever received *chemotherapy*?   ☐ Yes   ☐ No   ☐?
  - If so, how old were they when chemotherapy was administered? _____
  - Are they still receiving treatment?   ☐ Yes   ☐ No   ☐?
  - What type of cancer are they (or were they) being treated for? _____

*Note that although all the risk indicators listed require periodic audiologic monitoring, those in bold italics are of greater concern for delayed onset hearing loss and require more frequent assessment.

Pediatric Audiologic Evaluation Inquiries

- Did this child undergo a pediatric audiologic evaluation?   ☐ Yes   ☐ No   ☐?
  - If so, how old was the child when the audiologic evaluation was performed? _____
  - Where was the pediatric audiologic evaluation performed? _____
- Was a diagnostic ABR evaluation performed as part of this child's pediatric audiologic evaluation?   ☐ Yes   ☐ No   ☐?
- What were the results of the pediatric audiologic evaluation?
- **Right Ear:**   ☐ Normal hearing   ☐ Sensorineural hearing loss   ☐ Permanent conductive hearing loss   ☐ Transient conductive hearing loss   ☐ Mixed hearing loss with permanent conductive pathology   ☐ Mixed hearing loss with transient conductive pathology   ☐ Auditory neuropathy/auditory dyssynchrony   ☐ Results were inconclusive   ☐ Results unknown
- **Left Ear:**   ☐ Normal hearing   ☐ Sensorineural hearing loss   ☐ Permanent conductive hearing loss   ☐ Transient conductive hearing loss   ☐ Mixed hearing loss with permanent conductive pathology   ☐ Mixed hearing loss with transient conductive pathology   ☐ Auditory neuropathy/auditory dyssynchrony   ☐ Results were inconclusive   ☐ Results unknown
  - What follow-up recommendations were given as a result of the pediatric audiologic evaluation? _____

- Has this child undergone additional audiologic evaluations?   ☐ Yes   ☐ No   ☐?
- When was this child's last audiologic evaluation? _____
- Where was the last audiologic evaluation performed? _____
- Have there been any changes in this child's hearing since their initial audiologic evaluation?   ☐ Yes   ☐ No   ☐?
  - If yes, please specify the nature of the reported change in hearing: _____
- When are they scheduled for their next audiologic evaluation? _____   ☐?
- Where will they be receiving their next audiologic evaluation? _____   ☐?
- Has this child's siblings undergone audiologic evaluation?   ☐ Yes   ☐ No   ☐?
  - If yes, have any been diagnosed with hearing loss?   ☐ Yes   ☐ No   ☐?

Amplification Inquiries

- Has this child ever used hearing aids? Age at time of fitting: _____
- Has the child had more than one set of hearing aids?   ☐ Yes   ☐ No   ☐?
- Describe the hearing aid fitting by circling any of the following:
  - Ear: Right ear aided   Left ear aided   Binaurally aided
- Style:
  - Behind the ear hearing aid(s)   ☐ Right   ☐ Left   ☐ Binaural
  - Bone-anchored hearing aid: nonsurgical   ☐ Right   ☐ Left   ☐ Binaural

- • Bone-anchored hearing aid: implanted (*for children over 5 years*)   □ Right   □ Left   □ Binaural
  - • Conventional bone conduction hearing aid: □ Yes   □ No
- Make/model/serial # of hearing aid (right ear): _____
- Make/model/serial # of hearing aid (left ear): _____
- Dispensing location: _____
- Are hearing aids used through all waking hours daily?   □ Yes   □ No
  - • If not, how many hours daily? _____ hrs
- What reasons can the family provide as to why this child is not a full-time hearing aid user?
  _____
- How long ago did this child receive their current earmolds? _____
- When was the last aided testing conducted with this child? _____
- What was the outcome of the most recent aided testing? _____

FM System Inquiries

- Does this child use an FM system?   Circle: Personal   School
- Make/model: _____ □ ?
- Does this child utilize an FM system in conjunction with their hearing aids?   □ Yes   □ No   □ ?
- Has this child undergone an FM system evaluation?   □ Yes   □ No   □ ?

Cochlear Implant Information

- Does this child have a cochlear implant?   □ Yes   □ No   □ ?
- Age of initial stimulation: _____
- Manufacturer: □ Advanced Bionics   □ Cochlear   □ Med-El
- Name of surgeon: _____
- Name of implant center: _____
- When was this child's last mapping appointment?_____
- What was the outcome of the last CI evaluation? _____
- When is this child scheduled for their next CI appointment? _____

Habilitation Inquiries

- Is this child currently enrolled in an early intervention program?   □ Yes   □ No   □ ?
- Is the program home based?   □ Yes   □ No   □ ?
- Is the program center based?   □ Yes   □ No   □ ?
- Indicate which of the following services this child receives as part of their EI program: □ Speech therapy
  □ Physical therapy   □ Occupational therapy   □ Sign language instruction
- Does this child participate in therapy for one of the following communication modes?
  □ Auditory verbal   □ Auditory oral   □ Cued speech   □ Total communication
  □ ASL   □ Augmentative communication   □ Bilingual/bicultural
- List the names of specialists providing EI services:

  _____

  _____

  _____

  _____

- If this child is not receiving EI services, why not?

  _____

Otolaryngology Inquiries

- Has this child been evaluated by an otolaryngologist?   ☐ Yes   ☐ No   ☐ ?
  - If so, what is the name/address of the otolaryngologist? _____   ☐ ?
  - When did the examination take place? _____   ☐ ?
  - What were the findings for the evaluation? _____   ☐ ?
- Was otolaryngology follow-up recommended?   ☐ Yes   ☐ No   ☐ ?
- Is there a history of ear infections?   ☐ Yes   ☐ No   ☐ ?
- When was the last ear infection: _____   ☐ Right ear   ☐ Left ear   ☐ Both ears
- Has this child undergone surgery for placement of PE tubes?   ☐ Yes   ☐ No   ☐ ?
  - If so, when: _____   Where did surgery take place? _____
  - If so, which ear(s):   ☐ Right ear   ☐ Left ear   ☐ Both ears
- Does this child have seasonal allergies?   ☐ Yes   ☐ No   ☐ ?
- Has this child ever experienced dizziness?   ☐ Yes   ☐ No   ☐ ?
  - If yes, provide details:

  _____

Genetics Inquiries

- Has this child been referred for a genetic counseling evaluation?   ☐ Yes   ☐ No   ☐ ?
  - If so, when did the genetic counseling evaluation take place? _____   ☐ ?
  - Where did the genetic counseling take place? _____   ☐ ?
- Did this child undergo genetic testing?   ☐ Yes   ☐ No   ☐ ?
- Has this child been diagnosed with a syndrome?   ☐ Yes   ☐ No   ☐ ?
  - If yes, provide details: _____
- Does this child present with any other health conditions other than hearing loss?   ☐ Yes (if yes, specify condition(s): _____   ☐ No   ☐ ?
- What were the findings of the genetics evaluation?_____☐ ?
- What recommendations were made as a result of the genetics evaluation?

  _____☐ ?

- Has this child had to return to the geneticist since their initial evaluation?
  ☐ Yes   ☐ No   ☐ ?
  - If so, when? _____☐ ?
  - What was the outcome of the follow-up visit? _____☐ ?

Ophthalmologic Inquiries

- Has this child had their vision assessed by an ophthalmologist?   ☐ Yes   ☐ No   ☐ ?
  - If so, when was this assessment performed? _____
  - Where was this assessment performed? _____
  - What was the outcome of this assessment? _____
- Does this child wear glasses?   ☐ Yes   ☐ No   ☐ ?
- At what age did they begin wearing glasses? _____
  - Has this child had a follow-up examination?   ☐ Yes   ☐ No   ☐ ?
    - If so, when was this reassessment performed? _____
  - Were any changes noted in this child's vision?   ☐ Yes   ☐ No   ☐ ?
- What recommendations were made at the follow-up evaluation?
- When is this child's next eye examination? _____

Medication Inquiries

- Does this child currently take any medications?   □ Yes   □ No   □ ?
    - If so, which medications does this child take, and for what purpose?

_____
_____
_____

Parent Support Service Inquiries

- Has this family been referred for parent support services?   □ Yes   □ No   □ ?
    - If so, when? _____
- What is the name of the parent support agency? _____
- When was the last contact this family had with a parent support agency? _____

Counseling Services Inquiries

- Has this family been referred for counseling?   □ Yes   □ No   □ ?
- If so, when? _____
- What is the name of the counseling agency? _____
- Is this an agency with specific experience in working with children with hearing loss and their families?
    □ Yes   □ No   □ ?
- When was the last contact this family had with their counselor? _____

Additional Medical Referral Inquiries

- Has this child been evaluated by any other medical specialists?
- If so, list name, specialty, and details below:

_____
_____
_____
_____

Be certain to obtain signed release of information in order to obtain pertinent records as well as to have the parent's permission to speak with the professionals who have provided services to this child.

Appendix 13-C: Early Intervention

As a practicing speech-language pathologist, you will come to realize that state and federal regulations regarding service provision for individuals who are deaf or hard of hearing are living documents. By that, we mean that such documents are in a constant state of review and revision. A new document, *Part C Eligibility Considerations for Infants and Toddlers Who Are Deaf or Hard of Hearing* (2011), is now available from the National Center for Hearing Assessment and Management (NCHAM) and the IDEA Infant and Toddler Coordinators Association (ITCA). The purpose of this document is to provide information that will assist people responsible for state Part C systems in:

- Making informed evidence-based decisions as they develop or review eligibility criteria related to infants and toddlers who are deaf or hard of hearing
- Determining the appropriate personnel to participate in eligibility determination and the development of an individualized family service plan (IFSP) to address service needs of the child and family
- Providing resource information to families of children who do not meet the eligibility criteria established by the state's Part C program

It is available at www.infanthearing.org/earlyintervention/part_c_eligibility.pdf.

Chapter 14

Audiology Services in the School System

Cheryl DeConde Johnson, EdD, FAAA, Board Certified in Audiology
with Pediatric Audiology Specialty Certification

Key Terms

504 Plan
Child Find
Deafness
Hearing impairment
Highest qualified provider

Identification
Individualized education
  program (IEP)
Individual Family Service
  Plan (IFSP)

Response to intervention
  (RtI)
Reverberation
Reverberation time
Signal-to-noise ratio (SNR)

Objectives

- Explain the different ways in which a student can potentially receive services through the public education system
- Illustrate the various components of IDEA as it applies to a child with hearing loss
- Understand the main acoustical characteristics of a classroom and the deleterious effects they have on the hearing-impaired child
- Determine the school district's responsibility for the purchase and maintenance of assistive technology

Introduction

This chapter is intended to assist the speech-language pathologist in understanding and supporting appropriate school-based audiology services. Audiology services in an educational setting are different from those in a clinical setting. In hospitals and other medical facilities, a medical model of service provision is utilized for the continuity of patient care. In education, service provision is driven by local, state, and federal administrative codes. To effectively support students with hearing impairment, the speech-language pathologist should expect school audiology services to align with the Individuals with Disabilities Education Act (IDEA), No Child Left Behind (NCLB), and your state's administrative code on special education. It is important that the speech-language pathologist be provided with the information and tools necessary to align services in the classroom for deaf and hard of hearing students, as well as for students with auditory processing disorder, with special education law.

Whether educational audiology services are provided in-house or contracted through a local audiologist or other entity, they must address the individual's listening skills, language learning abilities, and communication access as well as the various parameters of the classroom and educational environment that impact communication. The primary goal of school-based audiology services is to level the playing field by minimizing the impact of hearing impairment on communication and learning so that children who are deaf or hard of hearing have the same learning opportunities as their hearing peers.

To do so, these services must adhere to the following:

- Identify and assess children/youth with hearing and listening problems

- Provide appropriate habilitation, including amplification and other accommodations that ensure full access to communication and the learning environment
- Provide counseling so that children/youth understand their hearing and communication situation, communication options, relevant accommodations, and rights, and are able to take personal responsibility for self-managing their needs
- Create and administer programs for the prevention of hearing loss
- Train teachers and staff and monitor the learning environment to ensure that it is structured to support students with hearing impairment

In this chapter, we will dissect the federal laws pertaining to the definition of audiology services [34 CFR 300.34(c)(1)], educational service provision [34 CFR 300.113], and assistive technology for students with hearing loss in public schools from ages 3 through 21 [34 CFR 300.5].

The provision of audiology services in a public school is considered a related educational service under IDEA, along with other services such as speech-language pathology, occupational therapy, physical therapy, psychological services, counseling, interpreting, parent counseling and training, and transportation. Educational audiology services that are considered "related services" in the individual education program (IEP) may include, but are not limited to, classroom listening assessment, classroom acoustics, assistive technology and devices, self-advocacy and habilitation, and a resource for the general management of children with hearing impairment in a classroom. These responsibilities in some cases may be assigned to the

---

34 CFR 300.34(c)(1)

Audiology includes—

(i) Identification of children with hearing loss;

(ii) Determination of the range, nature, and degree of hearing loss, including referral for medical or other professional attention for the habilitation of hearing;

(iii) Provision of habilitation activities, such as language habilitation, auditory training, speech reading (lip-reading), hearing evaluation, and speech conservation;

(iv) Creation and administration of programs for prevention of hearing loss;

(v) Counseling and guidance of children, parents, and teachers regarding hearing loss; and

(vi) Determination of children's needs for group and individual amplification, selecting and fitting an appropriate aid, and evaluating the effectiveness of amplification.

Reproduced from Office of the Federal Register, National Archives and Records Administration. (2006). Rules and Regulations. Federal Register, Monday, August 14, 2006. 71(156), 46760.

speech-language pathologist in the absence of a school system employing an educational audiologist. Within IDEA, specific terminology is used to refer to the **highest qualified provider** within a local education agency (LEA). When it comes to providing audiology services in the school setting, the speech-language pathologist may be considered as the qualified service provider. However, delegation of audiology responsibilities to a speech-language pathologist is not appropriate for all areas. Decisions regarding services for hearing screening, counseling, habilitation, and hearing loss prevention, should be determined by the multidisciplinary team, which includes an audiologist and a teacher of the deaf, based on their qualifications, and the experience of the speech-language pathologist to address the needs of each individual child. It is in the best interest of the speech-language pathologist to refer to professional standards of practice to address these issues with a supervisor specific to the municipality or state in which they are employed.

Identification

The **identification** of children with hearing impairment features several roles for the audiologist or speech-language pathologist. Identification does not explicitly mean screening of all children, but rather screening as a step in the process toward identification of hearing impairment. Resources and regulations generally dictate the level of involvement of the audiologist or speech-language pathologist at this stage, and may vary from state to state. At this point, let us clarify for a moment some processes and programs you will encounter when working in the school setting.

Hearing screening of all children in schools generally is the responsibility of a health and/or education agency that guides the screening processes and procedures. Therefore, basic hearing screening is considered a *population-based* activity, not a program under IDEA. Hence, nurses, health aides, volunteers, or other individuals designated by the responsible agency provide the services.

Population-based screening should not be confused with **Child Find**, which is the special education program under IDEA that requires schools to seek out and identify children from birth to 21 years of age with disabilities. Child Find programs primarily target at-risk early childhood groups by providing developmental screenings that also include vision and hearing. Procedures for screening hearing within the Child Find program should be designed and managed by the educational audiologist. Depending on local procedures, resources, and expertise, the speech-language pathologist

may also conduct or participate in the screening and assist in securing follow-up appointments for children who require additional assessment.

Screening procedures should include measures to target specific populations of students. For example, tympanometry may be part of a screening protocol for young children to identify middle ear problems; the addition of 6000 and/or 8000 Hz to a pure tone protocol for middle school- and high school-age students might identify potential noise-induced hearing loss (NIHL).

Children who are very young or unable to respond with traditional pure tone screening methods may require special behavioral screening techniques and technologies that require the expertise of an audiologist. Automated otoacoustic emissions (OAE) screeners have enabled widespread screening of young children by nonaudiologists. However, misuse is a concern; OAEs are not a substitute for pure tone measures and should not be used as a sole screening tool (American Academy of Audiology [AAA], 2011a). It is critical that you consult with an audiologist to manage screening programs, guide the development of the screening procedures, and provide training and supervision, if necessary. The speech-language pathologist may find himself or herself in charge of managing required screenings (preschool and school age) and Child Find screening following state policies and procedures. As part of this process, the speech-language pathologist may also be responsible for conducting follow-up activities to ensure that those referred have received the prescribed service, facilitate transition between early intervention and educational programs and services, and provide nonbiased information regarding communication options, service options, and community resources.

Putting Education in the Audiologic Assessment: The Classroom Listening Assessment (CLA)

Audiologic assessment for children with identified auditory disorders should include a combination of standard clinical measures and functional classroom-based measures to yield a comprehensive profile of auditory and communication abilities. Although you may find yourself with a diagnostic evaluation report from a clinical audiologist, the information may be lacking as to how the hearing loss may or may not impact the child's education. As we refer back to the laws of IDEA, Section 504 of the Rehabilitation

Act of 1973 (which is where 504 Plans originated), and the Americans with Disabilities Act (ADA), there are slightly different interpretations which make one eligible to receive services for a child with a physical disability (in this case, hearing loss). Under IDEA, eligibility for services requires an "educational manifestation" of the disability, i.e., there is evidence that the disability adversely affects a child's educational performance. Under Section 504, the impact on education is defined as "substantially limiting one or more major life function." Imagine, for example, a child with a broken leg. He is on crutches, but displays normal cognitive function. One could understand accommodations for participation in his physical education classes, but you would not automatically place him in a special education program because of his limited mobility. Accommodations for participation could be made easily to his physical environment within the general education setting, rather than developing an IEP for special education services.

Likewise, a student with hearing loss is not automatically eligible for special education and related services. It is the educational audiologist or, in many cases, the speech-language pathologist who must make the case for eligibility and service provision during the child study team evaluation process. Throughout your career, you will more than likely encounter individuals who are under the misconception that hearing aids correct hearing loss equivalent to eyeglasses correcting a vision problem. Especially in the educational realm, this statement could not be further from the truth. Unfortunately, this mindset must be overcome so that these students are serviced appropriately within their educational programs.

Many measures are available for evaluating the function of a student with hearing loss and determining how that hearing loss may or, in rare cases, may not manifest itself in the classroom environment. These measures include objective and subjective assessments from the perspectives of the student, his or her teachers, and, if desired, parent(s). In addition to the student, the classroom environment is also assessed to determine how well it supports communication access and learning. This comprehensive assessment leads the practitioner to the evidence for accommodations, including such assistance as hearing aid technology, assistive listening devices, or other accommodations within the classroom. It may also lead the practitioner to information regarding the appropriateness of program placement decisions, particularly the components falling under the special factors reflected in the IDEA (see text box: Development, Review, and Revision of the IEP, Consideration of Special

Factors) for further discussion related to the development of the **individualized education program (IEP)**.

Table 14.1 summarizes the protocols used in the classroom listening assessment. A detailed discussion of each assessment area follows. Ideally a Classroom Listening Assessment (CLA) is performed as part of the IEP assessment on all students with hearing impairment who have auditory potential. However, the time required to conduct the CLA generally limits its use to students who require the information for programming decisions or specific protocols within the assessment. The speech-language pathologist should work in collaboration with an educational audiologist (or the child's private audiologist if there is not a school-based audiologist) and teacher of the deaf to determine when the CLA is needed, identify the areas assessed, and determine who will complete each of them. The components of the CLA are not restricted in scope of practice to audiologists because they are classroom-based assessments that provide functional information regarding how communication and learning are impacted by hearing loss. Therefore, the speech-language pathologist in the educational setting may, in fact, be the responsible member of the child study team to complete these assessments.

Classroom Observation

A classroom observation provides a snapshot about the physical parameters of the classroom and the flow of communication. Information about the classroom design, seating arrangements, classroom acoustics, how a teacher manages instruction, expectations for student participation, and management of student behavior are useful when determining the classroom listening needs for a student. For example, a classroom that seems excessively noisy requires acoustic measurements before a recommendation can be made for the most appropriate type of hearing assistance technology (HAT). A predominantly lecture style format requires different accommodation strategies than a teacher who facilitates small group learning. A classroom seating arrangement in a U-shape or circle might provide good visual access but still not meet the acoustical needs of a student. Classroom participation expectations might not include sufficient "wait time" for a student with hearing impairment to hear and process information before being ready to respond.

Information about the student is equally important. What is the student's hearing impairment and functional listening abilities? How does noise influence the child's ability to respond? Was speech-in-noise testing part of the audiologic

Table 14.1   Classroom Listening Assessment Protocols

Type	Tool	Author	Where to Get It
Observation	Placement Checklist from Placement and Readiness Checklists (PARC) for Children Who Are Deaf and Hard of Hearing	Johnson, 2011b	www.ADEvantage.com
	Listening Inventory for Education–Revised (LIFE-R)	Anderson, Smaldino, & Spangler, 2011	www.successforkidswithhearingloss.com
	Screening Instrument for Targeting Educational Risk (SIFTER): Elementary (1989), Preschool (1996), Secondary (2004)	Anderson, 1989, 1996, 2004	www.successforkidswithhearingloss.com
	Children's Auditory Processing Scale (CHAPS)	Smoski, Brunt, & Tannahill, 1998	www.edaud.org
Classroom acoustics	Classroom Acoustics Appraisal, Clinical Practice Guidelines: Remote Microphone Hearing Assistance Technologies for Children and Youth from Birth to 21 Years. Supplement B: Classroom Audio Distribution Systems—Selection and Verification	AAA, 2011	www.audiology.org
Functional assessment	Functional Listening Evaluation (FLE)	Johnson, 2011a	www.ADEvantage.com
	Ling Six-Sound Test	Ling, 2002	http://www.cochlear.com/files/assets/Ling-6%20sound%20test%20-%20how%20to.pdf
Self-assessment	Listening Inventory for Education–Revised (LIFE-R)	Anderson, Smaldino, & Spangler, 2011	www.successforkidswithhearingloss.com
	Classroom Participation Questionnaire (CPQ)	Antia, Sabers, & Stinson, 2007	Educational Audiology Handbook, 2nd ed., Delmar Cengage Learning
	Self-Assessment of Communication–Adolescent (SAC-A); Significant Other Assessment of Communication–Adolescent (SOAC-A)	Elkayam & English, 2003	Guide to Access Planning (GAP) www.phonakonline.com/MyGAP/GAPMain_atl2.html

assessment? Are language and academic performance at grade level, or is the student behind? Are there attention or hyperactivity concerns, or other learning or physical problems, impacting communication and learning? What hearing instruments are currently being used? Are there concerns about self-esteem and personal acceptance of hearing impairment? Can the student self-advocate for his or her own communication access? Is the student motivated to work hard?

Observation tools should include consideration of these physical and instructional properties of classrooms as well as student characteristics. Some components of these areas can be determined through checklists completed by teachers about their classrooms and about the student; however, actual observation of the classroom environment provides an invaluable perspective when determining instructional style, accommodations, and amplification that might be necessary for a student. It also creates the context for training and coaching for the teacher. Tools from Table 14.1 should be chosen that are best suited to the student's developmental abilities as well as the intended purpose of the

assessment (e.g., SIFTER for general learning, LIFE for HAT efficacy, CHAPS for auditory skill development). These tools may also be used as pre-/postvalidation and monitoring measures for use and implementation of accommodations including HAT.

Classroom Acoustics Appraisal

A traditional classroom, as with any other room, possesses its own acoustic characteristics; each classroom, even within the same school building, will vary. Classrooms are like snowflakes—no two are exactly the same. Let us, for a moment, examine the variability of traditional classrooms. There are (at least) four walls. Of what are the walls fabricated? Is there a full wall of windows? Do the windows open? (Not all windows do, and some only open an inch or two.) Are the walls covered with bulletin boards, interactive whiteboards, chalkboards, or student work? Is there a full wall of coat closets? Each classroom should have a door. Is it the school policy that the doors remain open or closed during the school day? Is the door solid or does it have a window? Is there an air vent above the door that remains open to the hallway even if the door is closed? What covers the classroom floor? Is the floor hardwood, rubber tile, or carpeted? Are there area rugs? Of what is the ceiling made? Is it acoustic tile, a drop ceiling? How high is the ceiling? In the case of older schools, is the school plumbing exposed on the ceiling? While we are looking up, of what are the floors in the classroom above this one made? Can student activity be heard through the ceiling? Is there a heating/ventilation/air conditioning (HVAC) system in the classroom? Does it run continuously throughout the day? What type of lighting is used in the classroom? Do the lights emit a sound when they are on or when they are overheated? Are they bright enough for the students to clearly see the main area of instruction in the room? What other electronics are routinely used in the classroom? Is there a class pet? Aquarium filters and hamster wheels make a lot of noise. What type of student seating is used in the room, and what is the configuration of that seating? Individual desks and chairs within a classroom pose an interesting problem. Normal movement within the classroom requires desks and chairs to move on the floor. Are the legs of the desks and chairs covered to reduce this noise? Where does the child with hearing loss (or auditory processing deficits [APD]) sit in respect to where the teacher spends most of his or her time instructing? Is the child in question sitting next to one of the major noise sources in the classroom? How many other students are in the classroom? Is the student enrollment a mix of general education and special education students, or is it a self-contained special education environment? Are there special education students in the classroom who require external ventilation or other medical equipment? How many adults are in the classroom—teacher, inclusion teacher, personal aide, teacher's assistant, school nurse aide, and the like? What are their roles within the classroom? How have their instructional roles been defined? When you put all of these factors in motion at the same time, you can see the many variables that impact classroom acoustics and why evaluation of each classroom environment is necessary.

When assessing classroom acoustics, three aspects of sound must be evaluated. (1) The *direct sound* or primary signal is basically the information that should be the student's focus. Whether this is the teacher's voice, a teacher's aide providing supplemental instruction, or some type of recorded material, it is our goal for that signal to be clear and intelligible to the student. (2) *Reverberation* is the reflection of sound that varies according to the surfaces that it is reflected off of; softer surfaces generally have more absorption

ability and therefore less sound reflection. Conversely, hard surfaces will generally have less absorption ability and therefore more sound reflection. Sound that is reflected off of a surface or multiple surfaces takes longer to reach the listener's ears than direct sound. This time delay to a normal auditory system, known as *reverberation time*, is usually inaudible but has a significant effect on speech intelligibility in an impaired auditory system. Speech intelligibility is further decreased as a result of the interaction of multiple reflections in highly reverberant classrooms. For children using personal hearing instruments alone in the classroom, reverberation time creates an amplified, distracting "echo," further decreasing the intelligibility of the primary signal. (3) *Background noise* is perhaps the greatest classroom offender when it comes to children with hearing loss or APD. Outside of the primary signal, any unwanted sound generated by either internal or external sources is considered background noise. Within the classroom, a measurement is made of the intensity (loudness) of background noise compared to the intensity of the direct sound and is referred to as the signal (direct sound) to noise (background noise) ratio (SNR).

In a classroom, background noise levels (also referred to as ambient noise levels) and reverberation times should comply with American National Standards Institute (ANSI) s12.60-2010 (Acoustical Society of America, 2010); however, at present, this standard is voluntary unless there are state or local regulations that make it mandatory. The only mandatory compliance with this standard is for new school construction. However, with appropriate assessment of the student's listening requirements for communication and instructional access and the classroom acoustical environment, evidence can be acquired that substantiates a student's need for instruction in a classroom that meets the ANSI standards.

Determining Signal-to-Noise Ratio

What You Need to Know

An educational audiologist typically performs classroom noise-level measurements using a device known as a sound level meter. Sound-level meter applications for handheld devices, such as Audio Tools by Studio Six Digital (www.studiosixdigital.com), are now available that make noise-level measurements simple to perform. Readings are taken using a decibel scale that is acoustically modified for speech communication; it is known as the dBA weighted scale. Taking measurements from a variety of points in the classroom may also help in determining the appropriate seating of the student with hearing loss or APD.

Technically Speaking

The Classroom Acoustics Survey Worksheet (AAA, 2011b; see Appendix 14-B) contains observation considerations as well as a guide for making classroom acoustical measurements to identify whether classrooms meet ANSI noise and reverberation time standards (e.g., 35 dBA and 0.6 seconds for classrooms less than 10,000 cubic feet, which may be reduced to 0.3 seconds for children with special listening needs). Noise measurements should be made from several room locations with and without the HVAC system on, and with and without students in the room. Measurements should be repeated while the teacher reads a standard passage to establish SNRs for the same room locations. If a classroom audio distribution system (CADS) is used, measurements should be repeated to demonstrate the improvement in SNR. Children with hearing impairment generally require a +15 dB SNR, which means that the talker's voice is 15 dB greater than the background noise at the student's ear. Speech-in-noise assessments conducted as part of the audiological assessment, such as the BKB-SIN (Etymotic Research, 2005), identify specific individual SNR requirements and, thus, are an important part of the audiologic assessment battery for children with hearing impairment. More sophisticated measurements using a conventional type 2 sound-level meter (a weighted scale, slow response, and a minimum lower limit of 35 dBA) should be performed when acoustical alterations are necessary, such as modifications to ventilation systems or installation of acoustical panels.

Determining Reverberation Time

What You Need To Know

Reverberation time can also be measured with an app, or special reverberation time measurement equipment. Remember, for a student with hearing loss, reverberation is sound reflections amplified through a personal hearing instrument, creating a hollow echo-like sound. Depending on the classroom design, the echo and the time this echo takes to reach the ear (reverberation time) cause distortions of the speech signal and therefore may result in significant auditory fatigue for the child. Constantly seeking out a clear primary signal in the classroom through this myriad reverberation becomes an arduous task for a child with hearing loss or APD.

Technically Speaking

Reverberation time can be measured using conventional reverberation time meters or applications for handheld devices (similar to those used for **noise measurement**), or it can be extrapolated by calculating known absorption coefficients of common wall, floor, and ceiling surfaces. Critical distance marks the maximum point at which the listener receives the speech signal from the

---

34 CFR 300.6

Assistive technology service means any service that directly assists a child with a disability in the selection, acquisition, or use of an assistive technology device. The term includes

(a) The evaluation of the needs of a child with a disability, including a functional evaluation of the child in the child's customary environment;

(b) Purchasing, leasing, or otherwise providing for the acquisition of assistive technology devices by children with disabilities;

(c) Selecting, designing, fitting, customizing, adapting, applying, maintaining, repairing, or replacing assistive technology devices;

(d) Coordinating and using other therapies, interventions, or services with assistive technology devices, such as those associated with existing education and rehabilitation plans and programs;

(e) Training or technical assistance for a child with a disability or, if appropriate, that child's family; and

(f) Training or technical assistance for professionals (including individuals providing education or rehabilitation services), employers, or other individuals who provide services to, employ, or are otherwise substantially involved in the major life functions of children with disabilities.

Reproduced from Office of the Federal Register, National Archives and Records Administration. (2006). Rules and Regulations. Federal Register, Monday, August 14, 2006. 71(156), 46756.

talker directly, i.e., direct sound, without additional sound reflections from room surfaces. Therefore, optimal speech understanding requires that the listener is located within the estimated critical distance from the talker. Critical distance is determined by room size and reverberation.

Hearing Assistance Technology (HAT)

Now that we have examined the classroom acoustics, we will return to IDEA to review its content in terms of the school system's responsibility for providing amplification and hearing assistance technology. One of the primary roles of an educational audiologist in the school setting is providing services related to amplification; however, in the absence of a full-time or consulting audiologist, the highest qualified provider may become the speech-language pathologist or the teacher of the deaf. Again, it is imperative that the speech-language pathologist working with a child with hearing loss or APD provide services that are only within his or her scope of practice. A good rule of thumb in this area is that any device that comes into school as the personal property of the child be serviced only if specified in the IEP that it is assistive technology to be used at school and only for the services described. However, as will be discussed further, schools are responsible for monitoring the functioning of personal devices to ensure that they are functioning properly, and when there is a problem or malfunction the parents (or guardian) must be notified so that the child's personal audiologist can obtain the instrument to perform the necessary repairs or modification.

Amplification

The use of hearing instruments in conjunction with HAT, or in some cases HAT alone, in the classroom can be an integral part of service provision for a student with a hearing loss or auditory processing disorder. Although it is outside of the speech-language pathologist's scope of practice to apply 34 CFR 300.6 to "selecting, designing, fitting, customizing, adapting . . ." to personal hearing instruments and hearing assistive technology, maintaining/repairing (listening checks, changing the batteries, etc.) does fall within the interventions of auditory rehabilitation. In the absence of an educational audiologist, speech-language pathologists may find themselves in situations in which a wide variety of school personnel have been or are currently in charge of HAT. The school-based speech-language pathologist should work with the student's audiologist (private), the teacher of the deaf and his/her supervisor to determine how the management of HAT can best be accomplished within the requirements of IDEA and professional scopes of practice. Selection of appropriate HAT devices, fitting, and management of HAT is a primary responsibility of audiologists; as such schools may need to contract with audiologists to perform these duties.

Cochlear Implants and Monitoring Personal Instrument Function

As the number of students with cochlear implants increases in our schools, the speech-language pathologist must be acutely aware of what is in and what is outside of his/her scope of practice. Also what is the legal responsibility of the

---

34 CFR 300.113 Routine checking of hearing aids and external components of surgically implanted medical devices

Hearing aids. Each public agency must ensure that hearing aids worn in school by children with hearing impairments, including deafness, are functioning properly

External components of surgically implanted medical devices.

(1) Subject to paragraph (b)(2) of this section, each public agency must ensure that the external components of surgically implanted medical devices are functioning properly.

(2) For a child with a surgically implanted medical device who is receiving special education and related services under this part, a public agency is not responsible for the post-surgical maintenance, programming, or replacement of the medical device that has been surgically implanted (or of an external component of the surgically implanted medical device).

Reproduced from Office of the Federal Register, National Archives and Records Administration. (2006). Rules and Regulations. Federal Register, Monday, August 14, 2006. 71(156), 46764.

school system for maintaining a cochlear implant and what is not the responsibility of the LEA. The exclusion for cochlear implants was added in IDEA 2004 in order to limit the growing demands on schools to provide cochlear implant programming. IDEA 2004 also strengthened the responsibility of schools to monitor personal hearing instruments including the external components of cochlear implants and their function. As a result, schools should always include a monitoring plan that specifies who monitors the personal hearing instrument, when it is conducted, the procedures used, and what will happen if a problem is identified. It is recommended that this plan be included in the IEP. A sample amplification monitoring plan is located in Appendix 14-D.

Functional Assessment

Now that we have discussed the classroom environment, the responsibility of the school system to provide technology—in the form of HAT—and a system by which that device is monitored, we must now look at the student's ability to function in the classroom. The assessment of a child with hearing loss or APD in their classroom environment provides objective performance data that reflect functional listening capabilities. The goal of this step in the CLA is to address the acoustics of the classroom (e.g., noise and reverberation) and the communication characteristics (distance from the teacher and other talkers, audibility of the teacher/talker's and student's voices) encountered by children as these classroom dynamics change. For children who use HAT, the assessment should also be performed with the HAT to document the benefit provided by the assistive technology.

Conducting the assessment live in a child's classroom is challenging. The mere presence of a new adult in the room with special test equipment requires explanation and acclimatization until the novelty diminishes. Assessing a child in the presence of his or her peers to capture the typical auditory and visual atmosphere is even more difficult. Therefore, it may be necessary to compromise some components of the real-world assessment by using tools that build in or simulate those situations.

The Ling Six-Sound Test

The Ling Six-Sound Test is a simple procedure to determine the audibility of six sounds that represent the speech frequency spectrum of 1000–4000 Hz. The test can be used to determine detection, discrimination, and identification skills with and without amplification, and is an effective quick validation tool, especially for young children. Procedures and materials for the administration of the Ling Test are available from the Cochlear Americas website, as indicated in Table 14.1.

Self-Assessment

Children and youth should always have a role in the evaluation of their classroom listening performance as part of their annual assessment. Investing in self-perception increases knowledge of one's skills and needed accommodations as well as one's self-determination and self-advocacy development. Review of self-assessment results reveals issues that often open the door for further discussion and counseling about communication and/or listening problems and the development of strategies for addressing problem situations.

As with other parts of the CLA, self-assessment should be chosen based on the developmental considerations of the child/youth, and the information desired from the assessment. For children who are unable to read the questions or statements, self-assessments can be read to the student and explanations of terminology or concepts provided. However, the evaluator should never try to influence the response choice of the student. The Listening Inventory for Education (LIFE) and the Classroom Participation Questionnaire (CPQ) are generally appropriate for children beginning in elementary grades; the Self-Assessment of Communication for Adolescents (SAC-A) is designed for older children. Often, comparison of self-perceptions to those of an observer is helpful. The Significant Other Assessment of Communication-Adolescents (SOAC-A) is designed as a companion tool to the SAC-A to gain this added perspective. This additional information is particularly instrumental in the counseling process.

Each of these tools is also useful for pre/post efficacy for accommodations, including HAT, and to monitor their implementation. The CPQ (see Appendix 14-C) is particularly useful to gain information about communication access and ease of communication in the classroom and to initiate discussion of accommodations and self-advocacy during individual therapy sessions.

Parent Counseling and Training

Parent counseling and training is a separate, related service in IDEA. The law specifies that there are to be goals related to parent services as a component of the IEP when parents need assistance and information as well as acquiring skills to help their children accomplish their IEP goals in order to receive a free and appropriate public education (FAPE). Parents can choose whether they desire the support, but it must be made available by the LEA. Unfortunately, this service is underutilized and can be difficult to implement due to confusion about how to include the service in the IEP, how to provide the service, and how to promote and monitor parent compliance.

Prevention

As we further review the definition of audiology services within the school system, the portion of the IDEA that is most often overlooked, but is becoming increasingly important within the educational setting, is the prevention of hearing loss. Concern in this area is growing based on some of the following issues:

- Schools, as government entities, are exempt from the U.S. Occupational Safety and Health Administration's (OSHA's) standards unless there are state OSHA-like requirements; however, shop class noise levels have been reported to range from 85 dB to 115 dB (Lankford & West, 1993).
- Noise regulations that do exist in schools apply primarily to classified staff (e.g., grounds, facility, print shop, cooking staff).
- Insurance companies for schools have limited knowledge of noise exposure hazards.

- School hearing screening is not mandated in all states; thus, a mechanism to identify children with potential noise-induced hearing loss is not consistently available. When screening programs do exist, they generally are not designed to identify students with noise-induced hearing loss.

Based on the results of the Third National Health and Nutrition Examination Survey (NHANES III), Niskar and colleagues (2001) estimated that 12.5% of children 6 to 19 years of age demonstrate hearing loss that can be directly attributed to high levels of noise exposure. Shargorodsky, Curhan, and Eavy (2010) reported that the incidence of noise-induced hearing loss had increased in adolescents 12–19 years of age from 1984 to 2005–2006. In recognition of the evidence, the U.S. Department of Health and Human Services (2010) in its Healthy People 2020 goals includes the following objectives related to hearing loss prevention in adolescents:

- Objective ENT-VSL 6.2 Increase the proportion of adolescents 12–19 years who have ever used hearing protection devices (earplug, earmuffs) when exposed to loud sounds or noise.
- Objective ENT-VSL 7 Reduce the proportion of adolescents who have elevated hearing thresholds, or audiometric notches, in high frequencies (3, 4, or 6 kHz) in both ears, signifying noise-induced hearing loss.

Although there are many resources available that provide hearing loss prevention education (e.g., Dangerous Decibels, www.dangerousdecibels.org; Crank It Down, www.hearingconservation.org; Wise Ears!, www.nidcd. nih.gov/health/wise/), the difficulty lies in coordinating efforts for implementing a systematic hearing loss prevention education program within the curriculum.

---

34 CFR 300.34(c)(8)

(i) Parent counseling and training means assisting parents in understanding the special needs of their child;

(ii) Providing parents with information about their child's development; and

(iii) Helping parents to acquire the necessary skills that will allow them to support the implementation of their child's IEP or IFSP.

(vi) Determination of children's needs for group and individual amplification, selecting and fitting an appropriate aid, and evaluating the effectiveness of amplification.

Reproduced from Office of the Federal Register, National Archives and Records Administration. (2006). Rules and Regulations. Federal Register, Monday, August 14, 2006. 71(156), 46761.

Recent reports (Hendershot, Pakulski, Dowling, & Price, 2011; Sekhar et al., 2012) suggest that the most effective method for identifying teens with NIHL is a combination of a high-risk screening questionnaire for noise exposure, followed by hearing screening of those who report noise exposure that includes pure tone threshold measurements at 1–8 kHz.

Because of the effort necessary to address this area for all students, it is imperative that this service be part of a larger agenda shared by health and general education services. Hearing loss prevention education needs a national focus as a preventable health condition. Educational audiologists and SLPs should support such an effort by promoting the following activities (Johnson & Meinke, 2008):

- Noise education activities that are embedded within school health and science curriculums at multiple grade levels
- Identification of "at-risk" and "dangerous" noise sources
- Mandatory noise safety instruction for classes with potentially hazardous noise exposure, including strategies to minimize noise exposure in those settings
- Mandatory use of hearing protection for all individuals who work in noise hazard areas
- Mandatory monitoring of hearing levels of classified employees and teachers who work in noise hazard areas
- Training for school employees in hearing loss prevention, proper use of ear protection, noise control strategies, and interpretation of hearing test results
- School policies to limit decibel levels and exposure time at school-sanctioned events
- Required hearing screening of students that includes protocols targeted to identification of noise-induced HL

Considerations for Service Provision

Several important areas must be addressed when considering educational services for children with hearing impairment. Eligibility, 504 plan, response to intervention (RtI), referral for evaluation for special education, special considerations for communication needs in the IEP, and

placement options each have specific implications. In the absence of an educational audiologist, the speech-language pathologist may have a greater role in advocating for the student along with the teacher of the deaf, to make sure that the IEP team (the Child Study Team, school personnel, and parents) understands the implications of the student's hearing loss, which may limit his or her access to communication and the educational curriculum.

504 Service Provision

When an IEP team determines that a child's hearing impairment does not adversely affect educational performance, making the child ineligible for special education, students should be considered for accommodations under Section 504 of the Rehabilitation Act using a 504 accommodation plan. Although 504 does not include the individual entitlements that are part of special education, it does provide protection through the Office of Civil Rights (OCR) under the U.S. Department of Education. A 504 plan is generally developed by a school-based team under regular education. This team is frequently composed of a school administrator and/or school counselor, and/or lead teacher, and/or the school nurse. Depending on local procedures, a representative from special education may also be involved. For an effective 504 plan, it is critical that the educational audiologist, SLP, or other specialist experienced with hearing loss in children, as well as the student, be involved in the development of the accommodations plan. Each student's 504 plan should be monitored annually and adjusted accordingly, even though there are no specific federal procedures that dictate the development of the plan, and how it is implemented or monitored. However, some states or local municipalities may have additional imposed timelines. It is imperative that the speech-language pathologist be familiar with the local policies regarding 504 accommodation plans.

Students with hearing impairment who have a 504 plan, as well as those not receiving any support services, should have their hearing and school performance monitored at least annually to determine if they are exhibiting educational problems that require a future referral for special education. Students with hearing impairment who are not receiving special education services are the most vulnerable for falling through the cracks and eventually falling behind in school. The speech-language pathologist should be aware of state and local procedures for special education eligibility and 504 plans so they can properly advocate for the hearing and learning needs of all of these students and prevent unnecessary failure.

Response to Intervention (RtI)

Response to intervention (RtI) is one method for monitoring school performance and ensuring that the recommended accommodations are implemented correctly and are meeting the needs of the child for academic success in the general education setting. The RtI initiative has added a new dimension to services within the general education classroom. This model, which could be considered a prevention program to reduce special education referrals, is based on applying a succession of increasingly more intensive interventions based on the individual needs of children as part of general education delivery. The hallmarks of RtI are that the program must be school wide (i.e., apply to *all* children), must provide high-quality instruction matched to individual student needs, must include frequent monitoring of student progress to inform of changes in instruction, and must utilize child response data to make educational decisions (National Association of State Directors of Special Education [NASDSE], 2005). The multitiered RtI model should integrate the resources of general education, special education, and gifted education as well as any other school student support programs.

The implications of RtI include greater emphasis on research-based interventions that benefit students within the multiple tiers of the model (NASDSE, 2005). For children with hearing loss and APD, these interventions include appropriate classroom acoustics and use of CADS, both well-documented accommodations for all children (Crandell & Smaldino, 2000; Iglehart, 2008) that can be implemented at the Tier-1 universal level. Tier-2 interventions are individualized and might include special flexible seating or use of a personal FM system—again, accommodations that are known to be effective for children with special listening needs (Anderson & Goldstein, 2004; Boothroyd, 1992, Schafer & Thibodeau, 2003). To support children and youth with hearing and listening problems, audiologists and SLPs should be involved with school multidisciplinary teams at each of these tiers to ensure that appropriate interventions and accommodations are instituted.

As the use of the school-wide RtI model increases, more will be learned about how general education and special education supports are integrated throughout the tiers of intervention to support students with hearing loss in special education as well as those who may be on 504 plans because they do not meet special education eligibility. It is important to remember that RtI is not special education.

An important distinction of RtI is its focus on *prevention* as compared to *failure* for special education services. Therefore, RtI opens the door for SLPs and audiologists to support the classroom listening needs of all students who might benefit from listening-based services, not just those who have IEPs. Although this support is important, SLPs are reminded that schools cannot use RtI strategies to delay or deny a timely referral and evaluation for children suspected of having a disability (U.S. DOE, 2011). Therefore, the speech-language pathologist may need to advocate for a child with hearing loss, making a direct referral to the child study team in order to address the academic needs of the student.

Eligible for Special Education and Related Services

The IDEA requires that a disability must have an adverse impact on learning for a student to be eligible for special education. Therefore, audiologic assessment must include the procedures required by individual states for eligibility determination. Some states use the federal definitions for hearing impairment and deafness, whereas other states have specific decibel and performance criteria. A child age 3 to 22 years with a hearing loss that manifests itself within the educational setting is eligible for special education and related services under the disability condition of deafness or hearing impairment (34 CFR 300.8 (b)):

1. *Deafness* means a hearing impairment that is so severe that the child is impaired in processing linguistic information through hearing, with or without amplification, that adversely affects a child's educational performance;
2. *Hearing impairment* means an impairment in hearing, whether permanent or fluctuating, that adversely affects a child's educational performance but that is not included under the definition of deafness in this section;

After reviewing these general definitions, one can see that interpretation can and does vary from state to state, or even from municipality to municipality. Typically, APD is not considered an auditory impairment under either of these definitions. APD may be addressed as an aspect of a specific learning disability or communication impairments under most state administrative codes for education. This variability has led some states to add additional "technical" information to their state education code to define hearing impairment as well as criteria for adverse affect.

Audiologic assessments are required for initial eligibility and review evaluations. Because audiologic assessments for children and youth are typically completed annually in order to monitor hearing thresholds, use and performance of hearing technologies, and functional performance, the audiologist should include annual hearing evaluations in the child's IEP.

Special Considerations

The IDEA regulation 34 CFR 300.324(a)(2), which includes consideration of special factors, is the heart of the IEP for students who are deaf or hard of hearing. IEP teams must consider various aspects of language and communication access for every student as part of each annual meeting. The review should consider each element of the regulation, allowing for discussion regarding the current status and recommendations that should be addressed in the IEP. For example, if a student is the only one at the school with a hearing impairment, a discussion about opportunities for direct communication with peers in that child's language and communication mode might result in bringing students in similar settings together a few times a year to provide peer social and learning opportunities. Ideally the special factors discussion occurs early in the IEP meeting so that the IEP goals and services reflect the issues discussed. Some states have documents or forms within the IEP that guide the discussion for this regulation. Other states have passed Deaf Child Bill of Rights legislation that has essentially the same purpose (i.e., ensuring communication access in the child's language and communication mode), but contains additional considerations and requirements. School-based speech-language pathologists must thoroughly understand this regulation and any comparable state regulations to ensure they are applied appropriately in the IEP process, while advocating for language and communication access.

There are a wide variety of services appropriate for a speech-language pathologist to include in an IEP for a student with hearing loss. Refer to Table 14.2 for an overview of suggested goals.

Student Service and Placement Options

Many factors influence decisions about the services provided to students with hearing loss and the location of those services. Services may be consultative, itinerant, or more direct instruction. The service options typically include the general education classroom, a resource classroom, a special day program such as a regional program for students who are deaf and hard of hearing, or a school for the deaf. While IDEA requires a continuum of options, federal law also specifies "free *and appropriate* public education" (FAPE). Not always do these two mandates marry. Often, the options are limited by resources and the number of students with "like disability" in that area. If our goal is to set students up for a productive school experience, then we owe them a thorough evaluation to assess their ability to be successful in the recommended classroom environment. Even if the most appropriate instructional situation is not available, knowing the student's limitations helps identify key supports that are needed to support their learning. The Readiness Checklists component of the Placement and Readiness Checklists (PARC) protocol (available at www.ADEvantage.com) covers the areas of inclusion, use of sign language interpreting, use of captioning, and competency for instruction in listening and spoken language, sign language, or both. The functional assessments within the CLA also provide information that should be used when determining services and placement. Data sources such as these keep the IEP team focused on the student's abilities and performance rather than assumptions about learning. The audiologist, SLP, and

---

34 CFR 300.324(a)(2). Development, Review, and Revision of the IEP
Consideration of special factors

The IEP must—

(iv) Consider the communication needs of the child, and in the case of a child who is deaf or hard of hearing, consider the child's language and communication needs, opportunities for direct communication with peers and professional personnel in the child's language and communication mode, academic level, and full range of needs, including opportunities for direct instruction in the child's language and communication mode;

(v) Consider whether the child needs assistive technology devices and assistive technology services.

Table 14.2 Suggested Audiology IEP Services

Service	Where to Include in the IEP
Training for students regarding use of their hearing aids, cochlear implants, and hearing assistance technology; self-advocacy development	IEP Goals and Objectives: Audiology Related Services: Habilitation Assistive Technology Services
Counseling and training for students regarding their hearing loss and associated implications for communication and learning	IEP Goals and Objectives: Audiology Related Services: Counseling
Recommending acoustic modifications based on classroom acoustic evaluations that structure or modify the learning environment	Accommodations
Educating and training teachers, other school personnel, and parents, when necessary, about the student's hearing impairment, communication access needs, amplification, and classroom and instructional accommodations and modifications	Assistive Technology Services Access Skills Audiology Related Services: Parent Counseling and Training Related Services
Monitoring the functioning of hearing aids, cochlear implants, and hearing assistance technology (by who, how often, where, procedures used to monitor, and what will occur when a problem is identified)	Routine Checking of Hearing Aids and External Components of Surgically Implanted Medical Devices Monitoring Plan Addendum to IEP

teacher of the deaf must be strong advocates to guide these decisions. Another useful tool when assessing the educational needs of a deaf or hard of hearing student is the Colorado Individual Performance Profile (CIPP). This tool allows the evaluator to collect a wide range of functional and standardized assessment data on an individual student. Based on the data collected, a profile for educational service provision is derived. Using a tool that allows the professional to collect data from a wide variety of sources, gaining more of a comprehensive profile of the student's strengths and weaknesses, will aid in establishing an *appropriate* educational program that may minimize bias about that student from school personnel.

Self-Contained Programs for Deaf and Hard of Hearing Students

Another employment setting that carries unique responsibilities for the speech-language pathologist is schools for the deaf. In most instances, these schools employ educational audiologists. In this environment, the educational audiologist and the speech-language pathologist work in collaboration to support the communication systems that are utilized by the student or that are the philosophy of the school. This collaboration should ensure auditory communication access for those students who utilize hearing and listening whether a primary means of communication or to supplement or accompany visual systems (e.g., sign language), while being sensitive to the preferences of the child, his or her family, and the culture of the school.

Help! I Need an Educational Audiologist

There are two primary methods that schools may utilize to deliver audiology services: (1) employment directly by the local education agency (LEA) responsible for providing special education and related services, or (2) a contract with an individual, organization, or agency for specified audiology services. Many districts that do not employ a full-time educational audiologist will consider many services provided within the school setting the responsibility of the speech-language pathologist and the teacher of the deaf who service that specific setting. Again, emphasis is placed on the determination of what is and is not within the scope of practice for the speech-language pathologist. At the very least, the district should be providing the speech-language pathologist with the resources to consult with an educational audiologist under these conditions.

Another avenue that may be available to the local educational agency is a consortium established by the state that provides special education services for a group of school districts. These consortiums are usually referred to as boards of cooperative educational services (BOCES), intermediate units (IU), or area education agencies (AEA), and they are structured under the respective state department of education to provide special education services. In the absence of the services of an educational audiologist, the speech-language pathologist may need to advocate for the local school district to establish such services to meet the needs of the children and ensure FAPE.

For more information about contracting audiology services, see the Educational Audiology Association's *Guidelines for Developing Contracts for School-Based Audiology Services* at www.edaud.org.

Resources Through the Educational Audiology Association

In addition to the contract guidelines mentioned previously, the Educational Audiology Association (EAA) has developed several resources to assist with the development and implementation of school-based audiology services. The School-Based Audiology Advocacy Series contains the following brief statements regarding typical audiology services in the schools:

- School-Based Audiology Services Overview
- Assessment
- Audiology Services Under 504

- Auditory (Re)habilitation
- Classroom Acoustics
- Classroom Audio Distribution Systems
- Counseling
- Educational Audiology Services Under IDEA: Pertinent Regulations
- Hearing Assistance Technology
- Hearing Screening
- Noise and Hearing Loss Prevention
- References and Resource Materials
- Response to Intervention
- The Educational and Clinical Audiology Partnership
- The Educational Audiologist's Role in EHDI and Ongoing Hearing Loss Surveillance in Young Children

These documents are particularly useful when discussing educational audiology with general educators, administrators, school boards, or other groups. A PowerPoint presentation based on this series provides an illustrated version of these statements. These resources are available at the EAA website, www.edaud.org.

Summary

Effective support and services are critical to all children and youth with hearing loss in the schools. Educational audiologists have distinctive roles and responsibilities to ensure that these students are identified, properly assessed, and managed so that they have the same opportunity to access their educational program as all students. The speech-language pathologist plays an important role in facilitating services and working collaboratively with the educational audiologist for the success of the student with hearing loss or APD. Students with hearing loss can be serviced within the educational setting through a number of federal and state laws. Services available to the student should be based on the severity of their disability and its impact on the child's access to information within the classroom. Hard of hearing students face an extra communication challenge due to their hearing loss; it is the job of the speech-language pathologist to work closely with not only the educational audiologist, but all school personnel to support deaf and hard of hearing students to minimize the impact of that impairment. Whether through a 504 plan or an IEP, the student with hearing loss can easily meet with academic success when appropriate services are in place.

Discussion Questions

1. Name two specific areas of service provision within 34 CFR 300 that are not within your scope of practice. Name three areas in which you may serve a child who is deaf or hard of hearing.

2. A child with a cochlear implant enters your program. For what portion(s) of the implant is the LEA responsible?

3. What are the major differences between a 504 accommodation plan and an individualized education program (IEP)?

4. List three ways you may access an educational audiologist. Choose one, and provide specific references and contact information for your geographic area.

References

Acoustical Society of America. (2010). *ANSI/ASA ANSI S12.60-2010 American national standard acoustical performance criteria, design requirements, and guidelines for schools, Part 1: Permanent schools, and Part 2: Relocatable classroom factors*. Available from https://asastore.aip.org.

American Academy of Audiology. (2011a). *Clinical practice guidelines: Childhood hearing screening*. Available from http://www.audiology.org/resources/documentlibrary/Pages/Pediatric Diagnostics.aspx.

American Academy of Audiology. (2011b). *Clinical practice guidelines: Remote microphone hearing assistance technologies for children and youth from birth to 21 years. Supplement B: Classroom audio distribution systems—Selection and Verification*. Available from http://www.audiology.org/resources/documentlibrary/Pages/HearingAssistanceTechnologies.aspx.

Anderson, K. (1989, 1996, 2004). *Screening Instrument for Targeting Educational Risk—Fillable & Emailable SIFTERs*. Available from http://www.successforkidswithhearingloss.com/catalog/sifters.

Anderson, K., & Goldstein, H. (2004). Speech perception benefits of FM and infrared devices to children with hearing aids in a typical classroom. *Language, Speech, and Hearing Services in the Schools, 35*: 169–184.

Anderson, K., Smaldino, J., & Spangler, C. (2011). *Listening inventory for education—revised (LIFE-R)*. Available from http://www.successforkidswithhearingloss.com/tests/life-r.

Antia, S., Sabers, D., & Stinson, M. (2007). Validity and reliability of the classroom participation questionnaire with deaf and hard of hearing students in public schools. *Journal of Deaf Studies, 12*: 158–171.

Boothroyd, A. (1992). The FM wireless link: An invisible microphone cable. In M. Ross (Ed.), *FM Auditory Training Systems* (pp.1–19). Timonium, MD: York Press.

Crandell, C, & Smaldino, J. (2000). Classroom acoustics for children with normal hearing and with hearing impairment. *Language, Speech, and Hearing Services in the Schools, 31*: 362–370.

Elkayam, J., & English, K. (2003). Counseling adolescents with hearing loss with the use of self-assessment/significant other questionnaires. *Journal of the American Academy of Audiology, 14*(9): 485–499.

Etymotic Research. (2005). *BKB-SIN*. [CD]. Available from http://www.etymotic.com/pro/bkbsin.aspx.

Hendershot, C., Pakulski, L., Dowling, J., & Price, J. (2011). School nurses' role in identifying and referring children at risk of noise-induced hearing loss. *Journal of School Nursing, 27*(Suppl.): 380–389.

Iglehart, F. (2008). Speech perception by students with cochlear implants using sound-field systems in classrooms. *American Journal of Audiology, 13*: 62–72.

Johnson, C. D. (2011a). *Functional listening evaluation*. Available from http://www.ADEvantage.com/Downloads.html.

Johnson, C. D. (2011b). *Placement and readiness checklists (PARC) for children who are deaf and hard of hearing*. Available from http://www.ADEvantage.com/Downloads.html.

Johnson, C. D., & Meinke, D. (2008). Noise-induced hearing loss: Implications for schools. *Seminars in Hearing, 29*(1): 58–65.

Langford, J., & West, D. (1993). A study of noise exposure and hearing sensitivity in a high school woodworking class. *Language, Speech, and Hearing Services in the Schools, 24*: 167–173.

Ling, D. (2002). *Speech and the hearing impaired child* (2nd ed.). Washington, DC: Alexander Graham Bell Association for the Deaf and Head of Hearing.

National Association of State Directors of Special Education. (2005). *Response to intervention*. Alexandria, VA: National Association of State Directors of Special Education.

Niskar, S., Kieszak, S., Holmes, A., Esteban, E., Rubin, C., & Brody, D. (2001). Estimated prevalence of noise-induced hearing threshold shifts among children 6 to 19 years of age: The third national health and nutrition examination survey, 1988–1994, United States. *Pediatrics, 108*(1): 40–43.

Schafer, E., & Thibodeau, L. (2003). Speech recognition performance of children using cochlear implants and FM systems. *Journal of Educational Audiology, 11*: 15–26.

Sekhar, D., Rhoades, J., Longenecker, A., Beiler, J., King, T., Widome, M., et al. (2011). Improving Detection of Adolescent Hearing Loss. *Archives of Pediatric Adolescent Medicine, 165*(12): 1094–1100.

Shargorodsky, J., Curhan, S., Curhan, G., & Eavey, R. (2010). Change in prevalence of hearing loss in US adolescents. *Journal of the American Medical Association, 304*(7): 772–778.

Smoski, W., Brunt, M., &Tannahill, C (1998). *Children's auditory performance scale*. Available from Educational Audiology Association, http://www.edaud.org.

U.S. Department of Education, Office of Special Education and Rehabilitative Services (January 21, 2011). OSEP 11-07 RTI memo: *A Response to Intervention (RTI) Process Cannot be Used to Delay-Deny an Evaluation for eligibility under the Individuals with Disabilities education Act (IDEA)*. Available from http://www2.ed.gov/policy/speced/guide/idea/memodcltrs/osep11-07rtimemo.doc

U.S. Department of Health and Human Services. (2010). *Healthy people 2020*. Washington, DC: Author. Available from http://www.healthypeople.gov/2020/default.aspx.

Appendix 14-A: IDEA 2004 Key Regulations Pertaining to Deaf Education and Audiology

Part B: Related Services, 34 CFR 300.34(b)

Exception; services that apply to children with surgically implanted devices, including cochlear implants.

(1) Related services do not include a medical device that is surgically implanted, the optimization of that device's functioning (e.g., mapping), maintenance of that device, or the replacement of that device.

(2) Nothing in paragraph (b)(1) of this section—

  (i) Limits the right of a child with a surgically implanted device (e.g., cochlear implant) to receive related services (as listed in paragraph (a) of this section) that are determined by the IEP Team to be necessary for the child to receive FAPE.

  (ii) Limits the responsibility of a public agency to appropriately monitor and maintain medical devices that are needed to maintain the health and safety of the child, including breathing, nutrition, or operation of other bodily functions, while the child is transported to and from school or is at school; or

  (iii) Prevents the routine checking of an external component of a surgically-implanted device to make sure it is functioning properly, as required in Sec. 300.113(b).

Part B: Definition of Audiology, 34 CFR 300.34(c)(1)

Audiology includes—

  (i) Identification of children with hearing loss;

  (ii) Determination of the range, nature, and degree of hearing loss, including referral for medical or other professional attention for the habilitation of hearing;

  (iii) Provision of habilitation activities, such as language habilitation, auditory training, speech reading (lipreading), hearing evaluation, and speech conservation;

  (iv) Creation and administration of programs for prevention of hearing loss;

  (v) Counseling and guidance of children, parents, and teachers regarding hearing loss; and

  (vi) Determination of children's needs for group and individual amplification, selecting and fitting an appropriate aid, and evaluating the effectiveness of amplification.

Part C: Definition of Audiology, 34 CFR 303.13(d)(2)

Audiology includes—

  (i) Identification of children with impairments, using at risk criteria and appropriate audiological screening techniques;

  (ii) Determination of the range, nature, and degree of hearing loss and communication functions, by use of audiologic evaluation procedures;

  (iii) Referral for medical and other services necessary for the habilitation or rehabilitation of children with auditory impairment;

  (iv) Provision of auditory training, aural rehabilitation, speech reading and listening device orientation and training, and other services;

  (v) Provision of services for the prevention of hearing loss; and

  (vi) Determination of the child's need for individual amplification, including selecting, fitting, and dispensing of appropriate listening and vibrotactile devices, and evaluating the effectiveness of those devices.

Part B: Interpreting Services, 34 CFR 300.34(c)(4)

Interpreting services includes—

(i) The following, when used with respect to children who are deaf or hard of hearing: Oral transliteration services, cued language transliteration services, sign language transliteration and interpreting services, and transcription services, such as communication access real-time translation (CART), C-Print, and TypeWell; and

(ii) Special interpreting services for children who are deaf-blind.

Part B: Assistive Technology, 34 CFR 300.105(b)

On a case-by-case basis, the use of school-purchased assistive technology devices in a child's home or in other settings is required if the child's IEP Team determines that the child needs access to those devices in order to receive FAPE.

Part B: Routine Checking of Hearing Aids and External Components of Surgically Implanted Medical Devices, 34 CFR 300.113

(a) Hearing aids. Each public agency must ensure that hearing aids worn in school by children with hearing impairments, including deafness, are functioning properly.

(b) External components of surgically implanted medical devices.

(1) Subject to paragraph (b)(2) of this section, each public agency must ensure that the external components of surgically implanted medical devices are functioning properly.

(2) For a child with a surgically implanted medical device who is receiving special education and related services under this part, a public agency is not responsible for the post-surgical maintenance, programming, or replacement of the medical device that has been surgically implanted (or of an external component of the surgically implanted medical device).

Part B: Development, Review, and Revision of IEP, 34 CFR 300.324

(2) Consideration of special factors. The IEP Team must—

(iv) Consider the communication needs of the child, and in the case of a child who is deaf or hard of hearing, consider the child's language and communication needs, opportunities for direct communications with peers and professional personnel in the child's language and communication mode, academic level, and full range of needs, including opportunities for direct instruction in the child's language and communication mode.

Part B: Assistive Technology Device, 34 CFR 300.5

Assistive technology device means any item, piece of equipment, or product system, whether acquired commercially off the shelf, modified, or customized, that is used to increase, maintain, or improve the functional capabilities of children with disabilities. The term does not include a medical device that is surgically implanted, or the replacement of such device.

Part B: Assistive Technology Service, 34 CFR 300.6

Assistive technology service means any service that directly assists a child with a disability in the selection, acquisition, or use of an assistive technology device. The term includes—

(a) The evaluation of the needs of a child with a disability, including a functional evaluation of the child in the child's customary environment;

(b) Purchasing, leasing, or otherwise providing for the acquisition of assistive technology devices by children with disabilities;

(c) Selecting, designing, fitting, customizing, adapting, applying, maintaining, repairing, or replacing assistive technology devices;

(d) Coordinating and using other therapies, interventions, or services with assistive technology devices, such as those associated with existing education and rehabilitation plans and programs;

(e) Training or technical assistance for a child with a disability or, if appropriate, that child's family; and

(f) Training or technical assistance for professionals (including individuals providing education or rehabilitation services), employers, or other individuals who provide services to, employ, or are otherwise substantially involved in the major life functions of that child.

Part B: Definitions, 34 CFR 300.8(b)

(2) Deaf-blindness means concomitant hearing and visual impairments, the combination of which causes such severe communication and other developmental and educational needs that they cannot be accommodated in special education programs solely for children with deafness or children with blindness.

(3) Deafness means a hearing impairment that is so severe that the child is impaired in processing linguistic information through hearing, with or without amplification that adversely affects a child's educational performance.

(5) Hearing impairment means an impairment in hearing, whether permanent or fluctuating, that adversely affects a child's educational performance but that is not included under the definition of deafness in this section.

Appendix 14-B: Classroom Participation Questionnaire–Revised

Deaf/Hard-of-Hearing Students

Student's Name _____ Date Completed _____
School _____ Grade _____
Teacher Administering Scale _____ District _____

ELEMENTARY STUDENTS 3RD GRADE AND ABOVE complete this form for the **regular education classroom.**

MIDDLE and HIGH SCHOOL STUDENTS complete this form for your **Language Arts/English** class. If you are not in the regular classroom for Language Arts/English, then complete the form for your Social Studies or Science class – whichever of these two classes has the most frequent discussions.

Form completed for: _____ Language Arts/English _____ Social Studies _____ Science _____ Other (Please specify)

AT HOME

1. How often does your family use sign language?   Never   Sometimes   Often   All the time

2. a. Are there any other family members who have a hearing loss?   No   Yes

   b. IF YES, circle who: Father   Mother   Brother   Sister   Other_____

IN SCHOOL- Please circle <u>one</u> answer for each question. If there are no other deaf/hard-of-hearing students in your class(es), ignore questions 7 and 8.

	Interpreter	Sign	Speech	Speech & Sign	Writing Notes
3. How do you like best to communicate with hearing students?	1	2	3	4	5
4. How do you like best for hearing students to communicate with you?	1	2	3	4	5
5. How do you like best to communicate with teachers?	1	2	3	4	5
6. How do you like best for teachers to communicate with you?	1	2	3	4	5
7. How do you like best to communicate with other deaf/ hard-of-hearing students?	1	2	3	4	5
8. How do you like best for other deaf/ hard-of-hearing students to communicate with you?	1	2	3	4	5

	Interpreter	Sign	Speech	Speech & Sign	Writing Notes
9. Do you typically use an interpreter in class?	No		Yes		
10. How many other deaf/hard-of-hearing students are in your class(es)?	0	1–2	3–4	5 or more	

Classroom Participation Questionnaire—Revised

DIRECTIONS:

- Read each sentence.
- Decide how often it happens for you.
- Circle the answer that is best for you.
- Be sure to circle an answer for each sentence.
- The word **"understand"** is used frequently in this questionnaire. **"Understand"** is defined as knowing the meaning of what is said or asked.

HERE IS AN EXAMPLE:

How often do you make your bed?

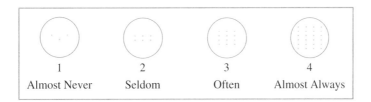

- Notice the circle pictures above each number. They are to help you think about how OFTEN you do something.
- Do you make your bed <u>almost always</u>? If so, you should circle number 4.
- If you <u>almost never</u> make your bed, you should circle number 1.
- If you <u>seldom (not very often)</u> make your bed, you should circle number 2.
- If you <u>often </u>make your bed, circle number 3.

NOW SELECT THE RESPONSE THAT IS BEST FOR YOU.

IF YOU HAVE ANY QUESTIONS PLEASE ASK THE TEACHER NOW!

If you use an interpreter, you understand what your teacher or classmates say through your interpreter. They understand what you say by listening to the interpreter.

If you do not use an interpreter, you understand what your teacher or classmates say by listening to them. They understand what you say by listening to you.

RESPOND TO EACH STATEMENT BASED ON THE WAY YOU USUALLY COMMUNICATE IN YOUR CLASS.

This questionnaire is not part of your schoolwork. It will not be graded. If the questions upset you, you can stop answering them at any time. We need your honest answers. Please read each question carefully. Thanks for your help.

	1 Almost Never	2 Seldom	3 Often	4 Almost Always
1. I understand my teacher.	1	2	3	4
2. I understand the other students in class.	1	2	3	4
3. I join in class discussions.	1	2	3	4
4. I feel good about how I communicate in class.	1	2	3	4
5. I feel frustrated because it is difficult for me to communicate with other students.	1	2	3	4
6. I get upset because other students cannot understand me.	1	2	3	4
7. I get upset because my teacher cannot understand me.	1	2	3	4
8. I feel relaxed when I talk to my teacher.	1	2	3	4
9. I understand my teacher when she gives me homework assignments.	1	2	3	4
10. I understand my teacher when she answers other students' questions.	1	2	3	4
11. I understand my teacher when she tells me what to study for a test.	1	2	3	4
12. I understand other students during group discussions.	1	2	3	4
13. I understand other students when they answer my teacher's questions.	1	2	3	4
14. I feel happy in group discussions in class.	1	2	3	4
15. I feel good in group discussions in class.	1	2	3	4
16. I feel unhappy in group discussions in class.	1	2	3	4

Classroom Participation Questionnaire—Revised

Summary Sheet

Student Name: Date: Grade: Class for which recorded:

Questions		Never	Sometimes	Often		All the Time
1	How often does your family use sign language?					
2	Are there any other family members who have a hearing loss?	No	Yes	List who:		
		Interpreter	Sign	Speech	Speech & Sign	Writing Notes
3	How do you like best to communicate with hearing students?					
4	How do you like best for hearing students to communicate with you?					
5	How do you like best to communicate with teachers?					
6	How do you like best for teachers to communicate with you?					
7	How do you like best to communicate with other deaf/hard-of-hearing students?					
8	How do you like best for other deaf/hard-of-hearing students to communicate with you?					
9	Do you typically use an interpreter in class?	No		Yes		
10	How many other deaf/hard of hearing students are in your class(es)?	0	1–2	3–4	5 or more	

Desirable ratings are in the 3–4 range.

1–Almost Never   2 – Seldom   3–Often   4–Almost Always

Subscale	Question Number	Questions	Ratings			
			1	2	3	4
Understanding Teacher (4)	1	I understand my teacher.				
	9	I understand my teacher when she gives me homework assignments.				
	10	I understand my teacher when she answers other students' questions.				
	11	I understand my teacher when she tells me what to study for a test.				
		Mean of the Subtotal	_____ / 4 = _____			
Understanding Student (4)	2	I understand the other students in class.				
	3	I join in class discussions.				
	12	I understand other students during group discussions.				
	13	I understand other students when they answer my teacher's questions.				
		Mean of the Subtotal	_____ / 4= _____			
Positive Affect (4)	4	I feel good about how I communicate in class.				
	8	I feel relaxed when I talk to my teacher.				
	14	I feel happy in group discussions in class.				
	15	I feel good in group discussions in class.				
		Mean of the Subtotal	_____ / 4 = _____			

Desirable ratings are in the 1–2 range.

Negative Affect (4)	5	I feel frustrated because it is difficult for me to communicate with other students.				
	6	I get upset because other students cannot understand me.				
	7	I get upset because my teacher cannot understand me.				
	16	I feel unhappy in group discussions in class.				
		Mean of the Subtotal	_____ / 4 = _____			

Reproduced from Stinson, M., Long, G., Reed, S., Kreimeyer, K., Sabers, D. & Antia, S.D. (2006).

Appendix 14-C: SAMPLE Personal Amplification Monitoring Plan

Student's Name: _Aiden Hears_ Date: _August 15, 2006_

Teacher: _Mrs. Nice_ Grade: _2_

Hearing Aid Brand/Model: RE-_PhonakSupero 411_ LE-_PhonakSupero 411_

Cochlear Implant: _____ ☐ RE ☐ LE

Hearing Assistance Device: Brand/Model: _PhonakCampus SX/MLxS_

1. Individual responsible for basic monitoring of device(s):

Teacher: _____ Nurse: _____

Aide: _Mrs. Health Aide_ Audiology Asst: _____

Self monitoring by student: _check battery_

2. Where will device(s) be monitored? General education classroom _____ Special education classroom _____ Nurse's office _____ Other: _____

3. When will device(s) be monitored (daily/weekly and time of day)? _Daily at beginning of school day_

4. Procedures used to monitor device(s):

Basic Check:
By: _Mrs. Health Aid_

1. Verify that HA/FM is turned on and working.
2. Conduct Ling 6 sounds test.

Troubleshooting
Strategies:
By: _Mrs. Health Aid_

Hearing Aid check: battery, earmold, tubing, intermittency and static
FM system check: battery, FM connection and channel, intermittency and static

Advanced Check:
By: _Dr. Audiology_

1. Verify status using basic troubleshooting strategies.
2. Conduct electroacoustic check.

5. What will occur if device is malfunctioning? _Audiologist will send hearing aid home with note indicating problem so that parents can take it to their dispensing audiologist for repair; school will continue to provide amplification access with FM system by adding a school-owned receiver._

Parent Approval of Plan:

I agree with amplification monitoring plan. Initials_____ Date_____

Courtesy of Cheryl DeConde Johnson.

Chapter 15

Aural (Re)habilitation

Ralph Moscarella, MA, FAAA, CCC/A
Educational Audiologist
Newark Public Schools

Cheryl DeConde Johnson, EdD, FAAA, Board Certified in Audiology
with Pediatric Audiology Specialty Certification

Key Terms

American Sign Language
(ASL)
Auditory/Oral Approach
Aural habilitation
Aural rehabilitation
Cued Speech

Deafened
Language
 acquisition
Listening and Spoken
 Language (LSL)
Manual communication

Manually Coded English
 (MCE)
Postlingually deaf
Prelingually deaf
(Re)habilitation
Total Communication (TC)

Objectives

- Recognize the difference between the concepts of aural habilitation and aural rehabilitation
- Understand and discuss models of aural habilitation for children
- Understand and discuss models of aural rehabilitation for adults

Introduction

In this chapter, the therapeutic area of aural (re)habilitation will be discussed, from its origins to its distinctive comprehensive team approaches. In between, we will discuss how hearing loss affects the patient and immediate family, the importance of early language acquisition, rehabilitation in the school setting, and methods used for adults and the elderly.

When working with an individual with hearing loss, the aural (re)habilitation process can be a rewarding experience for the speech-language pathologist and be most challenging as well. To take part in the progression of improving the quality of life for another is an amazing and gratifying part of a speech-language pathologist's career. Any functional progression a patient has, no matter how big or small, will inspire not only the patient and his or her family, but also the clinician. Of course you will encounter many challenges that may have you question and rethink your approach with a patient; however, when a breakthrough does occur, it will rejuvenate you and encourage you and your patient to continue on.

Aural (Re)habilitation Defined

Throughout this chapter the term **aural (re)habilitation** will be used as a generalized term. In fact, there are two major components that we, perhaps incorrectly, refer to within this single term.

Schow and Nerbonne (2007) have defined aural (re)habilitation as, "those professional interactive processes actively involving the client that are designed to help a person with hearing loss." Aural (re)habilitation is written in this way to give a definitive explanation of the differences in the populations with which you are working. **Aural habilitation** refers to the initial process of helping children born with prelinguistic congenital hearing loss, whereas **aural rehabilitation** refers to helping those affected by acquired hearing loss (children/adults/the elderly) after speech and language skills have been established. The aural rehabilitation process includes evaluation of hearing (including a thorough background history), diagnosis and effects of hearing loss, recommendation and selection of amplification devices (hearing aids/assistive listening devices/discussion/recommendation of cochlear implants), consideration of the type of rehabilitation setting (home/school/therapy room/hospital/long-term care facility), and counseling of the patient and the family about the impact of hearing loss and the need for rehabilitation.

Origins of Aural (Re)habilitation

Schools for the deaf were first established during the 1500s in Spain. Pedro Ponce de León worked with and taught deaf individuals; in the 1700s, schools in France and Germany were created. It was in France that Abbé de L'Épée first utilized finger spelling and sign language (**manual communication**). Another gentleman, Laurent Clerc' was a student at this school for deaf children in Paris. Following his formal education, he became a teacher there. In 1815, he traveled to England for a public speaking engagement and it was there that he met a young Thomas Hopkins Gallaudet. Clerc invited Gallaudet back to France and became his teacher. Together, Clerc and Gallaudet traveled to America and in 1817 started the first American school for the deaf in Connecticut. Its first classes were instructed in a room of an old hotel. This school remains today as the American School for the Deaf in Hartford, Connecticut.

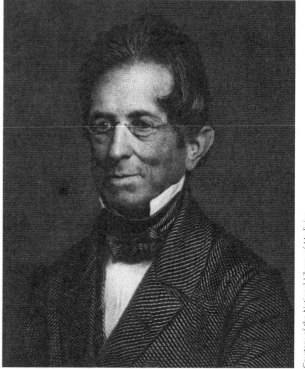

Courtesy of the National Library of Medicine.

Figure 15.1   Thomas Hopkins Gallaudet.

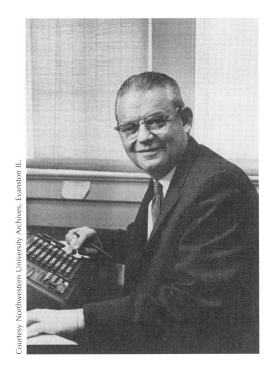

Courtesy Northwestern University Archives, Evanston IL.

Figure 15.2 Raymond Carhart.

Since that time, the debate over whether to use manual communication and/or speech-reading/oral approach utilizing residual hearing, a discussion which originated between Alexander Graham Bell and Edward Miner Gallaudet (son of Thomas Gallaudet), has raged. This is still a very polarizing and controversial topic today, with both camps very much at odds over which mode of communication is best for children with hearing loss and deafness. This philosophical debate is today, as it has always been, over the best way to communicate with and teach deaf students, with the major difference being the use of sign language (Winefield, 1987). The inception of amplification brought into play the idea that deaf individuals, once thought to be both deaf and cognitively impaired, could, in fact, be "assimilated into the hearing world" by the use of amplification and lip-reading. This sparked schools in the early 1900s to adopt an aural (ear and hearing)/oral (speech only) approach to deaf education. This controversy over the "best method" for educating deaf and hard of hearing students, in essence "to sign or not to sign; that is the question," still permeates the deaf community today (Schow & Nerbonne, 2007).

Although one may associate deaf education and audiology as working hand in hand, the field of audiology is actually much younger than that of deaf education; although both may be viewed as the (re)habilitation of hearing loss.

Audiology can be traced back to the end of World War II. Veterans who suffered noise-induced hearing loss/deafness while in battle were able to receive evaluations, amplification, and one-on-one and group aural rehabilitation therapy sessions. "What the government did was bring together a variety of specialists, tell them to organize an aural rehabilitation program, and essentially gave them a blank check" (Ross, 1997). These specialists included speech-language therapists, acoustic technicians, and auditory training instructors; the aural rehabilitation occurred in various military hospitals. The first of these facilities was the Walter Reed Hospital, which had on its staff the man who is considered by most to be the father of audiology, Raymond Carhart (American Speech-Language-Hearing Association [ASHA], 1981; see Figure 15.2). The main focus was on lip-reading/speech-reading strategies and utilizing listening techniques with very archaic hearing aids. Although the approach has improved today, we can thank the brave veterans who were the first patients for showing us how to improve the quality of life for those with hearing loss/deafness.

The Audiologic Evaluation

Aural (re)habilitation starts where the audiologic evaluation ends and hearing loss is identified. During the evaluation process, an audiologist will take an extensive background history, which will include general knowledge, medical history, hearing history, hearing aid history, and, if the patient is a child, developmental and educational histories should be included as well. As clinicians we are much like detectives; all the clues should add up. A good case history is the first and often the most important step in the audiologic evaluation because it provides information that will guide a clinician toward a correct and complete diagnosis.

With the advent of the newborn hearing screening, identification of hearing loss in infants has allowed the aural habilitation process to take place from the start of early language development. Benefits of early identification of hearing loss include improved communication development and access to hearing and language development (Fitzpatrick, Graham, Durieux-Smith, Angus, & Coyle, 2007). Decisions about amplification, form of amplification, types of therapy, and aural habilitation process can be decided on at a younger age, which greatly benefits the infant as well as the family.

Once a hearing impairment is diagnosed, the counseling of the patient, family, and friends begins. Very often a patient will bring a family member (spouse, sibling) for support. Children are accompanied by their parents, grandparents, and/or guardians. Remember, counseling is not just for the patient, but also for the family members involved. The consequences of hearing loss do not affect just the patient, but also the individuals around that person. Be aware that this could possibly be the initial diagnosis for the patient/family, or this evaluation is a second opinion and the audiologist is confirming an initial identification. Whichever the situation, during review of the test results with the family, the audiologist must be sensitive to the feelings of the patients and their family members. In addition, the clinician must be ready to act accordingly, whether that is to hand the person(s) tissues, give them water, or perhaps let them shout in disbelief. It is important to remember to give them a safe place to express their emotions toward the diagnosis and provide them the proper information, when they are ready for the next (re)habilitative steps. Never take words or actions from a patient or their family members personally; and always act in a professional manner.

At this point, the speech-language pathologist should be asking himself or herself, "Okay, so this is the job of the clinical audiologist. Why are you getting me involved?" Two factors come into play when you are discussing the earliest diagnosis of hearing loss, whether that patient is an adult or a child. First, to what extent did the patient (or parent) actually understand the initial diagnosis? Second, to what extent did the patient (or parent) own the diagnosis? Many times, a patient or parent will not even begin to accept the hearing loss until the therapeutic process begins. The speech-language pathologist may find himself or herself explaining the audiogram and the impact the hearing loss will have on communication function all over again, as if it were the first time the patient or parent has heard the diagnosis. Other times, the information will have to be reviewed several times, and by several different professionals, for it to actually be "owned" by the patient or parent regarding the diagnosis of hearing loss.

Knowing and Understanding the Hearing Loss

Hearing impairment is the most frequently diagnosed sensory deficit in human populations, affecting more than 250 million people in the world. Consequences of hearing impairment include inability to interpret speech sounds, often producing a reduced ability to communicate, delay in **language acquisition**, economic and educational disadvantage, social isolation, and stigmatization (Mathers, Smith, & Concha, 2001).

Knowing and understanding the type or types of hearing loss and their impact and being able to interpret individual results

for your patient or parent is critical. As a speech-language pathologist, understanding the hearing loss your patient has (severity, type, and degree) is the first step in serving their therapeutic needs. What sounds are missing, how is their audibility impacted by noise and lack of visual cues and unfamiliar language context, and, and what is their ability to function with amplification?

Counseling with Proper Terminology

It is important when you are working with an individual with hearing loss that the proper terms are used, by both the clinician and the patient, to describe their condition. Hearing loss is defined by categories: **prelingually deaf** (congenitally deaf/deaf from birth), **postlingually deaf** (became deaf after a spoken language system had been established partially or in full), **deafened** (hearing loss occurred after completing education in the teens/twenties), and **hard of hearing** (experienced partial hearing loss either at birth or acquired) (Moores, 1996). Remember that hearing loss affects all patients differently. Although two different patients may have similar types and degrees of hearing impairment, the consequences will affect them in a distinctive way, meaning your aural (re)habilitation approach will be not be the same for every patient. Regardless, understanding the nature of your patient's hearing loss can assist the clinician in designing the aural (re)habilitation approach, as well as guide educational and/or vocational plans for the patient.

Effects of Hearing Loss/Deafness

In 1967, Helen Keller described deafness as follows: "Deafness is a much worse misfortune, for it means the loss of the most vital stimulus, the sound of the voice that brings language, sets thoughts astir, and keeps us in the intellectual company of man" (Northern & Downs, 2002). The most significant effect of any hearing loss is the impact it has on a person's ability to communicate with others. According to Schow and Nerbonne (2007), the secondary consequences to hearing loss are its impact or influence on a person's educational, vocational, psychological, and social functions.

Educational consequences can be significant for students with any degree of hearing loss; even a mild hearing impairment can reduce communication access and learning opportunities, limiting options for higher education and employment after high school. In an article that studied the percentage of men with hearing loss attending college, as compared with their normally hearing peers, the authors found that the "odds of not attending a senior college are about 1.4 times greater among men with mild hearing loss then among men with normal hearing, and among men with more severe hearing loss they are more than twice as great" (Teasdale & Sorensen, 2007). However, with the proper early intervention and educational programs (i.e., Individual Family Service Plans [IFSP], Individualized Education Programs [IEP], Section 504 Plans) and communication access accommodations (HAT, e.g., personal and assistive hearing technology, sign language, captioning) a child with hearing loss does have a better chance of achieving their didactic goals. It is therefore important, when providing aural (re)habilitation, for a school-based speech-language pathologist to incorporate into their goals realization of the disability and to discuss vocational and postsecondary aspirations and options with their students.

The perception of the hearing loss and its perceived impact on daily living skills will differ from person to person, but clinicians need to understand diverse philosophies about communication and collaborate with other professionals to provide the correct information and style of aural rehabilitation process to our students.

Communication Options for Young Children with Hearing Loss

As mentioned previously, there are ongoing debates about which communication options are best for children who are hard of hearing or deaf. According to Gravel and O'Gara (2003), "both spoken and visual language approaches over the years have had strong proponents, which have led to the development of separate programs for the training of deaf educators and separate schools/classrooms wherein one philosophy or method of training/educating children who are hard of hearing or Deaf has been practiced."

If not adequately addressed, the effects of hearing loss on the acquisition of language can be catastrophic, causing "a delay in expressive and receptive language skills, restrict academic performance (literacy skills) and soon after, hinder an individual's opportunities for vocational choice and advancement" (Gravel & O'Gara, 2003). The future of a child with hearing loss or deafness is just one of the primary fears that normal hearing parents of a child with hearing loss may have. "How will I be able to communicate with my child?" "How will my child survive in this world without hearing?" These concerns can cause tribulations when parents are choosing the communication option for their child. Professional and parent-to-parent support

through the IFSP is essential during the early intervention process to address these issues.

Since the introduction of early hearing detection and intervention (EDHI) programs in the United States, the speech-language pathologist involved in the early intervention IFSP process must take into consideration that parents whose infants were newly identified with hearing loss are still grieving and may not be thinking clearly about which communication mode to consider. Dreams for their children are initially crushed and the future looks bleak. Decisions about different types of amplification, communication modes, and early intervention occur quickly. During the counseling sessions, the clinician must be ready to answer questions, give options/advice, and refer the parents to the proper professionals (e.g., social workers, teachers, audiologists) and parent-to-parent support networks to help them decide the best choices for early intervention planning and proper educational settings for their child. A considerable amount of pressure is placed on families to make important decisions in a very short amount of time concerning the management of their child's hearing impairment and communication mode—well before many have come to terms with their emotions. The parents may not truly understand what they are deciding on (Moeller & Condon, 1994).

The speech-language pathologist involved in the aural habilitation of an infant or young child, has many variables to consider when counseling the family on which communication options are best for their child. Some of these factors include type and degree of hearing loss, mode of communication at home (spoken or **American Sign Language [ASL]**), age of child identified with hearing loss, which communication approach will allow all family members to communicate with the child, preferences and motivation of parents and family members, and type of amplification used (hearing aids/cochlear implants). Before decisions are made, all variables must be considered and discussed with the family as part of the IFSP process for infants and toddlers and the IEP process for children 3 years and older. Parents should never feel that they are locked into a decision or made to feel guilty for a decision they have made. The Centers for Disease Control (CDC) document, *Making a Plan for Your Child: IFSP Considerations for your Child who is Deaf or Hard of Hearing,* is an effective tool to guide parents and ensure that their family's preferences and child's communication needs are addressed (http://www.cdc.gov/ncbddd/hearingloss/freematerials/planforyourchild.pdf). The Joint Committee on Infant Hearing (JCIH) Supplement to the 2007 JCIH

Position Statement, *Principles and Guidelines for Early Intervention After Confirmation that a Child is Deaf or Hard of Hearing* (March 25, 2013) contains critical guidance for all professionals, including speech-language pathologists, serving these children and their families (http://pediatrics. aappublications.org/content/early/2013/03/18/peds. 2013-0008.citation).

Communication Approaches for the Deaf and Hard of Hearing

A number of communication approaches are available for children with hearing loss to learn speech and language. Although there is no data that clearly illustrates one communication approach leads to better educational outcomes than another, the speech-language pathologist may still find him or herself in the midst of a longstanding controversy about different educational philosophies for deaf and hard of hearing students. When discussing what is in the best interests and needs of the child, the new speech-language pathologist must put aside their own opinions and consider all factors that will influence this child's communication abilities. Don't ever let anyone tell you that this is easy. The prevailing wisdom espoused by the parent organization, Hands & Voices, is "what works for your child is what makes the choice right" (www.handsandvoices.org). When considering what is working for a child, clinicians need to use the child's developmental progress and trajectory data to guide parents with regard to communication and early intervention services.

The modes of communication are the auditory–oral approach, auditory–verbal (AV) (spoken language), now combined and referred to as **Listening and Spoken Language (LSL)**, Cued Speech (spoken language/visual cues), Manually Coded English (MCE), Total Communication (TC; spoken language/ signs/cues), and American Sign Language (only visual/ manual language). In the sections that follow we will discuss all but American Sign Language (exclusively).

Auditory–Oral

The *auditory–oral approach* is a spoken language concept to language development that incorporates the use of amplification (hearing aids/cochlear implants/HAT) utilizing the child's residual hearing to develop his/her speech/ language skills. This approach does not use sign language or finger spelling and places emphasis on the child wearing and using his or her devices all day, every day; however, the use of communication strategies such as speech-reading, lip-reading, and reading body language are encouraged,

but not the use of formal sign language or a sign system of manual communication. Family members are asked to participate in the therapy sessions; children learn how to use a natural aural approach in their homes as well as in the world.

As previously discussed, as early intervention is established a variety of services will be available for the child with hearing loss. Teaching, coaching, and one-to-one therapy sessions can be provided depending on the family preference and EI resources. As the child progresses, the setting of the therapy sessions may change to play groups and eventually preschool in order to allow the child to use his/her skills in group settings and in the presence of background noise. Socialization and instruction in the presence of their peers allows children to establish skills that will enable them to adapt and communicate in a variety of conditions and environments. This communication approach is recommended strongly to parents of children who have cochlear implants.

Auditory–Verbal

The *auditory–verbal (AV)* approach is another spoken language concept, but unlike the auditory–oral method, it does not permit the child to use lip/speech-reading and other nonverbal cues to facilitate communication, and there is no access to Deaf culture or to sign language. The AV approach will allow the child to utilize his or her residual hearing only through the use of amplification, hence, a very strict approach to the development of spoken language. During the therapy sessions clinicians often cover their mouths and have the child use their hearing aids/ cochlear implants to hear the speech sounds. As with the auditory–oral approach, the clinician teaches the parents the AV technique and encourages them to use only their voices to convey a message. The goal of the AV approach is twofold—to have the child always use his or her residual hearing, and to grant the child auditory access to the surrounding world (to successfully communicate with others in all environments).

Listening and Spoken Language (LSL)

Early intervention initiatives, the advances in digital hearing aid technology, and cochlear implantation have led to a desire expressed by families with a spoken language goal for their child, to have high expectations for therapeutic outcomes. With similar philosophies for clinical outcomes, we have seen the auditory–oral approach and the auditory–verbal approach merge into the LSL approach for communication. LSL certification and certification as an auditory–verbal therapist (AVT) have become increasingly popular in the field of speech-language pathology for professionals to gain a greater understanding of the auditory–verbal continuum of communication. Endorsed by the Alexander Graham Bell Association, these certifications are now available together as an "LSLS, Cert.AVT". For further information readers are directed to the website: www. Listeningandspokenlanguage.org.

Cued Speech

The **Cued Speech** approach is a spoken language/visual cue concept strategy that utilizes eight hand shapes in four different positions around the speaker's face (see Figure 15.3). The positions are considered cues. The visual cues are incorporated because many of the different-sounding vowels and consonants can appear the same when attempting to lip-read. The visual cues (hand pattern and location, mouth positioning) help the child to identify each sound. The use of amplification is encouraged (hearing aids/cochlear implants/HAT), and families are trained in the use of the speech cues by either the speech therapist or a Cued Speech specialist. Cued Speech can be considered a gateway for ASL users to learn English (Gravel & O'Gara, 2003).

Total Communication

The **Total Communication (TC)** approach is a spoken language/sign concept that incorporates many modalities (ASL, Manually Coded English, or a derivative such as Signing Exact English (SEE), finger-spelling, lip-reading, nonverbal cues, amplification) to communicate. The speaker uses spoken language simultaneously with manual/visual methods to successfully communicate with a child with hearing loss/deafness (Hawkins & Brawner, 1997). As with the other modalities, amplification to maximize on the child's residual hearing is encouraged. The fill-in-the-blank concept is often discussed when explaining the advantages of a TC program. When the child misses a word with spoken language, he or she can fill in the gap through visual cues or manual language.

Manually Coded English

The **Manually Coded English (MCE)** approach is made up of signs that are a visual code for spoken English. MCE incorporates finger spelling and signing and follows the rules of English syntax (grammar/sentence structure). Spoken language may or may not accompany MCE to fully convey a message. Finger spelling is used to transmit morphemes that do not translate with sign. Amplification is not always used with MCE. Parents and family members can be trained in the use of MCE by the clinician to use in a variety of environments. MCE can be advantageous in environments with high amounts of background noise when attempting to communicate orally with a child with deafness, because the visual input takes the place of the missed spoken word, making it easier for the child to understand the message. Signing Exact English (SEE2), Seeing Essential English (SEE1) and Conceptually Accurate Signed English (CASE) are variations of MCE.

Troubleshooting Amplification

For families with a spoken language goal, the use of the child's amplification must be emphasized; the clinician must be able to notice when a particular device is not functioning correctly. Knowledge about how various devices work and basic troubleshooting of a hearing aid/cochlear implant/HAT is very important. The role of the speech-language pathologist in routine monitoring of the proper functioning of a child's device is paramount. The therapist should have a secure ability to perform basic troubleshooting of any auditory device. If not, seek out an audiologist for assistance. The three most important troubleshooting steps for a hearing aid are checking and changing the batteries, checking the earmold for occlusion of earwax, and assuring proper fit of the device on and in the ear. A more extensive guide to troubleshooting amplification is available in Chapter 10 of this text.

For cochlear implants, there is no conventional method to perform a listen check, so a behavioral approach should be used. If you observe your client is not responding typically, you may want to first check whether the on light is active. This is a small flashing light found on the top of the processing unit (located near the ear hook). If the light is not flashing, the batteries may need to be replaced. It is important to note that the battery energy to drive a cochlear implant is greater than that of a hearing aid. Therefore, you may notice that your patient with a cochlear implant is replacing batteries far more often than a hearing aid user. The next items to inspect on a cochlear implant are the wire and magnet attached to the internal cochlear implant components. Are they appropriately attached? Are bare wires exposed? Have little fingers detached the magnet from the external unit? If all basic external components are found to be functioning appropriately, the problem may be internal, and the child should be seen by his/her implant center. Advise him or her to make an appointment with their

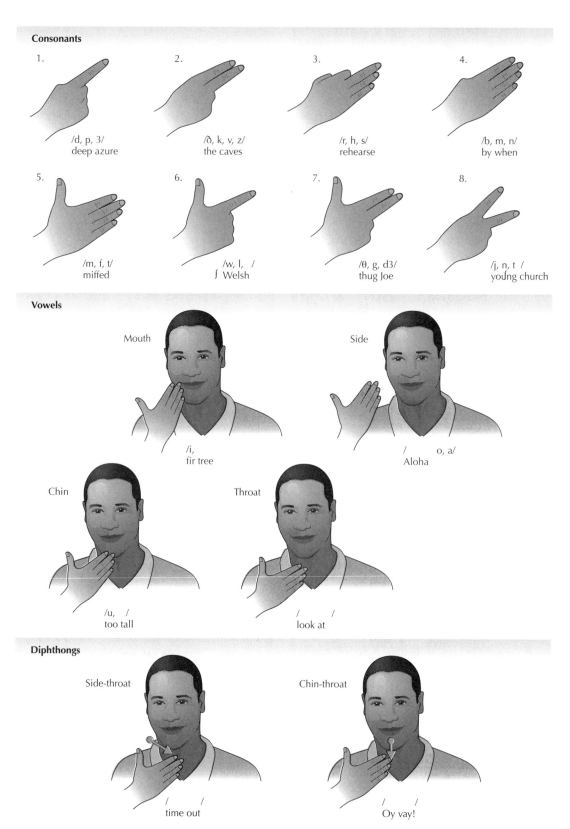

Figure 15.3   Cued speech chart.

implant audiologist as soon as possible. The absence of a fully functioning implant will greatly affect the child's progress during therapy sessions.

If a child with hearing loss is on your caseload, having size 13 (orange package) and 675 (blue package) batteries on hand, just in case, is a good idea.

Aural Habilitation in the Schools

Speech-language pathologists are part of a skilled group of professionals that provides a range of aural habilitation services to school-aged children with hearing loss. Depending on the school setting and degree of hearing loss, these individuals may include, but certainly are not limited to, a building principal/vice principal, a teacher of the deaf and hard of hearing, a general education inclusion teacher, an educational interpreter, a teacher's assistant or paraprofessional, a school social worker, a school psychologist, a learning disabilities teacher-consultant (LDT-C), and, hopefully, an educational audiologist.

Even though audiologists may receive more graduate preparation in auditory habilitation than speech-language pathologists or deaf educators, they are often the least likely to provide these services because of time and resource restrictions. Regardless of who delivers the services, you should be involving the educational audiologist in the development of habilitation activities. Both the speech-language pathologist and the audiologist must attend all annual and review IEP meetings for students with hearing impairment to support and advocate for appropriate intervention services across the students' various academic and extracurricular settings. The following list comprises specific areas that should be considered based on individual goals for each student:

- Auditory skill development and listening skill training.
- Language development (expressive and receptive): oral, signed, cued, and/or written language, including pragmatics.
- Speech production training, including phonology, voice, and rhythm.
- Visual communication systems and strategies, including speech-reading, manual communication, and Cued Speech.
- Selection and use of appropriate instructional materials and media.
- Use of assistive technologies, such as those necessary to access radio, television, and telephones, as well as pagers and alerting devices.
- Case management and care coordination with family/parent/guardian, school, and medical and community services.
- Habilitative and compensatory skill training to reduce academic deficits as related to, but not limited to, reading and writing.
- Social skills, self-esteem, and self-advocacy support and training.
- The transition between, but not limited to, levels, schools, programs, and agencies.
- Support for a variety of education options for children/students with hearing impairment and/or auditory processing disorder (APD).
- Along with the incorporation of some or all of the recommendations in Table 15.1, it is also important

Table 15.1 Suggested Audiology IEP Services

Service	Where to Include in the IEP
Training for students regarding use of their hearing aids, cochlear implants, and hearing assistance technology; self-advocacy development	IEP Goals and Objectives: Audiology Related Services: Habilitation Assistive Technology Services
Counseling and training for students regarding their hearing loss and associated implications for communication and learning	IEP Goals and Objectives: Audiology Related Services: Counseling
Recommending acoustic modifications based on classroom acoustic evaluations that structure or modify the learning environment	Accommodations
Educating and training teachers, other school personnel, and parents, when necessary, about the student's hearing impairment, communication access needs, amplification, and classroom and instructional accommodations and modifications	Assistive Technology Services Access Skills Audiology Related Services: Parent Counseling and Training Related Services
Monitoring the functioning of hearing aids, cochlear implants, and hearing assistance technology (by who, how often, where, procedures used to monitor, and what will occur when a problem is identified)	Routine Checking of Hearing Aids and External Components of Surgically Implanted Medical Devices Monitoring Plan Addendum to IEP

that IEP goals are aligned with the state's common core content standards. Standards addressing speaking and listening skills generally match well with hearing, listening, and speaking objectives for children with hearing impairment.

Counseling for the Student with Hearing Loss

The psychosocial implications of hearing loss can be easily overlooked, especially in mainstream classroom settings. Speech-language pathologists working in a program for students with hearing loss, or providing services privately outside of the school setting, must understand the connection between hearing loss and the resulting communication challenges that often isolate children from their hearing peers. It is important to probe students, as part of the assessment process, to uncover feelings and issues that need to be addressed through counseling.

Instruments such as the Classroom Participation Questionnaire (CPQ), Self-Assessment of Communication for Adolescents (SAC-A), and Significant Other Assessment of Communication for Adolescents (SOAC-A) often translate into counseling opportunities. The speech-language pathologist must be prepared to address issues that are identified by the student during the assessment or interview process. Sufficient time should be scheduled during the assessment period or shortly thereafter to give students the opportunity to at least briefly talk about their communication challenges and for the speech-language pathologist to begin to skillfully guide them through a problem-solving process. Anytime a student divulges sensitive information, it deserves at least acknowledgement and a response, even if brief. Scheduling of more in-depth counseling by the appropriately trained school personnel (i.e., social worker or school psychologist) can be scheduled once the "door has opened" (English, 2002).

Self-Advocacy

Self-advocacy is a growing area of habilitation focus for deaf and hard of hearing students. Students need to be able to describe their hearing impairment and the necessary accommodations they require for various learning and communication situations as part of the process of becoming responsible for their hearing and communication needs. Independence with hearing aids, cochlear implants, HAT, classroom amplification, and implementing accommodations should occur as early as possible, with expectations for basic self-advocacy beginning in kindergarten or sooner.

Guide to Access Planning (GAP) is an online learning guide available on the Phonak website (https://www.phonakonline.com/MyGAP/GAPMain_atl2.html) that promotes self-advocacy and personal responsibility. The curriculum includes materials regarding hearing loss, use of hearing and other assistance technologies, disability and access laws, accommodations, and other skills necessary for independence after high school. Tools for self-assessment of knowledge; communicating with teachers, employers, and others regarding accommodation needs; evaluating access services at colleges; and problem-solving difficult communication situations are examples of student-focused resources available in the guide. The GAP complements high school transition activities with materials designed specifically for teens and young adults who are deaf and hard of hearing.

Aural Rehabilitation Models for Assessment and Management in Adults

The World Health Organization uses two models for assessment and management of aural rehabilitation that concentrate on the importance of communication and the management procedures that follows. One model is for the assessment of hearing loss (CORE) and the other is for the management of hearing loss (CARE).

CORE (Assessment)

CORE stands for *c*ommunication status, *o*verall participation variables, *r*elated personal factors, and *e*nvironmental factors (Schow & Nerbonne, 2007). Communication status is identified through evaluation both diagnostically and by patient questionnaires. Audiologic testing is only one way of assessing the hearing loss; the clinician must obtain information from the patient about how the hearing impairment is affecting their ability to converse with others. This is achieved through patient questionnaires and the interview process with the clinician. In addition, inventories such as the Hearing Performance Inventory (HPI; Giolas, Owens, Lamb, & Schubert, 1979); Hearing Handicap Inventory for the Elderly (HHIE; Ventry & Weinstein, 1982); Client Oriented Scale Inventory (COSI), available at www.nal.gov.au/outcome-measures_tab_cosi.shtml (Dillon, James, & Ginis, 1997); and Abbreviated Profile of Hearing Aid Benefit (APHAB; Cox & Alexander, 1995), available at www.hearingutah.com/Aphab.pdf are just a few that can be used as helpful tools after the audiologic evaluation. Collectively, the results of the nonaudiometric assessment process are necessary to plan, implement, and evaluate any audiologic intervention program with adults and children (ASHA, 1998).

Consider, for example, a clinician looking at the configuration and overall word discrimination score who observes a bilateral sloping sensorineural hearing loss. On the questionnaire the clinician would expect to see that the patient has difficulties understanding people, especially in the presence of background noise; perhaps the patient has difficulty communicating with women because of the severity of the hearing impairment in the high frequency range. During the counseling session, the patient reveals that his hearing loss has been affecting his relationship with his family because he is constantly turning the television up. Using an inventory like the COSI can focus on the areas that are most important for improvement and help the patient; this information would not have emerged by audiogram alone.

Overall participation variables help to evaluate the characteristics of hearing impairment. What is the impact of the hearing impairment, and how is it affecting the patient, their family, and their friends? In addition, what are the educational, social, and vocational secondary consequences of hearing loss? Again, this information is obtained through questionnaires and counseling. How does our patient participate in the world with his or her hearing loss? How are his or her work relations affected by the hearing impairment? Does our patient hold a position where communication with others is not essential to his or her everyday occupation or routine?

Related personal factors directly relate to a person's attitude and motivation. When considering the prognosis of therapeutic intervention, this is perhaps the most important factor to consider. Once a hearing loss is diagnosed, a patient will have a variety of emotions towards their loss, especially toward the possibility of purchasing and wearing hearing aids. As the clinician, you must keep your patient motivated not only during your aural rehabilitation session, but also to have the patient follow through with the plan you have set forth. What good is all the work in the clinic if the patient and/or family members have poor attitudes about the patient's new devices?

Environmental factors will look at the individual's work, home, and social conditions they place themselves in. Which environments will be the most challenging? What strategies can be put in place to help our patient use their amplification to the fullest potential? Questionnaires again

are very useful, but the patient must be motivated to answer the form honestly.

CARE (Management)

CARE stands for *c*ounseling and psychosocial aspects, *a*udibility or amplification aspects, *r*emediation of communication activity, and *e*nvironmental participation (Schow & Nerbonne, 2007). Throughout aural rehabilitation sessions, the perceived psychosocial impact of a hearing loss will drive the course of therapy. Describing an audiogram is only the first step in a long journey of having our patients fully understand their hearing loss. As a speech-language pathologist, you must be aware of the audience in your office and the language you use during a therapy session. We all love our acronyms and high-tech words, but we cannot use them when the average patient does not even understand the markings on an audiogram. Taking the time to explain the results can be the difference between a motivated person and a disheartened one.

Often family members accompany an adult patient to the audiological evaluations, hearing aid evaluations, and therapy session. Many deep-rooted feelings about the hearing loss come out during these sessions. Many a newspaper cartoon has poked fun at the husband–wife relationship when both have a hearing loss, one with a hearing aid and one without, but in need of a hearing aid. A couple married for 50 years has fallen into a communication style, despite an unamplified hearing loss, and a hearing aid is about to change all of that. Clinicians should be sensitive to the relational dynamics, listen to all sides of the story, and explain how the hearing loss is impinging on everyone in the family; by doing this the clinician is opening the door to communication and laying the foundation for a positive home environment in which both husband and wife will aspire to work on communication strategies to improve their quality of life.

Proper fittings of all forms of amplification (hearing aids, assistive listening devices, cochlear implants) as well as introducing home amplification devices (fire/carbon monoxide detectors, amplified home/cell phones, and personal TV amplifying devices) is an integral part of aural rehabilitation. Properly fitting a hearing aid can be an arduous process in an adult ear, especially in older adults unaccustomed to change. Counseling patients about usage, care, and maintenance of the devices, both at home and when they are out and about, can be a tedious process, but perseverance will result in greater patient satisfaction. The speech-language pathologist must be mindful that family members and caretakers should also be included in this portion of the rehabilitation process because they are often the people responsible for the patient's devices. A clinician may find they are repeating the instructions of how and when to use the devices during the follow-up visits; this is where a hearing aid checklist and inventory can really come in handy for validation of the goals that were established for the patient (COSI, APHAB, HHIE).

The degree to which the patient with remediated hearing loss is able to interact with those around them is referred to as environmental participation. Remember, the hearing impairment affects not only the person, but also the people around them. Environmental participation considers the different types of settings (recreational/occupational) the person with hearing loss finds themselves in when interacting with others. This area of aural rehabilitation explores the use and flexibility of learned communication strategies and what type or types of amplification devices a person with a hearing impairment will use in different situations. For example, a patient will use one set of communication strategies at home with his or her spouse (turning down the volume of the television when conversing, wearing infrared headphones with the television) and use a different set of strategies when he or she is at a restaurant (sitting away from the kitchen, sitting in a well-lit area). The patient could also use similar strategies in different settings (maintaining eye contact, lip-reading, moving closer to the speaker). Knowing and understanding the lifestyle that the person with hearing loss desires to restore by the use of hearing aids will aid the speech-language therapist in designing appropriate goals for successful aural rehabilitation. It is very important that the patient sees success when using the strategies in different settings; this will motivate them to wear and work with their amplification as well as put more effort into using the communication strategies in and out of the therapy sessions.

Aural Rehabilitation and the Elderly

With the elderly population, acquired hearing loss is very common. There are many reasons for this; perhaps the patient has noise-induced hearing loss from serving in the military or was employed in a high noise environment. Perhaps it is due to presbycusis (hearing loss due to the aging process), ototoxicity (hair cell death due to medication), or physical pathologies (acoustic neuroma/middle

ear pathologies, cerebral vascular accident), to name a few. Each of these reasons carries with it a variety of hearing losses in terms of shape, type, and configuration. As mentioned before, the speech-language pathologist must take an extensive case history, asking questions about recent changes in medical conditions including any recent diagnoses, occupational and recreational activities, military experience, and prior audiologic evaluations. In addition, the speech-language pathologist should ask questions such as, "Describe your hearing loss," "In which situations do you have the most difficulty?" and "Which listening situations are easier for you?" Again, this information gives the clinician clues as to the possible type of hearing loss, level of acceptance of the hearing loss, and future recommendations to consider.

A hearing loss can signify aging to the patient (am I really that old?), which can be a very depressing concept. The patient may go through a grieving process. Venting these feelings is a natural occurrence during the counseling session, and should be allowed. Of course there are those patients who are ready to face their hearing loss and are motivated to start the rehabilitation process to improve their own quality of life.

Along with the audiogram, validation tools are necessary to determine the communication problem areas as well as the communication and listening goals of the patient. The COSI and APHAB are examples of validation tools that should be used to evaluate the patient's needs. According to ASHA (1998), these assessment tools provide individualized and situational information about the cause of the patient's communication breakdowns prior to the use of amplification.

The speech-language pathologist may be involved with providing aural rehabilitation services to the elderly in one-on-one sessions, group sessions, or as part of a comprehensive therapy plan with a secondary focus (e.g., a stroke patient with a hearing loss). Repair strategies for everyday life and communication situations such as handling conversations (self-advocating), using visual cues (facial expression, lip-reading, body language), dealing with background noise (requesting a table away from the kitchen at a restaurant), and making changes in the home (moving furniture away from noisy areas) can be explored during the one-on-one sessions. Group therapy meetings are helpful; they will demonstrate to the patient that he or she is not alone with their hearing loss challenges and that others have very similar issues. Having the patient bring family members to both the one-on-one and group sessions could be extremely beneficial to the patient. The family members can learn more about hearing loss, hearing aids, and what realistic expectations are. Once the family understands the difficulties that accompany hearing loss (even with the hearing aids), there will be less stress. Relationships can mend, and quality of life can improve.

Summary

The patient with hearing loss presents a unique challenge to the speech-language pathologist. Aural (re)habilitation can take on many forms because interventions and management cover all age ranges and degrees of hearing loss. The speech-language pathologist must have a solid understanding of the hearing loss and related technology used by the patient as well as the patient's and family's perception of that technology as part of the remediation process for successful therapeutic outcomes to be realized. It is only through this understanding and the collaboration with other professionals that the patient with hearing loss will meet maximum success with aural rehabilitation therapy.

Discussion Questions

1. How are aural habilitation and aural rehabilitation similar? How are they different?
2. What role can a self assessment inventory play in the rehabilitation process?
3. Why is it important to ensure that an individual's personal amplification or cochlear implant device is functioning properly, before each therapy session?
4. What are the communication models for the deaf and hard of hearing? Choose one approach and discuss.

References

American Speech-Language-Hearing Association. (1981); 23(11): 858.

American Speech-Language-Hearing Association. (1998). *Guidelines for hearing aid fitting for adults*. Available from http://www.asha.org/policy.

Cox, R. M., & Alexander, G. C. (1995). The abbreviated profile of hearing aid benefit (APHAB). *Ear and Hearing, 16*: 176–186.

Dillon, H., James, A., & Ginis, J. (1997). The client oriented scale of improvement (COSI) and its relationship to several other measures of benefit and satisfaction provided by hearing aids. *Journal of the American Academy of Audiology, 8*: 27–43.

Fitzpatrick, E., Graham, I. D., Durieux-Smith, A., Angus, D., & Coyle, D. (2007). Parents' perspective on the impact of the early diagnosis of childhood hearing loss. *International Journal of Audiology, 46*: 97–106.

Giolas, T. G., Owens, E., Lamb, S. H., & Shubert, E. D. (1979). Hearing Performance Inventory. *Journal of Speech and Hearing Disorders, 44*(2), 169–195.

Gravel, J. S., & O'Gara, J. (2003). Communication options for children with hearing loss. *Mental Retardation and Developmental Disabilities Research Reviews, 9*: 243–251.

Hawkins, L., & Brawner, J. (1997). Educating children who are deaf and hard of hearing: Total communication. Reston, VA:ERIC Clearinghouse on Disabilities and Gifted Education, the Council for Exceptional Children, 1997

Mathers, C., Smith, A., & Concha, M. (2003). Global burden of hearing loss in the year 2000. Global Burden of Disease (GBD) Working Paper, World Health Organization, Geneva. http://www.who.int/healthinfo/statistics/bod_hearingloss.pdf. Accessed June 23, 2013.

Moeller, M. P., & Condon, M. C. (1994). D.E.I.P.A collaborative problem solving approach to early intervention. InJ. Roush & N. D. Matkin (Eds.), *Infants and toddlers with hearing loss* (pp. 163–192). Baltimore: York Press.

Moores, D.F. (1996). *Educating the deaf: Psychology, principles, and practices*. Boston, MA: Houghton Mifflin.

Northern, J. L., & Downs, M. P. (2002). *Hearing in children* (5th ed.). Philadelphia, PA: Lippincott, Williams and Wilkins.

Ross, M. (1997). A retrospective look at the future of aural rehabilitation. *Journal of the Academy of Rehabilitative Audiology, 30*(1): 1–28.

Schow, R. D. & Nerbonne, M.A. (2007). *Introduction to audiological rehabilitation* (5th ed.). Allyn & Bacon, Boston.

Teasdale, T. W., & Sorensen, M. H. (2007). Hearing loss in relation to education attainment and cognitive abilities: A population study. *International Journal of Audiology, 46*: 172–175.

Ventry, I. M, Weinstein, B. (1982). The hearing handicap inventory for the elderly: A new tool. *Ear and Hearing, 3* (2), 128–134.

Winefield, R. (1987). *Never the twain shall meet: Bell, Gallaudet, and the communications debate*. Gallaudet University Press, Washington, D.C.

Chapter 16

Diagnosis and Treatment of (Central) Auditory Processing Disorders: A Collaborative Approach

Tena L McNamara, AuD, CCC-A/SLP
Department of Communication Disorders and Sciences
Eastern Illinois University

Annette E. Hurley, PhD, CCC-A
Health Sciences Center, School of Allied Health Professions
Louisiana State University

Key Terms

Amblyaudia
Attention deficit hyperactivity
  disorder (ADHD)
Auditory discrimination
Autism spectrum disorder
  (ASD)
Bellis/Ferre model
Binaural integration
Binaural interaction
Binaural separation

Buffalo model
(Central) auditory processing
  [(C)AP]
(Central) auditory processing
  disorder [(C)APD]
Comorbidity
Compensatory strategies
Dichotic listening
Electroacoustic
Electrophysiological measures

Environmental modifications
Formal auditory training
Informal auditory training
Low-redundancy speech
Metalinguistic
Monaural low-redundancy
Plasticity
Temporal processing/
  sequencing

Objectives

- To describe characteristics associated with a (central) auditory processing disorder [(C)APD]
- Associate specific tests used to assess (C)APD with specific auditory skills
- Identify intervention strategies associated with specific (central) auditory processing [(C)AP] deficits
- Discuss a collaborative model between the SLP and audiologist when addressing the diagnostic and intervention needs of an individual with a (C)APD

Introduction

There is an endless debate on the association between (central) auditory processing and language. Some professionals question whether a deficit in auditory processing skills is nothing more than a reflection of a delay or disorder in language. However, neuroscience research has linked difficulties with auditory processing tasks specifically to the central auditory nervous system (Musiek, Kibbe, & Baran, 1984; Musiek, Shinn, et al., 2005). Due to this evidence, it is inferred that deficits in auditory processing can be the basis for complications in language and learning. With that in mind, this chapter will review information on what constitutes a (central) auditory processing disorder and what type of treatment strategies are being used to address deficits in these areas. In addition, a model is presented that promotes a collaborative framework between the speech-language pathologist and audiologist when working with individuals with (central) auditory processing deficits.

Definition

In 2005, the American Speech-Language-Hearing Association (ASHA) created a task force to further define the diagnosis of and interventions for **(central) auditory processing disorders [(C)APD]**. The document that was generated from this collaborative effort was used to update the previous document (ASHA, 1996), which defines the role of the audiologist within the scope of practice for (C)APD. As a result, ASHA (2005) provided this definition, which is often referred to by many professionals:

> Central Auditory Processing [(C)AP] refers to the efficiency and effectiveness by which the central nervous system (CNS) utilizes auditory information. . . . (C) APD refers to difficulties in the perceptual processing of auditory information in the central nervous system and the neurobiologic activity that underlies that processing and gives rise to electrophysiologic auditory potentials. . . . Although (C)APD may co-exist with other disorders (e.g., attention deficit hyperactivity disorder [ADHD], language impairment, and learning disability) it is not the result of these disorders. (p. 2)

(Central) auditory processing [(C)AP] describes how information is processed after it leaves the peripheral auditory structures (outer, middle, and inner ear) and what happens to this information as it is transmitted along the central auditory nervous system (CANS). There are two core categories of evaluation protocols used to assess (central) auditory processing skills. The first category includes behavioral tests, which assess the functional capabilities of the auditory system. The second category for evaluating (C)AP is the use of electrophysiological measures.

Behavioral Testing

Behavioral tests are associated with the assessment of auditory-cognitive skills rather than true sensory processing abilities because it is often difficult to separate auditory sensory processing skills from various cognitive abilities. For example, speech-in-noise testing provides diagnostic information on how well an individual comprehends speech in the presence of competing messages or sounds. Many factors, such as attention, cognition, and/or language capabilities, can influence an individual's performance on speech-in-noise tests.

Electroacoustic and Electrophysiological Testing

Electroacoustic and electrophysiological measures include a variety of protocols that can range from otoacoustic emissions to auditory evoked response testing (i.e., auditory brainstem response, middle latency response, cortical event-related potentials) to functional imaging. Electrophysiological recordings of the central and peripheral neural auditory pathway and auditory cortex reflect neural functions and processes involved in neural coding for speech. Electrical potentials from the CANS are recorded in response to acoustic stimuli presented to the ear. They are beneficial in confirming a neurological disorder and identifying possible sites of lesion. By minimizing cognitive and language influences associated with performance on behavioral tests, these measures provide a clearer picture of the actual auditory–sensory processing capabilities of the CANS. This explains why abnormal electroacoustic and electrophysiological results do not give information on the skill level an individual possesses for various auditory behaviors.

Although these tests provide information on auditory–sensory capabilities of the CANS, information is still needed on the actual functional skill level and what auditory skill deficits are being experienced by an individual with abnormal nonbehavioral test results. This is where behavioral tests are needed because they reflect auditory–cognitive processes and can present a profile of functional auditory abilities. For example, you can take two individuals with known lesions in the same area along the CANS who may exhibit similar abnormal results on auditory evoked response tests, but each may exhibit varying severity and symptoms in behavioral skills related to audition.

Comorbidity of (C)APD

This quandary leads into the discussion of **comorbidity** of a (C)APD and language/learning disabilities. There are varying opinions regarding the relationship of auditory processing disorders and deficits in language. Some professionals believe (C)APD is nothing more than a reflection of a true language disorder or delay. However, a number of other professionals consider auditory processing difficulties to exist independently of language disorders or delays, but manifest themselves in a similar fashion. The latter is supported by research that has linked various auditory processing skills to specific anatomical sites along the central auditory nervous system (Barmiou, Musiek, & Luxon, 2001; Bocca, 1958; Bocca & Calearo, 1963; Bocca, Calearo, & Cassinari, 1954; Bocca, Calearo, Cassinari, & Migliavacca, 1955; Calero & Lazzaroni, 1954; Clarke, Lufkin, & Zaidel, 1993; Kimura, 1961; Musiek, 1983; Musiek, Kibbe, & Baran, 1984; Musiek, Shinn, et al., 2005). Abnormal function in one of these central auditory areas can lead to a (C)APD, triggering language and learning difficulties.

Language Delay/Deficit

It is evident that listening and language skills are interwoven and at times may be very difficult to separate in behavioral testing. Poor performance on listening tasks can be strongly reflected in language abilities, and vice versa. Thus, it is logical to assume that a child who has difficulty with behavioral tests may display symptoms of a language delay or deficit, thereby affecting academic performance. If auditory input is compromised, causing a child to receive degraded linguistic signals, the development of vocabulary, syntax, and semantics may be affected. Poor performance on behavioral tests may be described as an auditory–cognitive processing deficit, because it is so difficult to separate these domains with the use of behavioral assessments.

In light of these observations, it is more productive to spend less time focusing on whether poor performance on behavioral tests for (C)APD are specific to a (C)APD or to a language deficit. By taking a psychoeducational approach, less time can be spent debating the etiology of deficits for auditory-related skills and more time spent on the effects these auditory weaknesses have at home and at school. Then, intervention can begin sooner and more efficiently.

Attention Deficit Hyperactivity Disorder

Attention deficit hyperactivity disorder (ADHD) and learning disabilities are among the conditions that share many of the same behavioral characteristics as (C)APD and may coexist. As discussed earlier, differential diagnosis can be extremely difficult when using behavioral tests because of the influence of cognition, attention, motivation, and language skills on all of these disabilities. However, in spite of these influences, a behavioral (C)APD assessment battery can offer valuable information on specific auditory skills that may be difficult for a child. This information on auditory–cognitive processing, used in collaboration by a multidisciplinary team of educational professionals, can lead to the development of a finely tuned treatment plan that focuses on the individual needs of the child.

The Audiologist and the SLP: Working Together in Diagnosing (C)APD

Audiologists have the capability of investigating neurological components related to (C)AP skills. For example, Banai, Nicol, Zecker, and Kraus (2005) introduced speech-evoked auditory brainstem response (ABR) testing, which has shown neurological processing at the level of the brainstem for the temporal aspects of speech. Although this information is extremely valuable in detecting lesions for children who have difficulty discriminating speech sounds, diagnostic information still must be correlated to functional performance of that child in the home and school. In order to assess a child's educational needs, information about functional performance is needed. Behavioral tests for (C)APD reflect real-life skills and may be more practical when addressing the educational needs of a child. Evaluation tools used for the assessment of (central) auditory processing skills can be utilized to provide valuable information on a child's auditory–cognitive, functional listening abilities that may be inhibiting successful performance in school. However, testing should not stop here. The speech-language pathologist should also be involved in the diagnostic process in order to offer further insight into the child's language abilities affected by deficits in auditory skills.

Collaborative Model

The need for a collaborative model between the speech-language pathologist and the audiologist is truly justified. Although a multidisciplinary approach with a diverse group of medical and educational professionals is always preferred, (C)APD assessment should at minimum include a partnership between the audiologist and the speech-language pathologist. As stated earlier, if a child exhibits poor performance on functional tests that assess auditory skills, it is likely the auditory skill deficits may be associated with delays or deficits in language performance. However, it is unreasonable to make general judgments about a child's language skills based purely on his or her performance on tests that assess auditory skills. In return, it is unrealistic to assume poor performance on language tests can predict (C)AP skills. This is also a problem when clinicians try to categorize or infer language and learning deficits based on the results from a (C)APD evaluation alone. It is unfair to make recommendations for intervention based on a "profile" of the child, rather than actually focusing on the child's unique needs. A more efficient process would incorporate information provided by the audiologist on how deficits in auditory skills may be affecting the development of language, while the speech-language pathologist investigates how auditory deficits affect language skills. In turn, an intervention plan, reflecting the educational needs of the child, can then be established.

McNamara and Richard (2012) have recommended a collaborative diagnostic model to address children who are suspected of having a (C)APD (see **Figure 16.1**). The process would involve dialogue between the audiologist and speech-language pathologist at the point of initial referral. Once all information has been reviewed, deficit behaviors would then be categorized according to their characteristic patterns. Tagging behaviors under categories that directly correlate to specific problems in the classroom can be helpful. Categories would include language sorts such as phonology, semantics, syntax/morphology, reasoning, discourse, pragmatics, and literacy, because deficiencies in auditory skills would most likely be reflected in one or more of these language areas. From a qualitative analysis of the case history, a cooperative conclusion would be reached between professionals regarding the extent and type of testing needed. This may involve a team of professionals or just collaboration between the audiologist and speech-language pathologist. As Richard (2007) explains, the speech-language pathologist's role falls in the investigation of problems during the analysis of the acoustic signal, whereas the audiologist's role lies in the evaluation of the transference of the acoustic signal through the CANS.

Upon agreement regarding a diagnostic plan, the audiologist should initially complete the evaluation. These results can then be shared with the speech-language pathologist, because functional performance on auditory tests may provide further understanding of the effects on language. If completed in this manner, the speech-language pathologist will have available the auditory skills performance data, along with a behavioral profile of language concerns, to guide the speech-language evaluation process. Once the speech-language

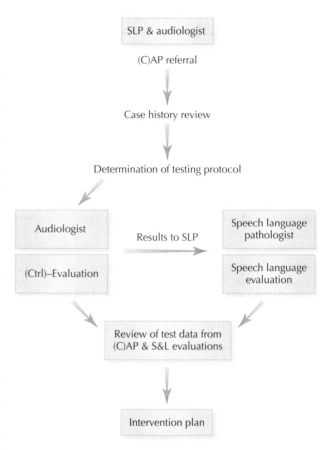

Figure 16.1   Referral and diagnostic process followed by the audiologist and speech-language pathologist for a child suspected of a (central) auditory processing deficit.

pathologist has completed an evaluation focusing on the specific deficits in the child's language, it is time again to discuss results and intervention strategies with the audiologist. This will ensure that the child receives a tailor-made strategic plan that will address areas of concern that are explicit to his or her needs. This model focuses on functional skill deficits and how these impact performance in school and daily living. With implementation of this cooperative model, functional skill deficits can be addressed in hopes that academic and psychosocial progress is realized.

In order for this model to work efficiently, several issues need to be discussed. First, it is important that the speech-language pathologist incorporate evaluation tools that not only address basic language skills, but also assess higher level language function. As with any child who experiences auditory deficits (deaf, hard of hearing, auditory processing), skills for abstract, critical thinking and language processing may pose challenges. This also includes **metalinguistic** analysis, due to problems in applying the rules of language to incoming auditory input. Furthermore, testing should involve phonological/phonemic awareness skills, because problems with discriminating speech may correlate with abnormal auditory processes (Banai & Kraus, 2007).

Second, because there is no gold standard for evaluating a (C)APD, the audiologist needs to clarify how and why to evaluate for this disorder. It is true that better reliability and validity is needed for evaluation tools used for assessing (C)AP skills (Friberg & McNamara, 2010). Many (C)APD tests do not meet the criteria for diagnostic accuracy and test validity. In addition, audiologists must establish the best standard for determining when a child falls within the clinical population for a (C)APD. Because of this, audiologists need to evaluate with the understanding that no one assessment tool is sufficient for the diagnosis of a (C)APD; rather, a variety of assessment tools need to be used to confirm the presence or absence of a (C)APD. This would include comprehensive case history information that provides insight into hearing, medical, educational, social, developmental, and communicative status (American Academy of Audiology [AAA], 2010). Questionnaires and surveys completed by the student, parent, and/or teacher include behavioral observations and are very useful as part of the diagnostic battery. The questionnaires include inquiries on how auditory behaviors affect academic, social, and communication abilities for the child referred for (C)APD testing. These surveys assist in planning for testing and in intervention protocols. Several commonly used auditory behavior observation tools are the Children's Auditory Performance Scale ([CHAPS]; Smoski, Brunt, & Tannahill, 1998), Fisher's Auditory Problems Checklist (Fisher, 1985), and the Listening Inventory for Education Revised ([LIFE]; Anderson, Smaldino & Spangler, 2012).

Behavioral tests assess auditory skills in the areas of sound localization/lateralization and binaural interaction, dichotic listening, temporal processing/patterning, low-redundancy speech tasks, and auditory discrimination (AAA, 2010). Through collaboration with other professionals and the interpretation of multiple cross-check testing data (including that gathered from nonbehavioral tests), a diagnostically accurate conclusion can be reached.

Who Should Be Referred for (C)APD Testing?

(C)APD can manifest itself in many different ways, and some of the same behavior patterns are shared with comorbid conditions such as ADHD, language difficulties, and/or learning disabilities. This makes it difficult to determine when a referral for (C)APD testing is appropriate. As with any other referral process, incorporation of a multidisciplinary team is helpful in navigating through behaviors or characteristics related to a variety of conditions. Screening is also difficult because there is no gold standard for screening protocols when assessing for (C)APD. There are screening tools available specifically dedicated to the rudimentary detection and referral of a suspected (C)APD (e.g., Differential Screening Test of Processing [Richard & Ferre, 2006]; Multiple Auditory Processing Assessment [Schow, Chermak, Seikel, Brockett, & Whitaker, 2006]). Nonetheless, the AAA (2010) has expressed the need for more efficient screening tools that accurately identify individuals at risk for (C)APD. This is difficult because there is some controversy about the definition of what truly constitutes a disorder in (C)AP skills; however, there is some consensus among professionals as to behaviors likely seen in individuals with a deficit in (C)AP skills (AAA, 2010; Johnson & Seaton, 2012; Keith, 2009a: Keith, 2009b). It is important to note that no one behavior exclusively represents a (C)APD, but a combination of characteristics would lead to the suspicion that an evaluation is warranted. Through self-reporting, behavioral observations, and preliminary testing by the teacher, speech-language pathologist, or audiologist, the following behaviors may be evident:

- Listening behaviors consistent with an individual who has a hearing loss; however, normal hearing has been confirmed
- Difficulty comprehending speech in the presence of noise or in poor acoustics due to reverberation
- Decreased attention to auditory information when compared to attention to visual information
- Inconsistent or inappropriate responses to auditory information or requests made by others
- Difficulty comprehending and following rapid speech
- Breakdown in following directions or remembering auditory instructions
- Regularly asks for information or directions to be repeated or rephrased
- Lack of ability to detect and produce changes in prosody of speech; can be reflected in poor musical abilities
- Poor phonological/phonemic awareness skills
- Poor auditory discrimination skills for speech sounds
- Difficulty localizing to the source of an auditory signal
- Weaknesses in speech-language or psychoeducational tests with an emphasis on auditory comprehension or auditory-related skills
- Difficulty learning a new language

Appropriate Age and Skills for Testing

When referring a child for (C)APD testing, it is recommended that test results for children under the age of 7 years be interpreted with caution because there is increased inconsistency and variability, and weaker reliability on performance for (C)AP tests (ASHA, 2005). In addition, normative data are limited for children under 7 years for a variety of behavioral tests used to assess (C)AP abilities. There are some tests available that provide norms for younger children (e.g., Staggered Spondaic Word [SSW; Katz, 1962]; SCAN-3:C Tests for Auditory Processing Disorders in Children [Keith, 2009b]). However, AAA (2010) recommends that these measures, along with behavioral surveys/checklists, be used as a flag to monitor children who could be considered at risk for (C)APD. These children should be followed and retested annually.

As with very young children, individuals with significant cognitive deficits may not be likely candidates for behavioral testing when assessing for (C)APD. Due to the complexity of test materials and the demands on language, memory, and attention, (C)APD testing may be inappropriate (ASHA, 2005; Bellis, 2003). If an individual has other global cognitive issues, a (C)APD would be difficult to segregate.

This same question may arise when a child diagnosed with **autism spectrum disorder (ASD)** is referred for a (C)APD evaluation. It is known that children with ASD can have difficulty receiving, filtering, organizing, and making use of sensory information, which includes the sensation of hearing. For children with ASD, it is evident that testing for (C)APD would not lead to a specific diagnosis in this area. Due to the characteristics associated with ASD, an etiology has already been identified that explains why the child may have difficulty comprehending auditory information. However, children with ASD can have varying degrees of cognitive function. If a child has adequate cognitive abilities to complete the demands of testing, the audiologists may be able to provide specific data on which auditory skills pose the most difficulty, and in turn may offer valuable insight on intervention strategies for the child. However, if the child cannot meet the demands for testing, a referral should not be considered. This is a decision best made by the multidisciplinary team, or at least with the cooperation of the audiologist and the speech-language pathologist.

The (C)AP Test Battery: What Does It Mean?

Historically, behavioral tests for (C)APD originated from studies on individuals with known sites of lesions within the CANS; for example, difficulty with dichotic listening tests has shown increased sensitivity for lesion studies of the CANS (Fifer, Jerger, Berlin, Tobey, & Campbell, 1983; Katz, 1962; Meyers, Roberts, Bayless, Volkert, & Evitts, 2002; Musiek, 1983). These studies have guided the conceptual framework for a majority of the tests utilized today for the assessment of (C)AP skills. However, a better protocol for the future development of behavioral tests that assess auditory–cognitive abilities may be to link reliability and validity measures to specific weaknesses in auditory skills that children may be experiencing; nonbehavioral tests, in contrast, may be used to provide auditory sensory processing information related to the status of the CANS.

Although the AAA (2010) and ASHA (2005) recommend the incorporation of electrophysiological measures when evaluating and diagnosing (C)APD, this is not feasible for all children due to cost and accessibility. Even though electrophysiological tests have the potential to provide a description of abnormal neurological function, this type of testing does not offer information on the type and degree of behavioral problems a child experiences, nor does it change the intervention plan. In turn, behavioral tests offer a characteristic profile on performance for auditory skills, which may be associated with academic, social, or communication abilities. This information, along with data on speech, language, and academic abilities, enables professionals to better address deficits in specific skill areas. Therefore, this section will focus on the explanation of specific categories of behavioral tests utilized for the evaluation of a suspected (C)APD. Likewise, much of the discussion will pertain to school-age children because this is the population in which symptoms initially occur and in which deficits in auditory processing are most noticeable. However, it is important to be aware that many of the characteristics discussed in children are also found in adults.

Dichotic Listening

Dichotic listening tests are useful for providing information on the function of the left and right hemispheres and the transfer of auditory information between hemispheres (Keith & Anderson, 2007). Dichotic tests involve the presentation of competing messages to each ear in a simultaneous manner. **Binaural integration** requires the participant to repeat back what is heard in both ears, whereas **binaural separation** tasks involve the repetition of stimuli presented to one ear while the stimuli in the opposite ear are ignored. Stimuli can range from digits to phonemes, words, or sentences (see Table 16.1).

Table 16.1   Behavioral Tests for (Central) Auditory Processing

	Dichotic Speech Tests	Age Range
Binaural Integration	Competing Environmental Sounds Test	3–12 years
	Dichotic Consonant-Vowel (CV) Test	7 years–adult
	Dichotic Digits Test	5 years–adult
	Dichotic Rhyme Test	8 years–adult
	Dichotic Sentence Identification Test	7 years–adult
	Multiple Auditory Processing Assessment (MAPA) Dichotic Digits	8 years–adult
	SCAN-3-C/A Competing Words Subtest	5 years–adult
	Staggered Spondaic Word Test (SSW)	5 years–adult
Binaural Separation	Competing Sentences Test	7 years–adult
	MAPA Competing Sentences	8 years–adult
	SCAN-3-C/A Competing Sentences Test	5 years–adult
	Synthetic Sentence Identification–Contralateral (SSI-CCM)	8 years–adult
	Monaural Low-Redundancy Tests	
Auditory Closure	Dept of VA High Pass Filter	adult
	Dept of VA Low Pass Filter	adult
	Dept of VA 45% Time Compressed Speech	adult
	Dept of VA 65% Time Compressed Speech	adult
	NU-6 Low Pass Filtered	7 years–adult
	NU-6 Time Compressed	7 years–adult
	NU-6 Time Compressed + Reverberation	7 years–adult
	SCAN-3-C/A Filtered Words Subtest	5 years–adult
	SCAN-3-C/A Time Compressed Sentences	5 years–adult
	Time Compressed Monosyllabic Word Tests	
	Time Compressed Sentence Test	6–11 years
Auditory Figure/Ground	Bamford-Kowal-Bench Speech in Noise Test (BKB-SIN)	4–14 years
	Discrimination of PB-K in Noise (PBKN)	grades K–5
	Listening in Spatialized Noise-Sentence Test (LiSN)	6–11 years
	Dept of VA Synthetic Sentences	adult
	MAPA Monaural Selective Auditory Attention Test (SAAT)	8 years–adult
	MAPA Speech-in-Noise for Children and Adults (SINCA)	8 years–adult
	Pediatric Speech Intelligibility Test (PSI)	3–7 years
	Quick SIN	adult
	SCAN-3-C/A Auditory Figure Ground Subtest	5 years–adult
	Selective Auditory Attention Test (SAAT)	5 years–adult
	Speech in Noise (SPIN)	
	Speech-in-Noise W-22 (Katz Battery)	5 years–adult
	Synthetic Sentence Identification–Ipsilateral (SSI-ICM)	8 years–adult
	Temporal Processing and Patterning Tests	
Temporal Resolution	Auditory Fusion Test–Revised	3 years–adult
	Gaps in Noise Test	6 years–adult
	MAPA Gap Detection Test (AFT-R)	8 years–adult
	Random Gap Detection Test	5 years–adult
	SCAN-3-C/A Gap Detection	5 years–adult
Temporal Ordering	Duration Pattern Test	8 years–adult
	MAPA Duration Patterns Binaural	8 years–adult
	MAPA Pitch Pattern Test	8 years–adult
	MAPA TAP test	8 years–adult
	Pitch Pattern Test	6 years–adult

(continues)

Table 16.1 *(Continued)*

	Binaural Interaction Tests	
Binaural Interaction	CVC Fusion Test	7 years–adult
	Intraural Intensity Difference Tonal Patterns (IID)	
	Masking Level Difference (MLD)	5 years–adult
	Rapidly Alternating Speech Perception (RASP)	5 years–adult
	Sound Lateralization & Localization	adult
	Spondee Binaural Fusion	7 years–adult
	Auditory Discrimination	
	Difference Limen for Intensity	adult
	Difference Limen for Frequency	adult
	Phonemic Decoding	
	Phonemic Synthesis Picture Test (PSPT)	4–7 years
	Phonemic Synthesis Test (PST)	6 years–adult
	Additional Behavioral Tests	
	Auditory Continuous Performance Test (ACPT)	6–11 years
	Auditory Processing Abilities Test (APAT)	5–12 years
	Differential Screening Test for Processing	6–12 years
	Functional Listening Evaluation (FLE)	4 years–adult
	Test of Auditory Processing Skills, 3rd ed. (TAPS)	5 years–adult
	Questionnaires and Checklists	
	Buffalo Model Questionnaire (BMQ)	6 and older
	Children's Auditory Performance Scale (CHAPS)	7 and older
	Children's Home Inventory for Listening Difficulties (CHILD)–Parent Version	3–12 years
	Children's Home Inventory for Listening Difficulties (CHILD)–Self Reporting	8–12 years
	Developmental Index of Audition and Listening (DIAL)	birth–22 years
	Early Listening Function (ELF)	4 months–3 years
	Fisher's Auditory Problems Checklist	5–12 years
	Listening Inventory for Education (LIFE)–Student Appraisal	grades 1–12
	Listening Inventory for Education (LIFE)–Teacher Appraisal	grades 1–12
	Scale of Auditory Behaviors (SAB)	8.9–10.11 years
	Screening Instrument for Targeting Educational Risk (SIFTER)–Preschool	3 years–kindergarten
	Screening Instrument for Targeting Educational Risk (SIFTER)–Elementary	grades 1–8
	Screening Instrument for Targeting Educational Risk (SIFTER)–Secondary	grades 9–12

Data from Educational Audiology Handbook, Summary of Common Behavioral Audiological Tests of Auditory Processing, Johnson & Seaton, 2012; Auditec, Inc.; Cacace & McFarland, 2009; Educational Audiology Association; Musiek & Chermak, 2007.

Dichotic listening tests are diagnostically significant in that during the transmission of the dichotic signal, information is transferred through the dominant contralateral pathways (Keith & Anderson, 2007). Many individuals have left hemispheric dominance for language, so dichotic testing offers valuable insight into the development and function of the right versus left hemisphere and of the corpus callosum, which connects both hemispheres (see Figure 16.2). This also clarifies why children often perform better on linguistically based right ear tasks versus left ear tasks during dichotic testing. When an auditory signal enters the right ear during dichotic testing, the signal travels the dominant contralateral pathway and crosses directly to the language-dominant left hemisphere, where it is perceived. In turn, when a linguistic signal is presented to the left ear, it crosses to the right hemisphere, which then must transmit the signal through the corpus callosum to the left hemisphere for comprehension.

In dichotic listening tests, there will often be a higher percentage of correct responses in the right ear versus the left ear (Jancke, 2002). This right ear advantage (REA) minimizes around adolescence when myelination increases in the corpus callosum, making it more efficient and speedier. A

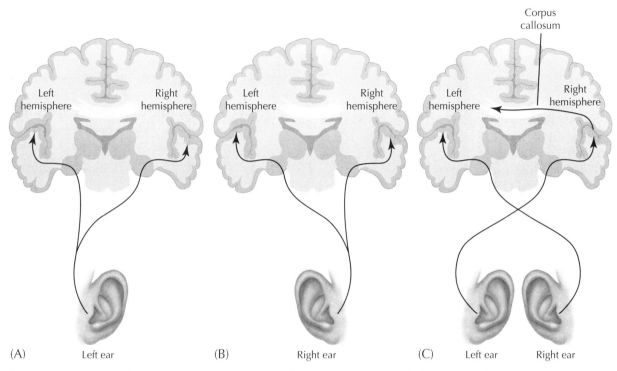

Figure 16.2   Model of Central Auditory Pathways for monaural versus dichotic stimulation.

significant REA in children—greater than normative data—may suggest a delay in maturation of the CANS, possibly within the corpus callosum. For these cases it is essential to monitor development of the CANS with annual testing for dichotic skills.

If test scores do not improve in the left ear with age, a disorder is suspected and further neurological testing is warranted. In turn, a left ear advantage (LEA) may reflect right hemisphere dominance or mixed right and left hemisphere governance for language (Keith & Anderson, 2007). Moncrieff (2011) coined the term **amblyaudia** to represent this atypical dominance in ear advantage. In addition, Obrzut, Boliek, and Obrzut (1986) found that when children were directed to repeat the right or left ear first on dichotic tasks, those participants with a language and/or learning disability revealed an abnormal REA for right-ear-directed tasks and an LEA for left-ear-directed tasks. In these directed ear dichotic tasks, children who were not identified with a disability scored within the expected "normal" range for an REA. For individuals that reflect an LEA in dichotic listening tasks, continued testing by a multidisciplinary team is necessary due to suspicion of other global problems.

Children who exhibit abnormal scores on dichotic listening tests may be at risk for difficulty interpreting speech in the presence of other competing messages. For example, listening to two speakers at one time is extremely problematic, a situation that children are exposed to multiple times throughout the day. More difficulty may also be noted in group discussions where the individual must divide auditory attention and comprehend multiple signals (Parthasarathy, 2006). When listening to multiple speakers, we have two choices—to block out one signal while focusing on another signal (binaural separation) or to listen to both signals simultaneously and interpret as much information as possible (binaural integration). Functionally, either of these skills is very taxing for a child who has shown poor performance on dichotic listening tasks.

Temporal Processing/Sequencing

Temporal is defined as time-based, and that is precisely how it relates to tests for (C)AP. Behavioral tests for **temporal processing/sequencing** assess the ability to recognize the timing aspects of acoustic stimuli (see Table 16.1). This is an important function for the processing of auditory signals, especially for the interpretation of speech. Intact and accurate temporal processing/sequencing is critical for the perception of rapidly altering speech sounds. Similarly, sufficient temporal skills are needed for the interpretation of prosodic aspects of speech (Johnson, Bellis, & Billiet, 2007).

Gap detection tests are generally used to assess temporal processing, the ability to recognize and distinguish auditory events over time (Shinn, 2007). Tests for gap detection assess an individual's ability to detect small intervals of time between two consecutive auditory stimuli. As an example, the Random Gap Detection Test (RGDT) requires an individual to indicate the lowest millisecond (msec) interval in which they are able to detect the presence of two similar tonal or click stimuli (Keith, 2000). Gap intervals for stimuli are varied from 0 to 40 msec. Individuals are asked to raise one finger if they hear one stimulus or two fingers if they perceive two stimuli. The Gaps-In-Noises (GIN) test is similar; however, the examinee is presented with a series of 6-second segments of a broadband noise (Musiek, Shinn, et al., 2005). Within these segments of noise, a silent interval or intervals may be present. The silent gap intervals vary from 2 to 20 msec. Again, the examiner records responses and calculates the shortest gap duration detected by the listener.

Temporal sequencing tests, also referred to as temporal ordering, involve the sequential discrimination of multiple auditory signals over time (ASHA, 2005). Temporal ordering requires efficient communication between the right and left hemispheres, thus making temporal sequencing/patterning tests sensitive to neuromaturation and dysfunction of the interhemispheric pathways (Musiek, Pinheiro, & Wilson, 1980). Two primary tests for temporal sequencing involve frequency recognition and duration recognition. The Frequency Pattern test consists of two frequencies (a high- and low-frequency tone) presented in three or four tonal patterns (Musiek, 1994; Schow et al., 2006). The listener is instructed to label the sequence of the tones and repeat the arrangement in the same order (e.g., high-low-high, low-low-high, high-low-low-high; low-high-low-high, etc.). The Duration Pattern Test (Pinheiro & Musiek, 1985) is structured in a similar manner as the Frequency Pattern test. Listeners are asked to label patterns of sounds, but instead of varying the frequencies, the duration of the stimuli fluctuates between two lengths (e.g., long-long-short, short-long-short, etc.). However, normative data are limited on children for most duration pattern tests.

Right hemisphere superiority is seen for such functions as the processing of prosodic features of speech, the analysis of facial expressions, and artistic talents such as musical abilities (Ross & Monnot, 2008), whereas interpretation of language is predominantly a role of the left hemisphere in right-handed individuals (Taylor & Taylor, 1990). Interhemispheric dysfunction may be reflected in poor performance on frequency and duration pattern tests. Problems with discrimination of speech, especially if it is rapid or presented in long segments with no breaks, may be observed in children who perform poorly on temporal processing tests. In addition, difficulty interpreting prosodic features of speech and trouble with gestalt may be observed (Bellis, 2003).

Low-Redundancy Speech

Low-redundancy speech tasks involve testing where the natural redundancy of speech is compromised by noise or poor signal quality. The ability to interpret degraded speech using auditory closure skills is a problem found in some listeners who experience (C)AP difficulties (Geffner & Ross-Swain, 2007). In order to make closure, a listener must be familiar with the speech signal and be able to fill in missing elements when speech is not clear. There are several means for assessing a listener's performance with degraded acoustic signals. The first is the most common method and employs identification of a speech signal while it is embedded in noise (AAA, 2010). Speech-in-noise tests, also referred to as auditory figure-ground tests, should be interpreted cautiously when used within the (C)APD test battery. Speech-in-noise tests are known for their lack of sensitivity when diagnosing a (C)APD. Other cognitive and attention influences may affect performance on speech-in-noise tasks. However, these tests are very useful in providing a description of how well an individual functions auditorily in excessive noise. This can be very valuable when developing a functional auditory profile for a child in the classroom. Speech-in-noise tests may be presented monaurally or bilaterally and require the listener to repeat an auditory signal in the presence of a competing message. Signal-to-noise ratios vary according to the criterion of the test, as do the stimuli (e.g., words versus sentences) and the type of competing noise (e.g., background noise versus speech competition). Varieties of tests normed for children are available and can provide insight on functional auditory abilities (see Table 16.1.)

A second method for assessing low-redundancy speech uses low-passed filter speech tests in which the speech signal is filtered, removing high-frequency spectral information. Several low-pass filter tests have been normed with cut-off filters at 500 Hz, 750 Hz, and 1000 Hz (Bellis, 2003; Keith, 2009a, 2009b; Wilson & Mueller, 1984); see Table 16.1. A list of low-pass filtered words are presented monaurally and listeners are required to repeat what they have heard. Low-pass filtered speech tests are associated with the ability to accurately make auditory closure when confronted with a poor acoustic speech signal.

Another procedure for evaluating auditory closure modifies temporal features of the speech signal. Time-compressed speech tests are presented at a rapid pace, without changing the frequency and intensity of the signal (Krishnamurti, 2007). Time-compressed speech tests are described by compression ratios; the percentage that the original stimulus is condensed with greater values equaling higher compressions. Stimuli can range from words to sentences. Normative data are available on several time-compressed assessment tools (see Table 16.1). Poor performance on time-compressed tests indicates decreased functional capabilities for processing rapid changes in acoustic stimuli, particularly fast speech.

Children who perform poorly on low-redundancy speech tasks may miss pieces of auditory information when the signal is distorted, indistinct, and/or degraded by noise. Although tests for low redundancy offer a questionable diagnosis for a true auditory sensory processing deficit, valuable information is given on auditory–cognitive abilities. This can be very useful when explaining poor listening skills in the classroom.

Binaural Interaction

Tests for binaural interaction reflect how auditory input works together from both ears at the level of the brainstem (see Table 16.1). These tests are very sensitive to intensity and timing differences between ears and are related to the localization and lateralization of sound (AAA, 2010). To date, there is no commercial test available that provides information concerning whether a listener has "normal" or "abnormal" abilities to accurately localize or lateralize to sound. There are tests that provide insight into the integrity of the lower brainstem, such as Masking Level Difference (Lynn, Gilroy, Taylor, & Leiser, 1981); however, these tests may not specifically provide a profile of localization/lateralization skills.

There are binaural interaction tests designed to measure binaural fusion of two signals presented simultaneously or interchangeably to both ears. For simultaneous signals, high-frequency information of a word is passed to one ear, while the low-frequency component is passed to the other ear. If the listener can adequately fuse the information, they are instructed to repeat the word that they hear. Binaural fusion tests also include tasks in which the listener hears rapidly alternating phonemes of a word or alternating words

in sentences between ears and is asked to repeat the whole word or the entire sentence. However, these tests have been effective only in identifying conspicuous pathologies within the brainstem (Bamiou, 2007). Because of the lack of sensitivity for tests of binaural fusion, an audiologist may not include this type of evaluation tool within the (C)APD test battery. However, there is growing research in this area, and new measures are being developed that examine binaural interaction functions. One such tool, the Listening in Spatialized Noise-Sentences Test ([LISN-S]; Cameron et al., 2009) was developed to measure how well the listener uses directional cues (spatial advantages) to interpret speech in noise. An individual is asked to repeat a target speech signal while noise is presented from different locations.

A child who performs poorly on tests of binaural interaction may possess problems comprehending speech in the presence of background noise. This is due to the inability to segregate the speech signal when there is a competing sound source (Parthasarathy, 2006). Thus, listening proficiency for sound localization and auditory performance in background noise is affected. If a child cannot quickly locate the teacher's voice in the room and has trouble understanding the teacher's message from the noise in the classroom, the opportunity for learning is compromised.

Auditory Discrimination

Discrimination of speech sounds involves the ability to identify the frequency, intensity, and duration of phonemes (AAA. 2010). **Auditory discrimination** would appear to be a very integral part of the (C)AP battery because perception of speech is necessary for the development of speech, language, and a host of other cognitive abilities. When a child cannot discriminate between sounds, especially those that have similar acoustic features, they will often misinterpret the message. However, deficits in auditory discrimination may show up on a number of behavioral (C)AP tests due to the multiple auditory skills needed for the interpretation of speech. In addition, auditory discrimination is an auditory cognitive function and is difficult to separate from a true auditory sensory pathology. Due to this, it is better for the speech-language pathologist to investigate behavioral skills related to phonological/phonemic awareness to get a profile of a child's ability to identify and manipulate sounds.

Electrophysiological Measures

Research has identified true auditory sensory deficits along the central auditory nervous system through the use of electrophysiological measures (Krause et al., 1996); however, these tests require intricate and expensive equipment that is not always readily available at all audiologic facilities. Electrophysiological measures currently cannot replace the behavioral test battery for (C)APD; however, in conjunction with behavioral tests, they provide valuable information about the physiology and integrity of the CANS. Positive changes between pre- and postauditory training recordings are an important, effective way to objectively monitor the progress of an auditory training program. Continued research of electrophysiological responses in children with (C)APD will further our understanding of auditory processing and the underlying auditory mechanisms that may be responsible for (C)APD.

Interpretation

The results of the (C)APD assessment should indicate whether a (C)APD is present. The diagnosis of (C)APD is based on reviewing all of the test results in the battery to determine whether there is a pattern of performance across different tests of auditory processing, possible interaural differences (ear weakness), and specific auditory processing deficits or weaknesses. Because (C)APD is a heterogeneous disorder, a description of the auditory weaknesses or

deficits should be detailed in order to implement a deficit-specific auditory rehabilitation plan.

One approach to test interpretation and auditory rehabilitation is to use models or profiles to further describe (C)APD deficits and associated underlying neurophysiological site(s) of dysfunction. It is important to note that although these models are widely accepted, they have not undergone peer review.

Models of (C)APD
Bellis/Ferre Model

The **Bellis/Ferre model** (Bellis, 2003; Bellis & Ferre, 1999) is one popular model that includes three primary subprofiles—Auditory Decoding Deficit, Prosodic Deficit, and Integration Deficit—and two secondary profiles—Associative Deficit and Output Organization (see Table 16.2). (For a detailed review, the reader is referred to Bellis [2003].) The *Auditory Decoding Deficit Profile* is characterized by auditory discrimination deficits and difficulty listening in noise. Children with this profile may behave similarly to a child with a hearing loss. This child will often have difficulty with reading and spelling and weak phonological skills. Performance on tests

Table 16.2   Bellis/Ferre Profiles of (C)APD and associated deficits

Primary Profile	Deficits	Targeted Skills for Remediation	Informal Games and Activities	Video Games
Decoding	Listening in background noise Spelling and reading difficulty Sound/symbol association Sound discrimination	Phoneme identification Phonological awareness Sound discrimination Sound blending Word attack skills	Red light–green light Telephone Wheel of Fortune Scrabble	Reader Rabbit Family Word Jong Story Hour Family Jump Start Games My Word Coach Wheel of Fortune
Integration	Combining multimodality information Reading comprehension Following auditory directions	Interhemispheric transfer Binaural skills Sound localization Auditory and visual information	Scrabble Bopit Simon Simon Says Card games	Sesame Street Family Reader Rabbit Nickelodeon Fit Jump Start Games Hasbro Family Game Night Pictionary Big Brain Academy Cosmic Family Dance Dance Revolution
Prosodic	Understanding the meaning Comprehending the main idea Frequency and temporal discrimination	Perception Temporal patterning Pragmatics	MadGab Singing Dramatic arts	Wii Music Disney Sing It Guitar Hero Dance Dance Revolution Karaoke Revolution Jump Start

of monaural low-redundancy speech will be abnormal. The *Prosodic Deficit Profile* describes deficits in temporal processing skills with abnormal performance in auditory pattern and temporal ordering tasks. Individuals with these deficits will have difficulty understanding the meaning of verbal messages because of difficulty with stress, rhythm, and intonation patterns. The *Integration Deficit Profile* is characterized by deficits in the ability to perform tasks requiring multisensory communication, such as incorporating both auditory and visual information simultaneously. The individual will have difficulty with tasks that require information processing from both the right and left hemispheres. Individuals with this profile will perform poorly on binaural integration tasks, dichotic listening tests, and linguistic labeling of temporals.

Buffalo Model

The **Buffalo model** of (C)APD (Katz, 1992) is another popular model and is strongly based on the individual's performance on the Staggered Spondaic Word Test. This model includes four categories: Decoding, Tolerance-Fading Memory, Organization, and Integration. The *Decoding* subtype describes individuals with difficulty synthesizing small parts of auditory information into larger parts. These individuals tend to respond slowly and have difficulty with spelling and reading. Remediation will focus on phonemic awareness skills. The *Tolerance-Fading Memory* subtype is characterized by short-term auditory memory deficits and difficulty listening to speech in poor acoustic environments. Remediation will incorporate speech-in-noise training and auditory memory strategies. The *Organization* subtype is characterized by inability to organize auditory information. An individual with this subtype will have difficulty retelling the sequence of a story. Speech-language intervention to

target sequencing is recommended. The *Integration* subtype is characterized by inability to integrate multisensory information, such as auditory and other modalities of information.

It is important to note that an individual may not fit into one particular profile and may have characteristics of more than one profile or subtype. For this reason, some clinicians will focus rehabilitation efforts on the specific areas of auditory weakness.

Process-Based Rehabilitation

Clinicians may use a process-based method to interpret the (C)AP testing results. This method identifies specific auditory deficits and weaknesses of auditory processing including such behaviors as temporal spectral and binaural processing, discrimination of speech in noise, and deficits in interhemispheric transfer of auditory information. Examples of interventions for process-based auditory remediation are shown in Table 16.3.

Monaural Low-Redundancy Training

Monaural low-redundancy training will help individuals who have difficulty hearing in background noise, understanding rapidly connected speech, or hearing when the auditory signal is not optimal. Clinicians may introduce background noise during therapy sessions; auditory closure activities and vocabulary building activities are often used in training.

Dichotic Listening Training

Dichotic listening training is an innovative therapy for the remediation of the compromised central auditory pathway (Musiek, Chermak, & Weihing, 2007). This is accomplished via dichotic listening tasks by decreasing the signal intensity

Table 16.3 Process-Based Auditory Remediations

Process Deficit	Process	Profile Deficit	Goal	Activities
Monaural low redundancy speech training	Auditory discrimination Auditory closure	Decoding	Train the listener to fill in missing or distorted auditory information	Vocabulary building enrichment Phonemic awareness activities
Dichotic speech tests	Binaural integration Binaural separation	Integration	Designed so the listener can integrate information from both hemispheres	Dichotic listening training Localization training Speech-in-noise training
Temporal processing Temporal patterning	Temporal resolution Frequency discrimination Intensity discrimination Duration discrimination Temporal ordering	Prosodic	Designed to enhance the ability of the listener to recognize prosodic aspects of speech such as intonation, stress, and rhythm	Prosody training Self-auditorization Key word extraction Word meaning

of the unimpaired pathway and slowly increasing the intensity level over time, as the weaker, impaired pathway grows stronger. This is referred to as the dichotic interaural intensity difference (DIID; Musiek et al., 2007). Dichotic listening training differs from traditional language therapy in which the acoustic signal (recorded speech, therapists voice, etc.) is presented binaurally. By contrast, dichotic listening training purports to specifically target the deficit ear and activate brain regions that receive auditory sensory input on the deficit side. Previous investigations have shown behavioral and electrophysiological evidence of improvement of the central auditory nervous system after dichotic listening training (Hurley & Billiet, 2008; Musiek, Baran, & Shinn, 2004).

Dichotic listening exercises are available commercially; however, dichotic training can also be accomplished by using recorded books. The signal (in this case, the story) will be directed to the target ear by an earphone, while noise such as a radio or television plays in the background. The intensity of the background noise can increase over time, or it may be transmitted to the nontarget ear via earphone.

Temporal Processing Training

Training for temporal processing deficits may include formal or informal activities. The Fast ForWord family of software is based on successful temporal processing training. Other training methods may include using nonspeech sound, involving "same/different" judgments of tones, or narrow or broadband sounds that differ in frequency and/or temporal gaps. Listeners can also imitate the rhythm of a series of claps or tones (such as notes on a keyboard) of increasing complexity and length.

Designing the Remediation Plan for (C)APD

Treatment of (C)APD generally focuses on three areas: (1) environmental changes to ease communication difficulties, (2) introducing compensatory skills and strategies for the disorder, and (3) remediation of the auditory deficit (ASHA, 2005). These include bottom-up skills that focus on enhancement of the auditory signal and training to utilize the auditory message, and top-down skills that teach strategies for how to utilize the auditory signal more efficiently (ASHA, 2005).

Environmental Modifications

Listening and learning can be adversely affected by the listening environment (Crandell & Smaldino, 2004. It is estimated that children spend approximately 50% of classroom time hearing and/or listening to instruction from their teacher (Berg, 1987) and approximately 45% of their time outside school hours involved in social activities requiring them to listen (Hunsaker, 1990). Creating an optimal acoustic environment for listening by making **environmental modifications** is important so that children with (C)APD will have access to auditory information.

An assessment of the auditory environment may include examination of acoustic factors such as background noise, reverberation, and distance from the signal, as well as non-acoustic factors such as lighting and supplemental visual information (Crandell & Smaldino, 2004). Technology to enhance the signal-to-noise ratio may be beneficial to some individuals with (C)APD, but may only be appropriate if the individual can adjust the unit. A general recommendation for an FM system is not appropriate for all individuals with (C)APD and should be considered only after positive improvements are noted during a trial period.

Compensatory Strategies

Listening is the most used language art, and the one taught the least (Jalongo, 2006). Good listening skills can be taught. **Compensatory strategies** are top-down skills and are an important part of teaching the child how to compensate for listening difficulties. These strategies teach techniques so an individual can become a better, active listener. Metalinguistic skills and metacognitive activities are top-down and equip the child to take responsibility for listening successes and failures.

Auditory Training

Auditory training takes advantage of the brain's lifelong capacity for **plasticity** and adaptive reorganization, which may be at least partially reversible through a deficit-specific training program (Musiek et al., 2007). Auditory training programs strengthen specific auditory skills, and programs may be formal or informal and active or passive. Passive music programs have become quite controversial in recent years. There is a lack of data to support such auditory integration treatments (ASHA, 2004), so they will not be discussed in this chapter. Active programs require participation from the patient and are probably more effective than passive programs (Bellis, 2003).

Formal Auditory Therapy

Formal auditory training programs are usually conducted by an audiologist, speech-language therapist, or other educational therapist. Clinicians should consider the patient's age, motivation, language ability, and ability to maintain attention throughout the therapy sessions. These factors should also be considered when choosing a training program. Therapy should be challenging, but not frustrating. Various tasks may be employed during sessions to prevent boredom. Examples of training include frequency discrimination (high vs. low frequency), intensity training (loud vs. soft), and duration training (long vs. short).

Computer-Mediated Auditory Training Programs

Computer-mediated auditory training programs are growing in popularity and have many advantages. They are convenient, they hold the interest of young children, there is a standardization of control of the stimulus, and the programs are adaptive. Thus, the stimulus or level may change based on the child's correct or incorrect response. It is important to recognize the individual's specific auditory deficit(s) and remember that no one single program will target every underlying auditory processing skill. New programs are introduced to the market continuously, so it is important for the clinician to be aware of new additions.

ForWord

ForWord is one popular software program based on the underlying temporal processing research of Tallal et al. (1996) and Merzenich et al. (1996). The Fast ForWord program is designed to develop temporal and acoustic skills to detect rapid transitions of speech. The exercises in the Fast ForWord program use acoustically modified speech. It is important to note an individual may not fit into one particular profile and may have characteristics of more than one profile or subtype. For this reason, some clinicians will focus rehabilitation efforts on the specific areas of auditory weakness.

In the beginning of the program, the exercises prolong and emphasize the sounds and are easier to distinguish. As the listener progresses, speech sounds approach the rate of normal speech. As the listener improves, the exercises become more challenging, and the participant develops enhanced language awareness and comprehension.

Earobics

The Earobics family of software products is another popular program for improving phonemic awareness, auditory processing, and phonics, as well as cognitive and language skills that may benefit auditory and listening comprehension. Earobics is available for home, clinic, and school use. It is available in three levels—prekindergarten, school age, and adolescents and adults.

Brain Train

Brain Train is another software program useful in aiding underlying language-processing skills, such as attention, sequencing, processing speed, and memory. Efficacy studies of this product have been limited to children with ADHD. This program is designed for patients age 6 years to adult.

Laureate Learning Systems

The Laureate Learning Systems include programs that address language-processing skills. The programs contain exercises for preverbal children up to adults. Exercises include categorization and syntax training, auditory discrimination, reading, and spelling.

Other Programs

Several other computer-mediated programs have been developed for individuals with hearing loss. These programs are appropriate for a wide variety of ages, from preschoolers through adults, and include exercises in sound identification, auditory discrimination, and speech-in-noise training.

New software programs targeting (C)AP skills are continuously introduced into the market. Clinicians need to routinely search for new product launches to remain current.

Informal Auditory Therapy

Informal auditory therapy activities may be done at home and are recommended to supplement formal auditory training. Engaging a young child at risk for (C)APD in auditory training or auditory enrichment may involve everyday routine activities. Reading to children is one very important auditory training activity. A child who listens to a story and then answers questions about the story, or retells the story, is practicing active listening and improving his or her listening skills.

There are numerous reports of superior auditory processing ability in musicians. Music and speech share many of the same acoustical properties, such as pitch, timing, and timbre, to convey meaning. Musicians have a superior ability to hear in background noise, and have better temporal, timbre, and pitch discrimination abilities. Kraus and Chandrasekaran (2010) reviewed the benefits of formal music training as an enjoyable auditory activity that sharpens one's sensitivity to pitch, timing, and timbre, and as a result aids the capacity to discern emotional intonation in speech and to learn native and foreign languages.

Another suggestion for informal auditory therapy is activities such as computer games, board games, or video games. Ferre (2002) provided a review of board games and activities targeting specific auditory processing skills (see Table 16.3). Dowell, Milligan, Davis, and Hurley (2011) reviewed current video games on the market to augment formal therapy. By incorporating skill development into everyday activities, auditory remediation may improve these deficit-specific areas. The use of popular, interactive games may be useful and convenient for audiologists, speech-language pathologists, early interventionists, or parents who wish to engage listening and auditory processing skills during play.

Conclusion: Working Together

Despite the controversy over auditory processing disorders, a cooperative team involving the speech-language pathologist and the audiologist is essential for addressing auditory skill deficits in children. Both the audiologist and the speech-language pathologist play an integral part in the diagnosis and treatment of children with (central) auditory–cognitive processing deficits. Audiologists provide a unique perspective as to why a child may not interpret auditory information accurately. In return, the speech-language pathologist offers insight into how language skills are affected by the breakdown in auditory-related skills. There are numerous disorders for which the true underlying etiology is unknown; however, this has not stopped our professions from treating behavioral deficits reflected by a disorder. It is time for the separate disciplines to work together to develop individualized and efficient intervention plans that meet the needs of children who have difficulty with the interpretation and comprehension of auditory information.

Summary

Despite the varying information in the literature concerning the etiology of (C)APDs, it is commonly described as an auditory diagnosis resulting from various dysfunctions of neural representation of auditory stimuli in the central auditory nervous system. This can manifest as a heterogeneous group of auditory deficits such as poor auditory discrimination for speech, decreased auditory attention, and difficulty comprehending rapid speech and/or speech in noise. A diagnosis of (C)APD cannot be made from one test, but rather must be made from looking at a pattern of performances across a test battery and is best identified while working in collaboration with other professionals as a multidisciplinary team. Collaboration among the audiologist, speech-language pathologist, and other relevant professionals will help to ensure the most accurate diagnosis and lead to a well-designed remediation plan that includes (1) environmental changes to ease communication difficulties, (2) compensatory skills and strategies to alleviate complications associated with the disorder, and (3) remediation of the auditory deficit (ASHA, 2005). These collaborative treatment plans may include bottom-up and top-down formal and informal activities and should be deficit specific to address the needs of the child.

Discussion Questions

1. Discuss how the collaborative model may be beneficial in the diagnosis and treatment of (C)APD.
2. Discuss other conditions that may coexist with (C)APD. How can these be distinguished?
3. Which auditory processes do dichotic speech tasks evaluate?
4. Discuss three temporal processing tests. Why is temporal processing important for understanding speech?
5. Briefly discuss methods used to reduce the redundancy of speech for (C)APD assessment.
6. Discuss the limitations of electroacoustic and electrophysiological testing in the (C)APD battery.
7. Briefly list behavioral, academic, and management approaches for the following subprofiles of (C)APD:
   - Auditory Decoding Deficit
   - Prosodic Deficit
   - Integration Deficit

8. What are three main categories of (C)APD treatment?
9. What are three advantages of computer-mediated auditory training programs?

10. What are some examples of informal auditory training programs?

References

American Academy of Audiology. (2010). *Guidelines for the diagnosis, treatment, and management of children and adults with central auditory processing disorder.* Available from http://www.audiology.org/resources/documentlibrary/documents/capd%20guidelines%208-2010.pdf

American Speech-Language-Hearing Association. (1996). *Central auditory processing: Current status of research and implications for clinical practice [Technical Report].* Available from www.asha.org/policy.

American Speech-Language-Hearing Association. (2004). *Auditory integration training.* Available from http://www.asha.org/docs/html/TR2004-00260.html.

American Speech-Language-Hearing Association. (2005). *(Central) auditory processing disorders—The role of the audiologist.* Available from http://www.asha.org/policy/PS2005-00114/

Anderson, K., Smaldino J. & Spangler, C. (2012) *Listening inventory for education revised.* http://lifer.successforkidswithhearingloss.com/

Auditec, Inc. (2014). *Catalog.* Available from http://www.auditec.com/cgi/Auditec2013Catalog.pdf.

Bamiou, D. E. (2007). Measures of binaural interaction. In F. Musiek & G. Chermak (Eds.), *Handbook of (central) auditory processing disorder: Auditory neuroscience and diagnosis* (pp. 257–286). San Diego, CA: Plural.

Banai, K., & Kraus, N. (2007). Neurobiology of (central) auditory processing disorder and language-based learning disability. In F. Musiek & G. Chermak (Eds.), *Handbook of (central) auditory processing disorder: Auditory neuroscience and diagnosis* (pp. 89–116). San Diego, CA: Plural.

Banai K, Nicol T, Zecker S, & Kraus N. (2005) Brainstem timing: Implications for cortical processing and literacy Journal of Neuroscience 25(43): 9850–9857.

Barmiou DE, Musiek FE, Luxon LM. An etiology and clinical presentation of auditory processing disorders: a review. *Archives of Disease in Childhood.* 2001; 85:361–5.

Bellis, T. J. (2003). *Assessment and management of central auditory processing disorders in the educational setting from science to practice.* Clifton Park, NY: Thomson Delmar Learning.

Bellis, T. J., & Ferre, J. M. (1999). Multidimensional approach to the differential diagnosis of auditory processing disorders in children. *Journal of the American Academy of Audiology, 10:* 319–328.

Berg, F. S. (1987). *Facilitating classroom listening: A handbook for teachers of normal and hard of hearing students.* Boston, MA: College-Hill Press/Little Brown.

Bocca, E. (1958). Clinical aspects of cortical deafness. *Laryngoscope, 68:* 301–309.

Bocca, E., & Calearo, C. (1963). Clinical aspects of cortical deafness. In J. Jerger (Ed.), *Modern developments in audiology* (pp. 337–370). New York: Academic Press.

Bocca, E., Calearo, C., & Cassinari, V. (1954). A new method for testing hearing in temporal lobe tumor. *Acta Otolaryngologica, 44:* 219–221.

Bocca, E., Calearo, C., Cassinari, V., & Migliavacca, F. (1955). Testing "cortical hearing" in temporal lobe tumors. *Acta Otolaryngologica, 42:* 289–304.

Cacace, A., & McFarland, D. (2009). Controversies in central auditory processing disorder. San Diego, CA: Plural.

Calero, C. & Lazzaroni, A. (1957). Speech intelligibility in relation to the speech of the message. *Laryngoscope, 67:* 410–419.

Cameron, S., Brown, D., Keith, R., Martin, J., Watson, C., & Dillon, H. (2009). Development of the North American listening in spatialized noise-sentences test (NA LiSN-S): Sentence equivalence, normative data, and test-retest reliability studies. *Journal of the American Academy of Audiology, 20*(2), 128–146.

Clarke, J. M., Lufkin, R. B., & Zaidel, E. (1993). Corpus callosum morphometry and dichotic listening performance: Individual differences in functional interhemispheric inhibition? *Neuropsychologica, 31:* 547–557.

Crandell, C., & Smaldino, J. (2004). Classroom acoustics. *Seminars in Hearing, 25:* 189–200.

Dowell, A., Milligan, B., Davis, B. D., & Hurley, A. (2011). Wii-habilitation for (central) auditory processing disorder [(C)APD]. *Journal of Educational Audiology, 17:* 76–80.

Educational Audiology Association. (2013). *EAA products.* Available from http://www.edaud.org/storeindex.cfm?startrec=1

Ferre, J. M. (2002). Managing children's central auditory processing deficits in the real world. *Seminars in Hearing, 4:* 319–326.

Fifer, R. C., Jerger, J. F., Berlin, C. I., Tobey, E. A., & Campbell, J. C. (1983). Development of a dichotic sentence identification (DSI) test for use in hearing impaired adults. *Ear and Hearing, 4*(6): 300–306.

Fisher, L. I. (1985). Fisher's Auditory Problems Checklist. *The Educational Audiology Association.*

Friberg, J. C., & McNamara, T. L. (2010). Psychometric validity of tests that assess (central) auditory processing abilities. *Journal of Educational Audiology, 16:* 59–72.

Geffner, D., & Ross-Swain, D. (2007). *Auditory processing disorders: A handbook of management and treatment for speech-language pathologists.* San Diego, CA: Plural.

Hunsaker, R. A. (1990). *Understanding and developing the skills of oral communication: Speaking and listening* (2nd ed.). Englewood, CO: Morton Press.

Hurley, A., & Billiet, C. (2008). *Dichotic interaural intensity difference (DIID) training: Auditory remediation after CVA.* Poster Presentation at the ASHA Convention, Chicago, IL.

Jalongo, M. R. (2006). *Early childhood language arts* (4th ed.). Boston, MA: Allyn & Bacon.

Jancke, L. (2002). Does "callosal delay" explain ear advantage in dichotic monitoring? *Laterality, 7:* 309–320.

Johnson, C. D., & Seaton, J. B. (2012). *Educational audiology handbook* (2nd ed.). Clifton Park, NY: Delmar Cengage Learning.

Johnson, M. L., Bellis, T. J., & Billiet, C. (2007). Audiologic assessment of (C)APD. In D. Geffner & D. Ross-Swain (Eds.), *Auditory processing disorders: Assessment, management, and treatment* (pp. 75–94). San Diego, CA: Plural.

Katz, J. (1962). The use of staggered spondaic words for assessing the integrity of the central auditory nervous system. *Journal of Auditory Research,* 2: 327–337.

Katz, J. (1992). Classification of central auditory processing disorders. In J. Katz, N. Stecker, & D. Henderson (Eds.), *Central auditory processing: A transdisciplinary view* (pp. 81–91). St. Louis, MO: Mosby

Keith, R. (2000). *Random gap detection test.* St. Louis, MO: Auditec.

Keith, R. (2009a). *SCAN-3: A tests for auditory processing disorders in adolescents and adults.* San Antonio, TX: Pearson.

Keith, R. (2009b). *SCAN-3:C tests for auditory processing disorders for children.* San Antonio, TX: Pearson.

Keith, R. W., & Anderson, J. (2007). Dichotic listening tests. In F. Musiek & G. Chermak (Eds.), *Handbook of (central) auditory processing disorder: Auditory neuroscience and diagnosis* (pp. 207–230). San Diego, CA: Plural.

Kimura, D. (1961). Some effects of temporal lobe damage on auditory perception. *Canadian Journal of Psychology,* 15: 157–165.

Kraus, N., & Chandrasekaran, B. (2010). Music training for the development of auditory skills. *Nature Reviews Neuroscience,* 11: 599–605.

Kraus, N., McGee, T. J., Carrell, T. D., Zecker, S. G., Nicol, T. G., & Koch, D. B. (1996). Auditory neurophysiologic responses and discrimination deficits in children with learning problems. *Science,* 273(5277): 971–973.

Krishnamurti, S. (2007). Monaural low-redundancy speech tests. In F. Musiek & G. Chermak (Eds.), *Handbook of (central) auditory processing disorder: Auditory neuroscience and diagnosis* (pp. 193–206). San Diego, CA: Plural.

Lynn, G. E., Gillroy, J., Taylor, P. C., & Leiser, P. C. (1981). Binaural masking-level differences in neurological disorders. *Archives of Otolaryngology,* 107: 357–362.

McNamara, T. & Richard, G. (2012). "Better together". *The ASHA Leader.* Vol.17:3, pp.12–14.

Merzenich, M. M., Jenkins, W. M., Johnston, P., Schreiner, C. E., Miller, S. L., & Tallal, P. (1996). Temporal processing deficits of language-learning impaired children ameliorated by training. *Science,* 271: 77–80.

Meyers, J. E., Roberts, R. J., Bayless, J. D., Volkert, K., & Evitts, P. E. (2002). Dichotic listening: Expanded norms and clinical application. *Archives of Clinical Neuropsychology,* 17(1): 79–90.

Moncrieff, D. W. (2011). Dichotic listening in children: Age-related changes in direction and Magnitude of ear advantage. *Brain and Cognition,* 76(2): 316–322.

Musiek, F. E. (1983). Assessment of central auditory dysfunction: Dichotic digits test revisited. *Ear and Hearing,* 4: 79–83.

Musiek, F. E. (1994). Frequency (pitch) and duration pattern tests. *Journal of the American Academy of Audiology,* 5: 265–286.

Musiek, F. E., Baran, J. A., & Shinn, J. (2004). Assessment and remediation of an auditory processing disorder associated with head trauma. *Journal of the American Academy of Audiology,* 15: 117–132.

Musiek, F. E., & Chermak, G. D. (2007). Auditory neuroscience and (central) auditory processing disorder: An overview. In F. Musiek & G. Chermak (Eds.), *Handbook of (central) auditory processing disorder: Auditory neuroscience and diagnosis* (pp. 3–12). San Diego, CA: Plural.

Musiek, F., Chermak, G., & Weihing, J. (2007). *Auditory training.* In F. E. Musiek & G. D. Chermak (Eds.), *Handbook of (central) auditory processing disorder: Comprehensive intervention* (Vol I; pp. 77–106). San Diego, CA: Plural.

Musiek, F. E., Kibbe, K., & Baran, J. (1984). Neuroaudiological results from split-brain patients. *Seminars in Hearing,* 5: 210–229.

Musiek, F. E., Pinheiro, M., & Wilson, D. (1980). Auditory pattern perception in "split-brain" patients. *Archives of Otolaryngology,* 106: 610–612.

Musiek, F. E., Shinn, J. B., Jirsa, R., Bamiou, D. E., Baran, J. A., & Zaidan, E. (2005). The GIN (gaps-in-noise) test performance in subjects with confirmed central auditory nervous system involvement. *Ear and Hearing,* 26: 608–618.

Obrzut, J. G., Boliek, C., & Obrzut, A. (1986). The effect of stimulus type and directed attention on dichotic listening with children. *Journal of Experimental Psychology,* 41: 198–209.

Parthasarathy, T. K. (2006). *An introduction to auditory processing disorders in children.* Mahwah, NJ: Lawrence Erlbaum Associates.

Pinheiro, M. L., & Musiek, F. E. (1985). Sequencing and temporal ordering in the auditory system. In M. L. Pinheiro & F. E. Musiek (Eds.), *Assessment of central auditory dysfunctions: Foundations and clinical correlates* (pp. 219–238). Baltimore, MD: Williams & Wilkins.

Richard, G., & Ferre, J. (2006). *Differential screening test for processing.* East Moline, IL: LinguiSystems.

Richard, G. J. (2007). Language processing versus auditory processing. In D. Geffner & D. Ross-Swain (Eds.), *Auditory processing disorders: Assessment, management, and treatment* (pp. 161–174). San Diego, CA: Plural.

Ross, E. D., & Monnot, M. (2008). Neurology of affective prosody and its functional-anatomic organization in right hemisphere. *Brain and Language,* 104: 51–74.

Schow, R. L., Chermak, G. D., Seikel, J. A., Brockett, J. E., & Whitaker, M. M. (2006). *Multiple auditory processing assessment.* St. Louis, MO: Auditec.

Shinn, J. B. (2007). Temporal processing and temporal patterning tests. In F. Musiek & G. Chermak (Eds.), *Handbook of (central) auditory processing disorder: Auditory neuroscience and diagnosis* (pp. 397–416). San Diego, CA: Plural.

Smoski, W. J., Brunt, M. A., & Tannahill, J. C.(1998). Children's Auditory Performance Scale. Tampa, FL: *The Educational Audiology Association.*

Tallal, P., Miller, S. L., Bedi, G., Byma, G., Wang, X., Nagarajan, S. S., et al. (1996). Language comprehension in language-learning impaired children improved with acoustically modified speech. *Science,* 271: 81–84.

Taylor, I., & Taylor, M. M. (1990). *Psycholinguistics: Learning and using language.* San Antonio, TX: Pearson.

Wilson, L. K., & Mueller, H. G. (1984). Performance of normal hearing individuals on Auditec filtered speech tests. *ASHA, 26,* 120.

Chapter 17

Acute, Subacute, and Nursing Home/Long-Term Care Facilities

Carol A. Ukstins, MS, CCC-A, FAAA
Educational Audiologist
Office of Special Education
Newark Public Schools

Deborah R. Welling, AuD, CCC-A, FAAA
Associate Professor and Director of Clinical Education
Department of Speech-Language Pathology
Seton Hall University

Key Terms

Acute care
Americans with Disabilities
   Act (ADA)
Consulting audiologist
Five stages of grief model
Hearing Handicap Inventory
   for the Elderly

In-service training
Medical model
Minimum Data Set
   for Nursing Home
   Residents Assessment and
   Care Screening
   Tool (MDS)

Omnibus Budget
   Reconciliation Act
   (OBRA)
Subacute care
Veterans Affairs facility

Objectives

- Understand the variety of services and responsibilities required of the speech-language pathologist in acute, subacute, and nursing home/long-term care facilities
- Define the role and responsibilities of the speech-language pathologist when working with an individual with hearing loss in an acute versus subacute setting
- Understand and describe the difference between the medical and educational model of service provision
- Discuss the different tools used to assess hearing and auditory communication status in the subacute and nursing home/long-term care settings
- Identify and describe the hearing aid issues and considerations for the patient in a nursing home/long-term care facility

Introduction

One of the most exciting aspects of being a speech-language pathologist is the wide variety of settings available to the professional. Although the majority of speech-language pathologists will find themselves employed in school systems (Lubinski, 2013) many will also seek employment in subacute facilities, rehabilitation centers, and long-term care facilities. Regardless of setting, eventually the speech-language pathologist will find him- or herself working with someone who is hearing impaired. The purpose of this chapter is to enable the speech-language pathologist to manage the resources available when working in such facilities, in the best interest of their patient with hearing loss.

Acute Care

Acute care settings deal with medically complex individuals; patients in this type of setting are usually treated for a sudden episode or illness. Speech-language pathologists (SLPs) in this setting provide evaluation and treatment for a variety of disorders, which may include, but not be limited to, swallowing, and speech and language deficits resulting from strokes, head injury, respiratory, and other issues. Additionally, according to the American Speech-Language-Hearing Association (ASHA, n.d., para.2), the top five primary medical diagnoses of acute care patients are cerebrovascular accident (CVA) or stroke, head injury, hemorrhage/injury, respiratory illnesses, and central nervous system (CNS) disease. Each of these disorders can cause and/or be associated with impaired auditory system function. Therefore, before the SLP does a speech-language evaluation on an acute care patient with a communication disorder of any type, finding out about the patient's hearing status will be very helpful.

In this section we will discuss different aspects of providing services in an acute care setting to patients who may experience hearing loss either comorbidly or as a direct result of the acute medical illness for which they are being treated.

The Medical Model of Health Care

In the United States and in many countries around the world, acute healthcare facilities provide care to their patients based on a **medical model** of service delivery. This model depends on an interdisciplinary group of trained professional and paraprofessionals working with a single patient. This interdisciplinary team is led by a primary physician who manages the overall care of the patient and forms this interdisciplinary team based on the needs of the patient. In this healthcare model, written requests for consultation by members of this team, otherwise known as doctor's orders, are required for all preventative, curative, consultative and rehabilitation services. No care can be provided to a patient without orders from the primary care physician (Zenzano et al., 2011).

As a speech-language pathologist working in an acute care facility, typically, your department will receive a written form (order) to provide consultation, evaluation, and rehabilitation within your scope of practice to the patient under the physician's care. This written process is carefully executed based on the liability of patient care and malpractice set forth by each hospital facility. In this employment setting, chances are that you will find yourself working side by side with one or more audiologist(s) in the same department or facility. Consulting with this individual on patient care becomes a routine part of the speech-language pathologist's day. If there is no full-time or part-time audiologist on staff at the hospital, find out who the **consulting audiologist** of record is. Alternately, if an individual has been identified in the patient chart as being hard of hearing or deaf, find out who the managing audiologist is and consult with that professional instead, or in addition.

Consulting Audiologists

In many rural healthcare facilities, audiologists may be hired as consultants rather than full-time employees of the healthcare facility. In this scenario, as the on-staff speech-language pathologist you may find yourself providing audiologic screening services, hearing aid maintenance, and the like based on your scope of practice (ASHA, 2007). In this setting you may be required to meet with the audiologist when that professional is on schedule for his or her assigned day(s) of consultation to the facility. In this case, it may be important (and useful) to establish a mutually agreeable time with that individual to review cases and update the audiologist on any new cases that have been admitted and any services that you have provided or may need to be prepared to provide in their absence. As acute care facilities attempt to keep a patient's stay as brief as possible, you may be asked to provide services that are not within your scope of practice at the urging of the facility in the absence of the consulting audiologist. It is therefore of utmost importance, when working in a medical facility with an audiologist on a consulting basis, that strict procedures are in place regarding each professional's responsibility to the patient with hearing loss.

Specialty Clinics

Acute care facilities that specialize in a specific disability, such as pediatric cochlear implants, cleft palate, or Down syndrome, may have established specialty clinics. When patients are seen in specialty clinics, a multidisciplinary team of medical and allied health professionals is gathered for a period of time. Typically clinics are run for a half day, either morning or afternoon, on a delineated day of the week or month (e.g., the third Tuesday of the month) when all patients are scheduled to arrive at a single time and are cycled through the specialty areas addressing the multiple needs of the patient. Because of the multiple conditions of the patient, hearing screenings may be a responsibility assigned to the speech-language pathologist as part of a comprehensive speech and language evaluation of the patient. The SLP should find out what the established protocol is for the screening and for referring a patient for a complete audiologic evaluation, should a patient fail the screening procedure. The SLP should then discuss with the multidisciplinary team that a speech and language evaluation should be postponed until hearing thresholds are established. Many hospitals running specialty clinics will have scheduled multidisciplinary team meetings following a clinic or at another scheduled time. This is the speech-language pathologist's opportunity to discuss the hearing concerns and recommendations for referral to an audiologist. If such meetings are not part of the particular hospital's clinic policy, then the SLP should find out what the hospital's system is for information sharing of this nature and the procedure for referring patients to the audiologist when a problem is suspected.

Veterans Affairs (VA) Hospitals

The U.S. Department of Veterans Affairs, also known as the VA, administers more than 1,700 hospitals, clinics, community living centers, domiciliary care centers, and readjustment counseling centers across the country. These facilities make up the largest integrated healthcare system in the United States. Services of the VA include a variety of medical and allied health benefits that are available to members of the armed services, veterans, their immediate families, and their survivors. Speech-language pathologists working in **VA facilities** will discover that audiologists are also widely employed by the VA to provide a range of services including the evaluation of hearing sensitivity, hearing aid dispensing, and aural rehabilitation services for military and veteran personnel as well as their families. As with acute and subacute facilities, the speech-language pathologist is encouraged to seek out the audiology department within the VA facility of employment,

understanding that he or she may not be associated with the department of speech-language pathology, but rather with the otolaryngology department of the hospital.

The following summarizes the long-term relationship between the VA and audiologists:

- The first VA audiology clinic opened in 1946 in New York.
- The VA is the largest employer of audiologists in the country.
- The VA is the largest single purchaser of hearing aids in the United States.
- The VA provides routine grant opportunities for research in the field of audiology.
- The first recorded materials for speech audiometry came from the Mountain Home VA Hospital in Tennessee (Jerger, n.d.).

Readers are encouraged to go the U.S. Department of Veterans Affairs at www.va.gov for additional information on healthcare settings and services available for patients who have served in the U.S. military.

Subacute Care

The definition of **subacute care**, as developed by several organizations (i.e., the American Health Care Association [AHCA], the Joint Commission, and the Association of Hospital-Based Skilled Nursing Facilities), states that subacute care is comprehensive inpatient care designed for someone who has an acute illness, injury, or exacerbation of a disease process. It is a goal-oriented treatment immediately after, or instead of, acute hospitalization (Kuchar, 2006). Patients are sent to the subacute facility once they have been stabilized in the medical facility (e.g., hospital), and no longer meet the criteria for that acute hospital setting. The subacute settings cover a wide range of services and may specialize in a specific type of care, either long term or rehabilitative in nature. The level of care provided in subacute units is generally for higher acuity conditions than care provided in long-term care units, but of lower acuity than in acute care hospital units (Kiresuk, 2010). The services are comprehensive and goal oriented, and many facilities may choose to use an interdisciplinary approach. These authors have found the collaborative approach to be most successful in our practice as communication disorders service providers.

The length of stay for a patient in subacute care depends on the individual patient's needs; however, it is likely to be longer, and in some cases considerably so, than the acute phase of care. As such, the speech-language pathologist will have more extensive contact with the patient, and have a greater variety of therapeutic experiences with them. The needs of the SLP in terms of understanding the nature, severity, impact of hearing loss, and hearing aids/assistive devices will be that much greater in this setting as well. Therefore, it is imperative that the speech-language pathologist establish whether there is an audiologist who consults with the particular subacute facility for the hearing health care of the patients while in residence. There may be a regularly scheduled day that the audiologist is there to see all patients referred for services. This person may be on call as needed and, as the speech-language pathologist, you may be the point person to identify and contact the audiologist when services are needed. The process for doing so must be clearly identified and, even better, documented in writing between the facility and the speech-language pathologist. Regardless, you must familiarize yourself with the policy of the facility. Likewise, a hearing aid dispenser may also be contracted to service the facility in a similar fashion. Again, good communication is the key to working with these individuals as partners in patient care. Many hospitals are affiliated with specific subacute facilities for the continuity of care for their patients. It is wise to make sure that you are aware of the facility's hospital affiliation(s), and the acceptable process of communication with that facility.

The Case History

If an established protocol for a relationship with the sending facility exists, this will enable you, as the speech-language pathologist on staff, to consult with the physician/specialist who may be familiar with the patient. If such a model of consultation is not available, then the patient records should be thoroughly reviewed. Always begin with a thorough case history. In such a facility you may encounter several stumbling blocks to a comprehensive case history, including records not being transferred properly with the patient, records being delayed but pressure to begin therapy being applied to you, the absence of family who can provide accurate information, the presence of a family member who is providing inaccurate information, and/or a patient who is unable, due to their medical condition, to provide an accurate self-report.

Case History Information Related to Hearing Loss

In many instances, when working in subacute care facilities, a significant emotional component regarding the overall status of the admitted patient may exist. Actual versus perceived medical condition, the family's emotional bond with the patient, their desire to see the patient return to full health and function, overall quality of life, and the reality of their loved one's prognosis, may all be factors that will stand in the way of an accurate case history (Adams-Wendling & Pimple, 2008). The patient and/or family and loved ones' reactions to some of the significant life changes that precipitate entry into the acute or subacute setting can resemble the stages that individuals have been observed to experience when faced with the prospects of death and dying (Long, 2011).

Dr. Elisabeth Kübler-Ross is well known for her methodology in the support and counseling of personal tragedy and grieving associated with death and dying. She also dramatically improved the understanding and counseling practices related to bereavement and hospice care. Her influential book, *On Death and Dying* (1969), mapped out a five-stage framework, known as the **five stages of grief model**, to explain the experience of dying patients, which progress through denial, anger, bargaining for time, depression, and acceptance (Columbia Electronic Encyclopedia, 2011). These stages are also observed in people and family members experiencing personal change and emotional upset resulting from factors other than death and bereavement.

This makes Kübler-Ross's model worth including when discussing the varied emotions the speech-language pathologist will encounter when working with both the patient and family members in acute and subacute care facilities. The model helps remind us that a person's perspective may be different from our own. Getting through this emotional component of patient care will allow the speech-language pathologist to better understand the patient's needs as a whole, understanding that family support is an important part of patient care as well.

Several key points may assist you in focusing case history questions that will allow you to proceed ethically with the care of your patient with hearing loss. First and foremost, you must know their diagnosis. What has led them to the facility? Was the event a stroke, car accident, or some other trauma? Even if you think the problem is not related to a hearing loss, it is most worthy of investigation. Often, a medical condition or diagnosis may not seem to be related to the auditory system, but there are conditions that can actually cause or exacerbate an existing hearing loss, and there also may be comorbidities. Again, your patient may or may not be the best historian. If the availability of records is limited, or if the family or the patient cannot be a reliable informant, try to answer the following questions:

- What is the patient's diagnosis?
- Is there a secondary or tertiary diagnosis?
- How long did the patient reside in an acute care facility?
- Is there anything in the chart that may be a red flag for hearing loss: notes from the physician that indicate the patient did not appear to comprehend instructions, nurse's notes indicating that the patient was speaking in a loud voice or patient was listening to the television too loud?
- Is there a pharmacological potential for hearing loss that may or may not have been discussed with the patient?
- Is the patient complaining of tinnitus?
- Do you see hearing aids? Remember, they may *not* be in the patient's ears; they may be with their belongings, or on an inventory list upon transfer from the acute care facility. Many times family members will take the hearing aids home, worried that they will be lost in the transition to a subacute facility. Do not assume that if a patient has hearing aids they will be in their ears.

Hard of Hearing Patients in Subacute Care

Beyond the legal rights of patient care and the **Americans with Disabilities Act (ADA)** laws of access, the speech-language pathologist may find him- or herself in a place of advocacy for appropriate communication between facility staff and the patient. One example may be creating and posting an advisement regarding hearing loss by a patient's bed or on the door of the patient's room to aid in communication.

In-service training, grand rounds, and patient review panels are examples of other avenues by which the speech-language pathologist can advocate for the hard of hearing patient. Other responsibilities may include counseling with the family members regarding follow-up for obtaining appropriate hearing evaluation/hearing aid purchase, tolerance when communicating with the family member, and/or encouragement for routine hearing aid use. Realistic expectations should also be set for the family regarding the benefit of amplification.

The Deaf Patient in Subacute Care

Rights of communication access become of paramount concern with the deaf patient in any medical facility. The denial of the ADA rights of access have led to many civil rights lawsuits across the United States between the deaf

Figure 17.1 Universal sign for deafness.

patient and healthcare facility. In reviewing the ADA rights, attention should be drawn to the word *obligated* in terms of providing interpreting services for the deaf patient and deaf family members as well. The purpose of this terminology is clear. Effective communication and a clear understanding of symptoms, medical diagnosis, and follow-up care are paramount to a patient's care. Failure to provide effective communication can result in misdiagnosis, delay in treatment, or even worse (i.e., inappropriate treatment). Again, the speech-language pathologist may find him- or herself in a position of being an advocate or facilitator of such services throughout their facility of employment.

Universal Sign for Deafness

Figure 17.1 shows the universal advisement sign for deafness. Posting of this sign on a patient's door or above the bed, with further directions on the ADA rights of communication (see previous section), may be beneficial to the prevention of facility liability.

Nursing Homes and Long-Term Care Facilities

The American Speech-Language-Hearing Association, Ad Hoc Committee of Audiology Service Delivery in Home Care and Institutional Settings, has published "Guidelines for Audiology Service Delivery in Nursing Homes" (ASHA, 1997). The document provides specific practice procedure recommendations for audiologists working in such facilities, but can also be used as a guideline for the speech-language pathologist servicing the hard of hearing or deaf patient. The speech-language pathologist should function only within his or her own scope of practice when providing services for the hard of hearing and deaf patients in such facilities.

Defining and Identifying Staff

Seeking out the appropriate professionals for providing care to the hard of hearing or deaf patient will be paramount to the success of patient care. Is there an audiologist on staff? Is that individual full time, part time, or available only on a consultative basis? Are the audiologist's services defined by the facility through a job description or an internal scope of practice?

Many long-term care facilities will also employ or have a working relationship with a local hearing aid dispenser. Whether licensed and credentialed as an audiologist or hearing aid professional will depend on the individual state regulations, which vary greatly from state to state. This person may or may not be the audiologist providing evaluation and follow-up care to the hard of hearing or deaf patient within the facility. Some facilities may use audiology technicians in lieu of a certified audiologist, in which case the speech-language pathologist may want to identify who the supervising audiologist is, and communicate with that person as well. Other facilities may employ no one at all, relying on the patient's family to provide such care. It is important that the speech-language pathologist determine the extent of service provision and work with the professionals in this area or make appropriate recommendations for the establishment of audiology services within the facility.

Minimum Data Set for Nursing Home Residents Assessment and Care Screening Tool (MDS)

The **Omnibus Budget Reconciliation Act** of 1987 (OBRA) requires all nursing homes receiving federal funding to assess each new patient using the **Minimum Data Set for Nursing Home Residents Assessment and Care Screening Tool (MDS)**. The MDS is part of the U.S. federally mandated process for clinical assessment that is to be administered to all nursing home patients in Medicare and Medicaid certified nursing homes within the first 14 days of admission. It covers a wide range of functional areas from behavior to special needs, including hearing acuity and hearing aid use (ASHA, 1997). The results of the MDS will drive the patient care program of the nursing home facility, which may include further evaluations involving the services of an audiologist.

Hearing Screening Tools

OBRA further addresses screening procedures for patients within the nursing home facility, including that of a hearing screening. As an audiologist, the term *screening* naturally refers to the use of calibrated electronic technology used to assess auditory thresholds. However, there are other tools, used inside and/or outside the field of audiology, that are used to help determine hearing and communication status and the need for further referral and interventions.

Audiometric Screening

If your information gathering, thus far, suggests that an audiometric screening has not been done, or cannot be located, then it is recommended that it be performed. Some of the audiometric screening devices that may be available and used to assess hearing acuity include audioscopes, otoacoustic emission screeners, and the traditional screening audiometer. These pieces of equipment may be available within the facility to more accurately assess auditory acuity versus perceived hearing status.

Questionnaires

In addition to the audiometric type of screening, other methods and tools, such as questionnaires and behavioral observation checklists, help determine hearing status and its concomitant impact on communication. These inventories rely on self-assessment and quality-of-life questions using the patient's or family's viewpoint of communication status (Lichtenstein, Bess, & Logan, 1988). An example of this type of measure is the **Hearing Handicap Inventory for the Elderly** (Ventry & Weinstein, 1982). This tool is a 25-item questionnaire that measures an individual's perceived activity limitation and participation restriction as a result of the hearing loss. Ventry and Weinstein also developed a screening version of this tool (1983), the Hearing Handicap Inventory for the Elderly–Screener version (HHIE-S), which is shown in **Figure 17.2**. This abbreviated version contains 10 questions, and can be easily and quickly administered to a patient.

As described by Thoren, Andersson, and Lunner (2012), there are other paper and pencil questionnaires that can be successfully used in this population; some of them address the patient's functional abilities with their hearing aids (or other device) in place, such as the International Outcome Inventory for Hearing Aids (IOI-HA), which is a seven-item questionnaire that measures the benefit of hearing aids (Cox & Alexander, 2001; Cox, Alexander, & Beyer, 2003; Cox et al., 2000), and the Satisfaction with Amplification in

Screening Version of the Hearing Handicap Inventory for the Elderly (HHIE-S)

ITEM	YES (4 pts)	SOMETIMES (2 pts)	NO (0 pts)
Does a hearing problem cause you to feel embarrassed when you meet new people?	_____	_____	_____
Does a hearing problem cause you to feel frustrated when talking to members of your family?	_____	_____	_____
Do you have difficulty hearing when someone speaks in a whisper?	_____	_____	_____
Do you feel handicapped by a hearing problem?	_____	_____	_____
Does a hearing problem cause you difficulty when visiting friends, relatives, or neighbors?	_____	_____	_____
Does a hearing problem cause you to attend religious services less often than you would like?	_____	_____	_____
Does a hearing problem cause you to have arguments with family members?	_____	_____	_____
Does a hearing problem cause you difficulty when listening to TV or radio?	_____	_____	_____
Do you feel that any difficulty with your hearing limits or hampers your personal or social life?	_____	_____	_____
Does a hearing problem cause you difficulty when in a restaurant with relatives or friends?	_____	_____	_____

RAW SCORE _____ (sum of the points assigned each of the items)

INTERPRETING THE RAW SCORE

 0 to 8 = 13% probability of hearing impairment (no handicap/no referral)

 10 to 24 = 50% probability of hearing impairment (mild-moderate handicap/refer)

 26 to 40 = 84% probability of hearing impairment (severe handicap/refer)

Figure 17.2   Screening version of the Hearing Handicap Inventory for the Elderly (HHIE-S).

Reproduced from Ventry, I. and Weinstein, B. (1983). Identification of elderly people with hearing problems. American Speech-Language-Hearing Association; July, 37–42.

Daily Life (SADL) (Cox & Alexander, 2001), which is a 15-item questionnaire that measures the benefits and positive effects of hearing aids on a seven-point scale.

Whispered Voice Screening Test

Another screening tool used is the Whispered Voice Screening Test (Swan & Browning, 1985). In this screening, the examiner stands 2 feet away from and behind the patient, in order to remove the ability to speech read, and whispers into the test ear; at the same time, the examiner occludes (using a finger) and simultaneously gently rubs the nontest ear, in an attempt to mask the nontest ear. A random set of three numbers or letters is then verbally presented, with the direction to repeat what the examiner has said. Despite the fact that it may be difficult to compare results of this test from examiner to examiner, within the same examiner it has been found to be a valid and reliable screen for hearing loss (Bagai, Thavendiranathan, & Detsky, 2006).

Hearing Aid Care in the Nursing Home

One of the greatest challenges the speech-language pathologist will face in a nursing home facility when caring for the hard of hearing patient is designing a plan for hearing aid use, care, safety, maintenance, and accountability. A care plan can be incorporated into therapy goals and can employ the participation of the patient, nursing services, family members, and housekeeping. What follows is a brief, non-exhaustive list of issues that should be considered when designing a care plan:

- *Patient's view of amplification:* Is the patient amenable to using the hearing aid(s)? What is the word discrimination ability of the patient? Are the hearing aids just making poor word discrimination louder? Remember, hearing aids make things louder, not always clearer. They cannot always correct the distortional aspect of a sensorineural hearing loss.

- *Hearing aid manipulation:* Can the patient manipulate the hearing aid? Does the patient know how it operates? Are the family members knowledgeable about the care and manipulation of the device(s) as well? The speech-language pathologist often has more regular contact with the patient than do the audiologist and/or hearing aid dispenser and therefore must become educated regarding care, manipulation, and functionality of each patient's hearing aid(s). The SLP would be well served to contact the audiologist, hearing aid dispenser, and also a representative from the hearing aid technology manufacturer for any necessary guidance.

- *When hearing aids aren't used for listening:* Is the patient spending most of the time sleeping in his or her room? Remember, feedback (a high-pitched electronic whistle) occurs when the seal between the ear and the hearing aid is broken and amplified sound leaks out of the ear and is reamplified. When a patient lies on their side and is wearing a hearing aid, the pinna is pushed back, creating this situation. Frequently, in a partially sleeping state, the hearing aid may be removed and placed on a side table or on the bed sheet.

- *Who is responsible for the hearing aid batteries?* As with small children, caution should be used with hearing aid batteries in patients with waning cognitive status. Hearing aid batteries can be mistaken for medication and ingested, causing significant internal damage. Should consideration be given to tamper-resistant battery doors on the devices (Cohen-Mansfield & Taylor, 2004)?

- *Vanity thy name is hearing aid:* Socially interactive patients who want to use their hearing aids also insist on looking their best. Hairspray is an arch enemy of a hearing aid, clogging the microphone, on/off switch, and volume control wheel of the device. Instructing the patient to put on jewelry and hearing aids after completing a hair care routine will extend the life of the hearing aid.

- *Cerumen management:* Cerumen, or ear wax, is another arch enemy of the hearing aid. During the aging process, ear wax tends to get drier and harder. In addition to clogging up the small components of the hearing aid, hearing aid's mere presence in the ear disturbs the body's natural process for moving the wax out of the ear canal. The growth of hair in the ear also contributes to the impaction of cerumen in the elderly patient. Although the saying, "Never stick anything smaller than your elbow in your ear" holds true, the elderly patient always seems to find small thin objects to use in an attempt to remove ear wax.

- *Consider other devices for terminal patients:* Small portable devices, frequently called *pocket talkers*, are available at local electronic stores and are an affordable alternative to hearing aids for improving the quality of life for terminally ill patients. These devices function as a small amplifier, and are the size of an iPod or old transistor radio. Earphones are attached via an earphone jack and the volume is controlled manually. Such devices can be used to communicate pertinent information to a patient and then can be removed for the comfort of the patient when not in use. **Figure 17.3** shows an example of a Pocket Talker Pro.

- *What is the plan for follow-up?* Routine hearing evaluations will indicate if there has been a change in auditory status that may or may not require reprogramming of the hearing aid(s). Cerumen management may have to be done on a routine basis to prevent issues of occlusion or interference with amplification usage. Whatever the case, a clear, routine plan for follow-up audiologic testing, medical management, and hearing aid maintenance should be discussed with the patient and the family.

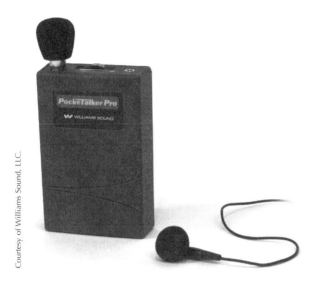

Figure 17.3   Pocket Talker Pro.

Aural Rehabilitation Groups

The speech-language pathologist may be requested, or required, to facilitate therapy groups for hearing-impaired patients within the nursing home facility. These groups might center on self-advocacy for the hard of hearing patient, hearing aid care, listening strategies with and without hearing aids, and understanding the nature of hearing loss. Specifics on running such a group will depend on the needs of the patients and their individual goals for therapy. There may also be local community resources such as the Hearing Loss Association of America (HLAA; available on the web at www.hearingloss.org), formerly known as Self Help for the Hard of Hearing (SHHH), which facilitate such services or work in conjunction with the speech-language pathologist servicing the patients. State agencies for the deaf and hard of hearing are also a useful resource. Frequently, publications from such agencies will provide information regarding support groups and interpreter services or social activities throughout the area.

Aural rehabilitation groups are also an excellent avenue to involve family members in the hearing health care of the nursing home patient. Information packets describing many of the care and maintenance issues can be disseminated at such meetings. Realistic goals and expectations can also be discussed in general terms, easing some of the frustration that the family members may be having in communicating with the patient. When issues such as these are discussed in group settings, there is less of a chance of confrontational issues coming up that may cloud the ability of

the family to understand the nature of the patient's hearing loss and communication needs.

In-Service Training

Perhaps the most valuable asset you will have in the nursing home is the other staff members with whom you will work. Training those staff members, nurses, nurses' aides, environmental engineers, and the staff responsible for linens and laundry will be crucial to the overall well-being and quality of life of the hard of hearing patient in a nursing home facility. **In-service training** may present a specific challenge with these staff members; the speech-language pathologist must make every effort to put aside the vocabulary of the field and break down the terminology to a level that can be understood by lay personnel. As professionals in the disciplines of audiology and speech-language pathology, we gain comfort in our terminology; however, discussing a "postauricular hearing aid fitting appropriately around the pinna" may cause the audience to lose attention to the material being taught. "This is a typical behind-the-ear hearing aid, and it is made to fit comfortably around this part of the ear" may be more user-friendly language that can be understood by all. A good rule of thumb is to practice any presentation on family members not trained in the field to determine if the instructional level of content is appropriate for your audience.

In-service training allows the speech-language pathologist to assist in staff team building, which benefits not only the atmosphere of the workspace, but also the attitude of patient care. Make sure that the material being covered is applicable to the current environment of the facility (i.e., don't train the staff on communicating with deaf residents if there isn't currently a deaf resident in the home). Keep training light-hearted and fun. Whenever possible, make training hands on, with lots of interactive exercises. Even the title of the training is important to spark an interest in the topic at hand (McLagan, 1978). "How to Spot a Hearing Aid in a Laundry Cart," "Do You Hear What I Hear?" "It's Not that I Didn't Hear You, I Was Ignoring You," are just some ideas of catchy titles that may motivate someone to attend your workshop.

We have all participated in continuing education forums and been asked to fill out a questionnaire before leaving. Have you ever wondered why? Judging the value and ultimate results of in-service instruction is also an important part of the training process. Feedback from the trainees is important for judging their understanding of materials, their attitude about the subject matter, and how receptive they will be in changing their current work behaviors. Feedback regarding the trainer's ability to instruct and hold their interest, and the trainees' desire to be trained further on similar topics, will allow the facility administration to plan for future trainings (Dopyera & Lay-Dopyera, 1980).

Most important, the goal of your training should be ongoing, not a one-shot deal, to better educate your coworkers on effectively communicating with the deaf and hard of hearing patient.

Summary

The speech-language pathologist providing therapeutic interventions to hard of hearing and deaf patients in an acute, subacute, or nursing home setting will face a wide variety of challenges; they may range from identifying the patient's auditory diagnosis to in-service education for all staff in a given facility. This chapter provides some guidance and suggestions for the practicing clinician for managing these challenging situations. Although some of these matters may at first seem intimidating, remember that your goal is to practice as an interprofessional collaborative team. The mutual sharing and collaboration among the speech-language pathologist, audiologist, hearing aid dispenser, and other involved healthcare professionals is in the best interest for optimal patient outcome.

The reader is encouraged to explore some of the resources provided in this chapter, and to seek out your "friendly local audiologist" with any questions or problems that may be better solved with the collaborative approach.

Discussion Questions

1. Describe the medical model of healthcare provision. How might this differ from an educational model?
2. What is the difference between a consulting audiologist and a staff audiologist? List three ways you could easily locate these professionals.
3. How has Veterans Affairs played an important role in the development of audiology services in the United States?
4. List three factors that might stand in the way of providing services to a hard of hearing patient in a subacute facility. How would you remedy each situation?
5. You have been assigned to a 75-year-old resident with hearing aids in the nursing home. Design either (1) a hearing loss advisement poster to place at the door of the patient's room, or (2) an outline for an in-service training for the nursing home staff.

References

Adams-Wendling, L., & Pimple, C. (2008). Evidence-based guideline: Nursing management of hearing impairment in nursing facility residents. *Journal of Gerontological Nursing*, 34(11): 9–17.

American Speech-Language-Hearing Association. (1997). *Guidelines for audiology service delivery in nursing homes*. Available from http://www.asha.org/policy.

American Speech-Language-Hearing Association. (2007). *Scope of practice in speech-language pathology*. Available from http://www.asha.org/policy.

American Speech-Language-Hearing Association. (n.d.). *Getting started in acute care hospitals*. Available from http://www.asha.org/slp/healthcare/start_acute_care/.

Bagai, A., Thavendiranathan, P., & Detsky, A. S. (2006). Does this patient have hearing impairment? *Journal of the American Medical Association*, 295(4): 416–428.

Cohen-Mansfield, J., & Taylor, J. W. (2004). Hearing aid use in nursing homes, Part 2: Barriers to effective utilization of hearing aids. *Journal of the American Medical Directors Association*, 5(5): 289–296.

Cox, R., Hyde, M., Gatehouse, S., Noble, W., Dillon, H., Bentler, R., et al. (2000). Optimal outcome measures, research priorities, and international cooperation. *Ear and Hearing*, 21(Suppl. 4): 106–115.

Cox, R. M., & Alexander, G. C. (2001). Validation of the SADL questionnaire. *Ear and Hearing*, 22: 151–160.

Cox, R. M., Alexander, G. C., & Beyer, C. M. (2003). Norms for the international outcome inventory for hearing aids (IOI-HA). *Journal of the American Academy of Audiology,* 14(8): 403–413.

Dopyera, J. E., & Lay-Dopyera, M. (1980). Effective evaluation: Is there something more? *Training and Development Journal,* 34(11): 67–70.

Jerger, J. (n. d.) A brief audiological journey. Microsoft PowerPoint AAA presentation. Available at www.audiology.org/documents/An2009handouts/FS111_Jerger.pdf

Kiresuk, T. B. (2010). Intermediate length of stay: Bridging the gap of care delivery. *Doctor of Nursing Practice Systems Change Project.* Paper 4. http://sophia.stkate.edu/dnp_projects/4

Kübler-Ross, E. (1969). *On death and dying.* New York: Touchstone, Simon & Schuster.

Kuchar, J. (2006, Feb. 5). What is subacute care? *Families of Loved Ones Magazine.* Available from http://www.familiesoflovedones.com/index.php?option=com_content@task=view@id=33@itemid=29.

Lichtenstein, M. J., Bess, F. H., & Logan, S. A. (1988). Validation of screening tools for identifying hearing-impaired elderly in primary care. *Journal of the American Medical Association,* 259(19): 2875–2878.

Long, T. G. (2011). Grief without stages. *Christian Century,* 128(13): 35.

Lubinski R. (2013). Speech Therapy or Speech-Language Pathology. In: JH Stone, M Blouin, editors. *International Encyclopedia of Rehabilitation.* Available online: http://cirrie.buffalo.edu/encyclopedia/en/article/333/

McLagan, P. A. (1978). *Helping others learn.* Reading, MA: Addison-Wesley.

Swan, I. R., & Browning, G. G. (1985). The whispered voice as a screening test for hearing impairment. *Journal of the Royal College of General Practitioners,* 35: 197.

Thoren, E. S., Andersson, G., & Lunner, T. (2012). The use of research questionnaires with hearing impaired adults: Online vs. paper-and-pencil administration. *Ear, Nose and Throat Disorders,* 12: 12. Available from http://biomedcentral.com/1472-6815/12/12.

Ventry, I. M., & Weinstein, B. E. (1982). The hearing handicap inventory for the elderly: A new tool. *Ear and Hearing,* 3(3): 128–134.

Ventry I. M., & Weinstein B. E. (1983). Identification of elderly people with hearing problems. *ASHA,* 25: 37–42.

Zenzano, T., Allan, J. D., Bigley, M. B., Bushardt, R. L., Garr, D. R., Johnson, K., et al. (2011). The roles of healthcare professionals in implementing clinical prevention and population health. *American Journal of Preventive Medicine,* 40(2): 261–267.

Glossary

Acceleration The speed (distance traveled per unit of time) of an object per unit of time, which is represented mathematically as length divided by time.

Accreditation norm A norm geared around competence, which includes standard operating procedures (SOP) that are evidence based and scientifically "validated."

Acoustic reflex decay Measures how long and how well the acoustic reflex is capable of sustaining itself. In the normal system, the acoustic reflex should be able to maintain its contraction for a period of time before it drops off; however, the auditory system whose reflex falls off too quickly is abnormal.

Acoustic reflex threshold The acoustic threshold at which the muscles of the middle ear contract in response to a high-intensity sound.

Acoustic stapedial reflex Involuntary contractions of the middle ear muscles, the stapedius (primarily) and the tensor tympani, which occur in response to high-intensity sound.

Acoustics The study of sound; a branch of physics.

Acquired hearing loss A hearing loss that is the result of an illness, disease, or disorder that was not present at birth.

Acute care Refers to a medical setting where patients are treated for a sudden episode or illness. A hospital stay in an acute care facility is typically brief, only until a patient is considered medically stable.

Air conduction The normal means of sound transmission to our ears in day-to-day situations. Sound transmitted through air reaches the outer ear and travels through the middle ear to the organ of hearing in the inner ear and then is sent along the central auditory pathway to the brain for interpretation.

Amblyaudia A term coined by Moncrieff (2011). Represents the atypical dominance in ear advantage, in which a left-ear advantage may reflect right-hemisphere dominance or mixed right- and left-hemisphere governance for language (Keith & Anderson, 2007).

American sign language A visual language system of communication that is based on hand shapes, hand movements, and gestures relative to their placement on the body.

Americans with Disabilities Act A federal civil rights law that protects individuals with disabilities, intended to prohibit discrimination in a broad range of contexts.

Assistive listening device (ALD) Devices that help an individual with hearing loss or disorders of auditory attention to more effectively communicate and participate in communication situations. These devices help an individual hear and understand what is being said more clearly, thus allowing access to sound and speech for personal communication, group situations, vocational and educational situations, and recreational situations. Examples of assistive listening devices include FM amplification systems, induction loop systems, and infrared systems.

Asymmetrical hearing loss A significant variation in a person's hearing sensitivity from one ear to the other. This could be a unilateral hearing loss or a different degree of loss in one ear versus the other.

Atresia A malformation of or misshaped pinna, which may also include the malformation or absence of an external auditory canal.

Attention Deficit Hyperactivity Disorder (ADHA) A chronic condition that may be a combination of difficulties including sustained attention, hyperactivity, and impulsivity.

Audiogram Graphic depiction of a person's hearing sensitivity; when pure tone thresholds are obtained, they are charted on this grid. The frequency is in Hertz (Hz) on the x-axis, and intensity in the decibel scale of hearing level (dB HL) is on the y-axis. Frequencies are in full octaves ranging from 125 Hz to 8000 Hz, and intensity is marked from -10 dB HL to 120 dB HL.

Audiometric zero The decibel level that is denoted as a solid black line on the audiogram and corresponds to 0 dB HL; this represents average normal hearing acuity. However, 0 dB HL may not be the lowest level that a person with superior hearing can detect.

Auditory access Ensuring that each child who is deaf or hard of hearing has optimal access to the speech signal through appropriate advanced hearing technology. This includes access to and consistent wearing of appropriate individual hearing instruments, monitoring the child's auditory learning through the hearing device(s), appropriate ongoing audiological management, and sufficient auditory input of language.

Auditory brainstem response study (ABR) Indirect measure of hearing that tests the neurological response to an auditory stimulus at the level of the brainstem.

Auditory comprehension A higher auditory skill level in which an individual can understand elements and meaning of a spoken message.

Auditory detection The ability to be aware of and detect the mere presence of sounds in the environment.

Auditory discrimination The ability to differentiate between words that differ in phonemic content.

Auditory environment The child's listening situation at home and at school. An optimal auditory environment incorporates reducing background noise, moving closer to the speaker, and being on the same level when speaking to the child.

Auditory labyrinth (also known as the cochlea) The sensory end-organ of hearing. The cochlea is a fluid-filled space within the temporal bone and is a snail-shaped spiral canal, with three chambers and inner and outer hair cells that help to analyze frequency and intensity of incoming sound signals.

Auditory masking When the introduction of one sound prevents the perception of another sound. In audiometric testing, it refers to the process whereby sound is introduced into the "nontest" ear to prevent the test sound from reaching that ear and, thus, being heard by that ear instead of the "test ear."

Auditory steady state response study (ASSR) Indirect assessment of hearing that yields electrophysiological results same general anatomical sites as ABR, but uses different stimulus; useful when distinction of a severe versus profound hearing loss is sought.

Auditory threshold The lowest hearing level at which a person responds in at least one half (50%) of a series of ascending trials (ASHA, 2005).

Auditory/oral approach Spoken language concept to language development, which incorporates the use of amplification utilizing the child's residual hearing to develop speech/language skills.

Aural atresia Congenital absence of the ear canal opening.

Aural habilitation Initial processes of therapeutic intervention to help children born with hearing loss, which begin at the start of early language development. Decisions about amplification, types of therapy and communication method, etc. can be decided at a younger age, which greatly benefits the infant as well as the family and are also considered to be part of the aural habilitation process.

Aural (re)habilitation The process of helping those affected by acquired hearing loss who have already attained language and require restoration of these skills. This includes evaluation of hearing, diagnosis and effects of hearing loss, recommendation and selection of amplification devices, consideration of the type of rehabilitation setting, and counseling of patient and families about the impact of hearing loss and the need for rehabilitation.

Autism spectrum disorder A developmental disorder characterized by difficulties in social interactions, receptive and expressive language skills, and may or may not be accompanied by repetitive physical behaviors (self-stimulation).

Automated auditory brainstem response (AABR) screening An electrophysiologic screening tool that can infer the presence of hearing loss by measuring auditory brainstem integrity.

Behind-the-ear hearing aid (BTE) Hearing device that is worn over the top of the ear. The components are housed in the casing that sits on the pinna, and an ear hook is connected to the earmold, which is placed in the ear canal.

Bel Unit of measurement used to describe human intensity differences. This is a relative measurement of intensity, which expresses the ratio of a measured sound intensity to a relative sound intensity.

Bellis/Ferre Model A model of (C)APD that includes three sub-profiles, or categories, of dysfunction: Auditory Decoding, Prosodic Deficit, and Integration Deficit, and two secondary profiles: Associative Deficit and Output Organization.

Best practice A management philosophy that asserts that there is a technique, method, process, or activity that is more effective at delivering a particular outcome than any other technique, method, process, or activity.

Binaural Of or pertaining to both ears together.

Binaural interaction Tests for binaural interaction reflect how auditory input works together from both ears at the level of the brainstem. They are sensitive to intensity and timing differences between ears and are related to the localization and lateralization of sound. Children who perform poorly on tests of binaural interaction may possess problems comprehending speech in the presence of background noise because of the inability to segregate the speech signal when there is a competing sound source.

Bone-anchored hearing aid (BAHA) Involves surgically anchoring a "screw" into the skull behind the ear, to which an external device is connected, and directly stimulates the cochlea by bone conduction, which bypasses the outer and middle ears. This style of hearing aid is typically used with conductive hearing losses associated with atresia, and other such pathologies when a traditional hearing aid and earmold cannot be utilized.

Bone conduction Sound transmitted through vibration of the skull, which directly stimulates the cochlea in the inner ear and then is sent along the central auditory pathway to the brain for interpretation.

Boyle's law For a fixed volume of vibrating air molecules, increased concentration (density) of air particles results in increased air pressure. Pressure and volume of a gas are inversely proportional if kept at a constant temperature.

Broca's area Located in the inferior frontal gyrus where motor production of language is located and processing of sentence structure, grammar, and syntax is located.

Brownian motion Random movement at high speeds, which results from the impact of molecules, found within a gas or liquid. This was named after Robert Brown, a Scottish botanist who described this motion.

The Buffalo model A model for the diagnosis of (central) auditory processing, which is strongly based on the individual's performance on the Staggered Spondaic Word Test. This model includes four categories: Decoding, Tolerance Fading Memory, Integration, and Organization. An individual may not "fit" into one particular profile and may have characteristics of more than one profile or subtype; therefore, some clinicians will focus rehabilitation efforts on the specific areas of auditory weakness.

CapTel captioned telephone A type of video telephone system that provides a display of a written text or caption of everything the caller says. This allows the user to hear and see what the speaker is saying.

(Central) auditory processing The efficiency and effectiveness by which the central nervous system utilizes auditory information. Describes how information is processed after it leaves the peripheral auditory structures and what happens to this information as it is transmitted along the central auditory nervous system. This can be assessed using behavioral tests and/or electrophysiological measures.

(Central) auditory processing disorder (C)APD refers to difficulties in the perceptual processing of auditory information in the central nervous system and the neurobiologic activity that underlies that processing and gives rise to electrophysiologic auditory potentials. Although this may co-exist with other disorders, it is not the result of these disorders (ASHA, 2005).

Certification norm A norm geared around management, which includes standard operating procedures (SOPs) that are "feasible."

Cerumen Earwax.

Child Find A portion of federal special education laws that requires the local education agency (LEA) to seek out and identify children with disabilities, aged from birth to 21 years. Child Find programs primarily target at-risk early childhood groups by providing developmental screenings, which also include vision and hearing screening.

Closed-set assessment An assessment that has a fixed number of stimuli from which the child chooses the correct answer.

Cochlea A fluid-filled space within the temporal bones that is a snail-shaped spiral canal. Within each membranous duct there are three fluid-filled chambers. The Organ of Corti is within the cochlear duct, which contains the sensory cells of hearing on the basilar membrane. The inner and outer hair cells analyze frequency and intensity of incoming sound signals at the basilar membrane.

Cochlear implant These surgically implanted amplification devices can enhance hearing and speech abilities for individuals with severe to profound hearing loss. A cochlear implant system has an external speech processor and an internal implant, which is placed under the skin. A cochlear implant device has four parts: a microphone; a speech processor, which selects and arranges sounds picked up by the microphone; a transmitter and receiver/stimulator, which receives signals from the speech processor and converts them into electric impulses; and electrodes, which collect the impulses from the stimulator and send them to the brain.

Comorbidity A condition occurring simultaneously with another, which may or may not have similar characteristics.

Compensatory strategies Techniques that are either learned or naturally developed to overcome weaknesses manifested in a specific function or skill.

Completely-in-the-canal hearing aid (CIC) Type of hearing aid style that is custom molded to fit the shape of the individual's ear, but is inserted deeper into the canal to be less noticeable than other in the ear (ITE) devices.

Condensation/compression (re: sound waveforms) Displacement passed from molecule to molecule creates areas of increased pressure and density.

Conductive hearing loss Hearing loss caused by an abnormality in the external or middle ear characterized by the reduction in the conduction of sound into the ear. Individuals with (purely) conductive hearing loss have normal sensorineural hearing.

Congenital hearing loss Hearing loss present at birth, which may or may not be associated with familial hearing loss.

Consulting audiologist Using a consultative model of service provision, audiologists may be hired on an as-needed basis rather than as full-time employees.

Cued speech Spoken language/visual cue concept that utilizes eight hand shapes in four different positions. The positions are considered cues, which are all located around the speaker's face. The visual cues are incorporated because of the many different sounding vowels and consonants that appear the same when lip-reading. The visual cues help identify each sound for the child, and the use of amplification is encouraged.

Deafened Hearing loss that occurs after completing education; teens/twenties.

Deafness (as defined by IDEA) A hearing impairment that is so severe that the child is impaired in processing linguistic information through hearing, with or without amplification, and that adversely affects a child's educational performance.

Decibel (dB) A ratio between the measured sound pressure and relative sound pressure, using logarithms. This unit is used in measurement of intensity of the range of human hearing.

Decibel hearing level (dB HL) This decibel reference level is used to audiometrically measure an individual's hearing level, and its reference varies with frequency according to minimum audibility curve.

Decibel sensation level (dB SL) The intensity level of stimulus presentation using the individual's threshold as reference. For example, a 30 dB SL sound for someone with a 20 dB HL threshold will result in a presentation level of 50 dB HL for that particular sound.

Decibel sound pressure level (dB SPL) Expresses the ratio of measured sound pressure to a reference sound pressure to indicate the intensity of a sound stimulus.

Dementia An age-associated syndrome with a negative impact on memory, cognition, attention, problem solving, and language.

Diagnostic audiometry A process by which ear-specific information and thresholds are established for individual frequencies. When air and bone conduction are tested, type of hearing loss and severity can be established.

Dichotic listening Both ears working together to process an auditory message. Dichotic tests provide information on the function of the left and right hemispheres and the transfer of auditory information between hemispheres. Dichotic listening tests are diagnostically significant in that, during the transmission of the dichotic signal, information is transferred through the dominant contralateral pathways.

Differential diagnosis Method used to clinically distinguish or differentiate one disorder from another that presents with many of the same or similar symptoms and characteristics. Key concerns include the correct diagnosis of hearing loss and the identification of possible additional comorbid conditions.

Direct audio input (DAI)   Circuitry included in many BTE hearing aids that allow an external source or device to be connected directly into the hearing aid as an input that bypasses the microphone. This allows the hearing aid to be connected to external devices for a direct signal transmitted directly into the hearing aid. For example, this can be used with a television, telephone, computer, or CD player; however, this circuitry is not available on smaller ITE, ITC, or CIC hearing aids.

Displacement (re: sound waveforms)   Movement of air molecules away from the rest position.

Distortion product otoacoustic emission (DPOAE)   A type of evoked otoacoustic emission (*see* evoked otoacoustic emission) that is measured by inserting a probe tip into the external auditory canal and presenting a stimulus that consists of two simultaneous tones of different frequencies.

Dynamic range   Mathematical difference between the lowest level that an individual begins to hear (threshold) and the upper limit of what the individual finds uncomfortable (UCL).

Ear canal volume   The volume, measured in cubic centimeters or ML, of the external ear canal.

Ear pit   Abnormality of the pinna characterized by a small hole typically located about the tragus.

Ear tag   Abnormality of the pinna characterized by a small additional piece of skin typically located about the tragus.

Early Hearing Detection and Intervention (EDHI)   National public health initiative that intends to maximize linguistic competence and literacy development for children who are deaf or hard of hearing by early identification of hearing loss through universal newborn hearing screening, timely audiologic and medical evaluations and monitoring, early intervention, and ongoing connections to family support services.

Elasticity   A tendency exhibited by molecules to resist deformity and return to their rest position, so there is no change in shape when they bump into each other and/or other objects.

Electroacoustic measures   An acoustic measurement of function that provides us with objective information about how portions of the peripheral auditory system function.

Electronystagmography   Evaluates the inner ear balance system and records a symptom called nystagmus. Nystagmus is an involuntary rhythmic oscillating movement of the eyes, which works in connection with the organs of the vestibular system to establish our sense of balance.

Electrophysiological measures   Evaluates functional integrity of various structures along the auditory pathway beyond the cochlea, at the level of the 8th cranial nerve and brainstem.

Endocochlear electrical potential   The difference in ionic concentration between endolymph and perilymph gives rise to this "cochlear battery."

Endolymph   Fluid found in the scala media, which has a higher concentration of potassium than sodium ions. The difference in ionic concentration between endolymph and perilymph gives rise to an endocochlear electrical potential that helps conduct neutral transmission of sound.

Environmental modifications   The use of HAT in the form of assistive listening devices to overcome the poor acoustical characteristics in a room.

Eustachian tube   Part of the middle ear anatomy that connects the middle ear space to the back of the throat. The Eustachian tube equalizes the pressure of the middle ear space with our environment (normal atmospheric pressure).

Evoked otoacoustic emissions   A type of otoacoustic emission (*see* otoacoustic emission) that is clinically useful as an electroacoustic measure (*see* electroacoustic measure) and that can be useful in the diagnosis of hearing loss as a nonbehavioral indirect estimate of peripheral hearing. The sounds are elicited by presentation of a stimulus via a probe tip inserted into the external ear canal.

External auditory canal   That portion of the ear that connects the pinna to the tympanic membrane and middle ear cavity.

External auditory canal atresia   *See* atresia.

External auditory meatus   See external auditory canal; also known as external ear canal.

Familiar sounds audiogram   A counseling tool that may be used to explain to patients and their families what kind of impact the hearing loss may have on the ability to function and respond to sounds that are routinely encountered in everyday life.

Five stages of grief model   Dr. Elizabeth Kübler-Ross's framework to explain the experience of dying patients, who progress through denial, anger, "bargaining for time," depression, and acceptance. These stages are also observed in people and family members experiencing personal change and emotional upset resulting from factors other than death and bereavement.

Force   A push or pull on an object with both magnitude and direction (vector). Force is mathematically determined to be the product of mass multiplied by acceleration.

Functional auditory assessment   An assessment of listening that encompasses observations of functional listening behaviors and abilities in addition to diagnostic assessments of the child's listening skills on a variety of tasks.

Guidelines   Any document that aims to streamline particular processes according to a set routine. Following guidelines/best practices is not mandatory.

Hearing age   Calculated from the date the child begins to consistently wear appropriate hearing technology, which helps put into perspective the child's listening skills progression over time.

Hearing assistance technology (HAT)   Terminology encompassing any technology that assists an individual with hearing loss, beyond the use of a hearing aid, BAHA, or cochlear implant.

Hearing handicap inventory for the elderly   A self-assessment tool that explores quality-of-life questions using the patient's or family's view of communication status. This tool is a 25-item questionnaire that measures an individual's perceived activity limitation and participation restriction as a result of hearing loss.

Hearing impairment (as defined by IDEA)   An impairment in hearing, whether permanent or fluctuating, that adversely affects a child's educational performance but that is not included under the definition of deafness.

Helicotrema   The point where the scalae vestibuli and tympani communicate in the cochlea.

High frequency sensorineural hearing loss (HF SNHL)   A hearing loss of greater severity in the higher frequencies than in the lower frequencies, where thresholds may be in the normal to near normal range. There may be normal or relatively normal hearing up to approximately 2000 Hz, and then a sloping hearing loss at frequencies of 3000 Hz and above.

Highest qualified professional   Terminology in education law (which may vary from state to state), which deems a hierarchy of professionals to speak on a specific discipline for which they are qualified.

In-the-canal hearing aid (ITC)   Custom molded hearing aids to fit the shape of the concha and outer ear canal portion of an individual's ear. In these devices, all components are housed within one hard shell.

Incus   The middle bone of the ossicular chain that comprises two parts: the short crus, which fits into a recess wall of the tympanic membrane, and the long crus, which is attached to the head of the stapes.

Individuals with Disabilities Education Act (IDEA)   Laws that ensure that services to special needs students throughout the United States are equal and homogenous. These laws include both part (C), early intervention, and part (B), children 3–21 years.

Inertia   All bodies remain at rest or in a state of uniform motion unless other forces act in opposition. The amount of inertia is directly proportional to a body's mass.

Inner hair cells   Cells that form a row in the proximity of the tectorial membrane, near the modiolus of the cochlea. More than 90% of these hair cells are neurologically connected to the brain via nerve fibers, and they encode sound and send it further along the auditory nervous system up to the brain for interpretation.

Interaural attenuation   The reduction, in dB, caused by the skull as sound travels from the test ear to the nontest ear. This dB level is what is absorbed by the skull.

Invisible in-the-canal hearing aid (IIC)   Type of hearing aid style that is custom molded to fit the shape of the individual's ear, but is inserted even deeper into the canal to be the least noticeable as compared with other in-the-ear (ITE) or completely-in-the-canal (CIC) devices.

Keloids   Abnormality of the pinna characterized by large growth irregular in shape, which is formed as a result of excessive collagen.

Linear scale   Measuring scale with a true zero point, each increment on this scale is equal to every other increment, and you can sum incremental units by addition.

Listening & spoken language (LSL)   A model of therapeutic intervention that combines aural/oral and auditory/verbal educational models to promote spoken language skills in children with hearing loss.

Logarithmic scale   Relative scale where there is no zero point, the zero point does not represent the absence of what is being measured, and each successive unit is larger than the one preceding it; therefore, each increment is not equal and represents increasingly large numerical differences.

"Look, play, talk"   Variation of the informal observation in which the clinician should look at the child for nonverbal communication behaviors, observe play behavior, and listen to the child talk. This will allow the clinician to earn the trust of the child and determine developmental level and abilities.

Loudness discomfort level (LDL)   *See* uncomfortable listening level (UCL).

Low-redundancy speech   Tasks that involve testing when the natural redundancy of speech is compromised by noise or poor signal quality. The ability to interpret degraded speech and make auditory closure is a problem found in some listeners who experience (C)AP difficulties (Geffner & Ross-Swain, 2006). In order to make closure, a listener must be familiar with the speech signal and be able to fill in missing elements when speech is not clear.

Malleus   The malleus is the most lateral of the three bones making up the ossicular chain and is embedded slightly into the tympanic membrane at the manubrium. When the tympanic membrane vibrates from sound energy impinging on it, the malleus also moves at the same vibratory speed.

Manual communication   Visual communication system used to convey a message, such as sign language.

Manually coded English (MCE)   Spoken language/sign concept that incorporates the use of finger spelling and signing to represent spoken English; MCE follows the rules of English syntax. Finger spelling is used to transmit morphemes that do not translate with sign, and the use of amplification is not always used with MCE.

Masking   Process where one sound is blocked out by another in order to prevent the test sound from being heard by the nontest ear.

Mass   The quantity of matter present that is unaffected by gravitational forces.

Medical home   Term used to describe the management and coordination of health care for an individual throughout a lifetime. This model of service provision enables a healthcare provider to coordinate and track infants and children who have failed their newborn hearing screening or are at risk for progressive/late-onset hearing loss to ensure that follow-up is routinely in place and that these infants and children are not lost in the follow-up process.

Medical model   A model of health care, used in an acute care facility, which depends on an interdisciplinary group of trained professional and paraprofessionals working with a single patient. This interdisciplinary team is led by a primary physician who manages the overall care of the patient and forms this interdisciplinary team based on the needs of the patient. Written requests for consultation by members of the team are required for all preventative, curative, consultative, and rehabilitative services. No care can be provided to a patient without orders from the primary care physician.

Membranous labyrinth   Soft-tissue, fluid-filled channels within the osseous labyrinth containing the end-organ structures of the auditory and vestibular systems.

Metalinguistics   Top-down skill that equips the child to take responsibility for his or her listening successes and failures. Metalinguistic analysis may be due to problems in applying the rules of language to incoming auditory input.

Microtia   Malformation of the pinna, such that when the pinna is visualized it appears smaller in shape and size than normal. This condition may or may not accompany atresia.

Middle ear   That portion of the ear that connects the outer ear anatomy to the inner ear anatomy and encompasses the ossicular chain, the Eustachian tube, middle ear cavity, and middle ear attic.

Middle ear implant   Hearing aid in which the receiver or entire hearing aid is inserted into the middle ear. For sensorineural hearing loss, it delivers vibratory mechanical energy to the ossicular chain located in the middle ear system and then sends mechanical energy to the cochlea at the round window via motion of the stapes. For conductive or mixed hearing loss, mechanical energy is sent directly to the cochlea through direct bone conduction circumventing the ossicular chain in the middle ear.

Minimal hearing loss   That classification of auditory impairment that, although the very nature of its term is to be "minimal," can have significant manifestation in children's speech, language, and communication development including phonological, vocabulary, and language delays; difficulty understanding speech presented with background noise; difficulty localizing the source of a sound; problems with reading comprehension; and educational difficulties.

Mixed hearing loss   A hearing loss that is a combination of a conductive component plus a sensorineural component. Bone conduction thresholds are outside of normal (sensorineural component), and air conduction is even further abnormal (conductive component), showing an air-bone gap on the audiogram.

Monaural   Of or pertaining to one ear individually.

Monaural low redundancy   Speech that is unfamiliar (open set) to the listener, which is presented to each ear individually. Monaural low redundancy training will help individuals who have difficulty hearing with background noise, understanding rapid connected speech, or when the auditory signal is not optimal. Clinicians may introduce background noise during therapy sessions and may introduce auditory-closure activities and vocabulary-building activities in training.

Most comfortable listening level (MCL)   The dB level that is mutually decided on by the audiologist and patient as being the most comfortable level for the patient when listening to connected speech.

Omnibus Budget Reconciliation Act   Requires all nursing homes receiving federal funding to assess each new patient using the MDS. The MDS is part of the U.S. federally mandated process for clinical assessment that is to be administered to all nursing home patients, in Medicare- and Medicaid-certified nursing homes, within the first 14 days of admission. OBRA further addresses screening procedures for patients in the nursing home facility, including procedures of a hearing screening.

Open-set assessment   Assessment containing items on the test that are unknown to the child and in which there is no defined set (for example, 4 to 6) of answer choices from which the child may choose; thus increasing the difficulty level.

Organ of Corti   Contains the sensory cells of hearing, which lie on the basilar membrane within the cochlear duct.

Osseous labyrinth   The bony structure of the inner ear, which lies within the temporal bone and houses both the auditory and vestibular labyrinth.

Ossicles   *See* ossicular chain.

Ossicular chain   Three connected bones in the middle ear that form a chain. From lateral to medial these bones are the malleus, the incus and the stapes; and they are collectively responsible for taking the acoustic energy at the tympanic membrane, converting it to mechanical energy, and delivering it to the oval window.

Ossicular discontinuity   Disruption (or break) of the ossicular chain.

Otitis media: An inflammation of the middle ear system, which may or may not include the collection of fluid in the middle ear cavity, primarily due to a dysfunctional Eustachian tube. When fluid is present, it typically becomes infected. This condition is also known commonly as an "ear infection."

Otoacoustic emission screening   Electroacoustic screening tool that can infer the presence of hearing loss by measuring cochlear integrity.

Otoacoustic emissions (OAEs)   Sounds that emanate from the ear, thought to be the product of outer hair-cell activity in the cochlea. In some forms, this sound can be measured clinically and can be useful in the indirect measurement of hearing sensitivity.

Otosclerosis   A condition that causes fixation of the stapes bone in the middle ear, resulting in a conductive hearing loss.

Otoscope   An instrument that provides magnification and a light source to examine that portion of the ear from the external auditory canal to the eardrum.

Otoscopy   Process of examining the external auditory meatus, especially the eardrum, which allows the examiner to identify several common problems that preclude the sound from entering the ear.

Outer hair cells   Hair cells that form three rows. The base of the cells sit on top of the basilar membrane and the stereocilia at their tops of the cells embed themselves in the tectorial membrane above; they connect with the cochlear branch of the 8th cranial nerve (vestibulocochlear). The vibration of the basilar membrane causes the cilia of the outer hair cells to bend, and the length of the outer hair cells increases to generate an electrical response created by the incoming stimulus. Outer hair cells are tuned to sound intensity to act as transducers by changing fluid energy into electrical energy.

Outer ear   Comprising two structures, the pinna (or auricle) and the external auditory meatus (ear canal), to collect sound and amplify it for the middle ear.

Oval window   One of the two tissue-covered openings found on the cochlea, which is covered by the stapes footplate.

Pars flaccida   More compliant, smaller section of the tympanic membrane located superiorly to the pars tensa.

Pars tensa   Stiffer, larger, section of the tympanic membrane located inferiorly to the pars flaccida.

Pascal   A linear unit of measurement that describes sound pressure (Pa).

Perilymph   Fluid found in the scalae vestibuli and tympani that has a higher concentration of sodium ions than potassium ions. The perilymph wave displaces the scala media, setting up a wave on the basilar membrane, which moves from the base to the apex.

Phonemically balanced (PB)   Words that have been statistically analyzed for their phoneme content and compared with a sampling of spoken discourse.

Pinna   The visible part of the ear, also called the auricle, which is shaped like a funnel to collect and send sound waves through the ear canal. The pinna also assists in sound localization and helps protect the entrance to the external auditory canal.

Postlingually deaf   Refers to a person who becomes deaf after a spoken language system had been established partially or in full.

Prelingually deaf   Congenitally deaf or deaf from birth.

Pressure wave   When air molecules are set into vibration, they produce a pressure wave. When air molecules near a vibrating object are displaced, adjacent air molecules are also displaced, and so on. This wave motion is propagated through the air to the human ear.

Propagation   Movement of a disturbance (vibration), which is generally represented as a wave.

Pseudohypacusis   False, exaggerated, or psychogenically motivated hearing loss.

Pure tone   The resultant pressure wave formed by areas of alternating condensation/compression and rarefaction changing at a steady rate. Pure tones move in simple harmonic motion and are represented graphically by a sine wave.

Rarefaction (re: sound waveforms)   Thinning of air molecules, which creates areas of decreased air pressure and density.

Response to intervention (Rti)   A portion of the federal education laws, which require school systems to put in place interventions that attempt to meet the needs of a child for academic success in the general education setting and emphasize prevention through special education services rather than failure. RTI must be school wide and provide high-quality instruction matched to individual student needs, include frequent monitoring of student progress to inform changes in instruction, and utilize child response data to make educational decisions.

Retrocochlear pathology   Pathological condition that is located beyond (retro) the level of the cochlea.

Reverberation   Characteristic of sound when it is reflected off of a (usually hard) surface rather than absorbed by a (usually soft) surface.

Reverberation time   The time delay to a normal auditory system caused by sound reflected off of a surface, which is usually inaudible but has a significant effect on speech intelligibility in an impaired auditory system.

Round window   One of the two tissue-covered openings found on the cochlea that is between the scala tympani and middle ear.

Saccule   One of the two organs of balance housed within the vestibule.

Scala media   One of three chambers within the cochlea, in which endolymph circulates.

Scala tympani   One of three chambers within the cochlea, in which perilymph circulates.

Scala vestibule   One of three chambers within the cochlea, in which perilymph circulates. When the stapes footplate rocks back and forth in the oval window, a wave is established within the scala vestibuli.

Screening audiometry   Pass/fail paradigm used with air conduction audiometry to determine if further evaluation is necessary.

Section 504 (504 Plan)   A portion of the Rehabilitation Act of 1973, which protects individuals from discrimination based on a disability via a written document specifying service provision. 504 Plans were reauthorized by the ADA in 1990.

Semicircular canals   Sensory end-organ of balance within the vestibular labyrinth.

Sensorineural hearing loss   Hearing loss in the inner ear due to damage to the cochlea and/or retrocochlear pathway, resulting in alterations of perception of sound frequency and intensity. This hearing loss also results in a loss of speech clarity due to damage to the neural fibers located in the cochlea.

Shadow curve   Responses of the normal hearing ear are recorded falsely as responses of the "bad" ear, caused by cross hearing.

Signal-to-noise ratio   The mathematical ratio between a primary signal (for example, speech) and the measurement of simultaneous noise.

Simple harmonic motion   The type of motion characteristic of pure tones, which is due to areas of alternating condensation and rarefaction occurring at a steady rate of change. When pure tones move in SHM, they take the same amount of time to complete each cycle of vibration, or are periodic.

Sound   Physical phenomenon described as the movement or propagation of a disturbance (i.e., a vibration) through an elastic medium (e.g., air molecules) without permanent displacement of the particles. Three prerequisites are necessary for production of sound: a source of energy, a vibrating object, which generates an audible pressure wave, and a medium of transmission.

Speech audiometry   Formal measurements of an individual's ability to hear and/or understand speech.

Speech awareness threshold (SAT)   *See* speech detection threshold (SDT).

Speech banana audiogram   A counseling tool used to convey the significance and impact of a person's hearing loss. The speech banana audiogram is a typical audiogram with a shaded "banana shape" area representing the approximate area where speech sounds typically occur, with the individual phonemes placed where they will fall on the audiogram based on their frequency and intensity.

Speech detection threshold (SDT)   Minimum hearing level for speech at which an individual can just detect the presence of speech stimuli.

Speech discrimination testing   *See* word discrimination testing (WDT).

Speech reception threshold (SRT)   Measurement of person's threshold for the recognition of 50% of simple speech (spondee) stimuli. This indicates how loud speech has to be for a person to just barely recognize it as a speech signal and repeat the word(s) accurately.

Speech recognition threshold (SRT)   *See* speech reception threshold (SRT).

Spondee   Words made up of two syllables in which equal emphasis is placed on both syllables when spoken (i.e., hotdog, downstairs, baseball, toothbrush).

Spontaneous otoacoustic emissions   Sounds that are generated by and emitted from the inner ear spontaneously, without stimulation. Spontaneous otoacoustic emissions are not present in all people, and therefore hold little clinical application.

Standards   A design or format applicable because it is recognized by an official organization or because it is used by a majority of users. Following standards is mandatory.

Stapedius muscle   Muscle of the middle ear that contracts bilaterally in response to high-intensity sounds to stiffen the ossicular chain, which protects the inner ear from intense sounds. This contraction results in attenuation of sound pressure reaching the inner ear.

Stapes   The stapes is the most medial bone in the ossicular chain and looks like a stirrup; it fits very neatly in the oval window of the cochlear wall to help push sound (as mechanical energy) into the inner ear.

Subacute care   Comprehensive inpatient care designed for someone who is recovering from an acute illness, injury, or exacerbation of a disease process. It is goal-oriented treatment immediately after, or instead of, acute hospitalization (Kuchar, 2006). Patients are sent to the sub-acute facility once they have been stabilized in the medical facility and no longer meet the criteria for that acute hospital setting. These settings cover a wide range of services and may specialize in a specific type of care either long term or rehabilitative in nature.

Tectorial membrane   A gel-like membrane that forms the roof over the basilar membrane. The outer hair cells are embedded into the tectorial membrane, with the inner hair cells in close proximity.

Telecoil (T-Coil)   Circuitry within a hearing aid device that is designed to pick up an electromagnetic signal. Such circuitry is most often found in the ITE- and BTE-style hearing aids. The T-coil is useful for amplifying sound from older model telephones and also useful in some designs of assistive listening technology.

Telecommunication device for the deaf (TDD)   *See* text telephone (TTY).

Telescope vocal production   Progression from immature verbalizations to the production of the entire range of vocal behaviors.

Temporal processing/sequencing   Ability to recognize the timing aspects of acoustic stimuli. This is an important function for the processing of auditory signals, especially for the interpretation of speech. Intact and accurate temporal processing/sequencing is critical for the perception of rapidly altering speech sounds and is needed for the interpretation of prosodic aspects of speech.

Tensor tympani muscle   Muscle of the middle ear that runs parallel to the Eustachian tube and assists in its function. When the tensor tympani muscle contracts, it pulls the malleus to draw the tympanic membrane inward, which increases the pressure in the middle ear and Eustachian tube.

Text telephone (TTY)   System of communication via telephone using typewritten messages instead of speaking and listening. TTY has a keyboard for typing out messages and a display for the incoming messages.

The Minimum Data Set for Nursing Home Residents Assessment and Care Screening Tool (MDS)   Part of the U.S. federally mandated process for clinical assessment that is to be administered to all nursing home patients in Medicare- and Medicaid-certified nursing homes within the first 14 days of admission. It covers a wide range of functional areas from behavior to special needs, including hearing acuity and hearing aid use, and results of the MDS will drive the patient-care program of the nursing home facility.

Threshold of discomfort (TD)   *See* uncomfortable listening level (UCL).

Tonotopic organization   The auditory nerve fibers are arranged on the basilar membrane in this fashion, meaning nerve fibers at the apical end of the cochlea respond preferentially to low-frequency stimuli, and high-frequency sounds are encoded at the base. The auditory nerve is tonotopically arranged so that low-frequency sounds are found in the core of the auditory nerve and high-frequency sounds are arranged around the periphery.

Total communication   A philosophy of education for the deaf that encompasses spoken language/sign concepts, which can use many modalities to communicate, such as ASL, Sign Exact English, finger-spelling, lip-reading, nonverbal cues, or amplification. The speaker will use spoken language with manual/visual methods simultaneously to successfully communicate with a child with hearing loss/deafness.

Transducer   Object that changes one form of energy to another form. For example, the ear is a transducer because acoustic energy is changed to hydro/electrical energy via mechanical energy of the middle ear, which allows the ear to analyze various physical parameters to perceive in the brain what the ear has heard.

Transient evoked otoacoustic emission (TEOAE)   A type of evoked otoacoustic emission (*see* evoked otoacoustic emission). The sound used to elicit a response with this testing is a transient, click sound, stimulus of brief duration.

Tympanic membrane   Anatomic boundary between the outer and middle ear, which comprises multiple layers of tissue that are both concentric and radial. Also commonly known as the eardrum.

Tympanogram   Graphic display reflecting the volume, compliance, and pressure of the outer and middle ear systems.

Tympanometric compliance   The amount of mobility (movement) the eardrum demonstrates.

Tympanometric pressure   The measure of pressure in the middle ear cavity referencing normal atmospheric pressure measured in daPa.

Tympanometry   An evaluation of the physical working properties of the middle ear system based on the mathematical principles of pressure, compliance, and volume.

Uncomfortable listening level (UCL)   Limit at which the patient would find sound to be unacceptably loud, or painful to listen to, for any significant period of time.

Uniform circular motion   Projected movement of an air molecule if it were to move around the circumference of the circle, formed by the trough directly beneath the peak of a sine wave, at a constant rate.

Universal Newborn Hearing Screening (UNHS)   Ensures that all infants have equal access to early hearing loss identification. UNHS is supported by the passage of national and state legislation that has resulted in a significant decrease in the age at which children are diagnosed with hearing loss.

Universal precautions   Recommendations developed by the Centers for Disease Control and Prevention to control the spread of infectious diseases.

Utricle   One of the two organs of balance housed within the vestibule.

Vector   Object that has magnitude (some amount greater than zero) and direction.

Vestibular labyrinth   The portion of the ear that includes the semicircular canals and the vestibule, which houses the saccule and utricle. This sensory end-organ of ear, in conjunction with the vision and proprioception, is responsible for maintaining our balance system.

Vestibular membrane   The membranous roof of the cochlear duct.

Vestibule   This connects the two end-organs of hearing and balance (the cochlea and semicircular canals) and houses the saccule and utricle.

Veteran's Administration Hospital   Service provider of choice for medical and allied health benefits for members of the armed services, veterans, their immediate families, and their survivors.

Videonystagmography   An evaluation of the inner ear balance system that records a symptom called nystagmus. Nystagmus is an involuntary rhythmic oscillating movement of the eyes, which work in connection with the organs of the vestibular system to establish our sense of balance. Video goggles are used that incorporate a camera to record and measure the person's eye movements.

Wave form equilibrium (re: sound waveforms)   Resting state of air molecules (no vibration).

Wavelength   A graphic representation of the disturbance created by the sound wave in a medium, which is measured in units of length and represented by the Greek letter lambda (λ).

Wernicke's area   That area of the brain within the lower temporal lobe, where speech perception is located.

Word discrimination testing   Procedure by which phonemically balanced word lists are used to estimate how well a person is able to understand speech once it has been made comfortably loud enough for them.

Word recognition testing   *See* word discrimination testing (WDT).

Index

Note: Page numbers followed by *f* or *t* indicate material in figures or tables, respectively.